Peri...
Anesthesia
AND *Critical*
Care

Perinatal Anesthesia AND *Critical Care*

James H. Diaz, MD, MHA

Clinical Associate Professor of Anesthesiology
Tulane University School of Medicine;
Director of Pediatric Anesthesia
Co-Director, Intensive Care Unit
Ochsner Clinic and Alton Ochsner Medical Foundation
New Orleans, Louisiana

W. B. Saunders Company
Harcourt Brace Jovanovich, Inc.
Philadelphia   London   Toronto   Montreal   Sydney   Tokyo

W. B. SAUNDERS COMPANY
Harcourt Brace Jovanovich, Inc.

The Curtis Center
Independence Square West
Philadelphia, PA 19106

Library of Congress Cataloging-in-Publication Data

Perinatal anesthesia and critical care/[edited by] James H. Diaz.

p.   cm.

ISBN 0–7216–1874–X

1. Anesthesia in obstetrics.   2. Anesthetics—Physiological
effect.   3. Infants (Newborn)—Effect of drugs on.
4. Surgical intensive care.   I. Diaz, James H. [DNLM:
1. Anesthesia—in infancy & childhood.   2. Anesthesia—in
pregnancy.   3. Critical Care—methods.   4. Fetus—drug
effects.   5. Infants, Newborn, Diseases—surgery.
6. Surgery, Operative—in pregnancy.   WO 450 P4454]

RG732.P474   1991

617.9′682—dc20

DNLM/DLC   90–9122

Editor: Richard Zorab
Designer: Paul Fry
Production Manager: Ken Neimeister
Manuscript Editor: Kate Troemel
Illustration Coordinator: Lisa Lambert
Indexer: Ruth Low

PERINATAL ANESTHESIA AND CRITICAL CARE   ISBN 0–7216–1874–X

Printed in the United States of America.

Last digit is the print number: 9   8   7   6   5   4   3   2   1

Contributors

J. Sherman

N. Scott Adzick, M.D.
Associate Professor of Surgery and Pediatrics, University of California, San Francisco, School of Medicine; Attending Pediatric Surgeon, University of California, San Francisco, Medical Center, San Francisco, California
Perioperative Management of the Fetus Undergoing Surgery in Utero

Robert M. Arensman, M.D.
Professor of Surgery and Pediatrics, University of Chicago Pritzker School of Medicine; Surgeon-in-Chief, Wyler Children's Hospital, Chicago, Illinois
Perioperative Management of Neonatal Emergencies; Postoperative Critical Care Management of Neonates

B. Wycke Baker, M.D.
Assistant Professor of Anesthesiology and Obstetrics and Gynecology, Baylor College of Medicine; Attending Anesthesiologist, Ben Taub General Hospital, Houston, Texas
Maternal and Fetal Effects of Anesthesia

Haywood L. Brown, M.D.
Associate Professor of Obstetrics and Gynecology, Indiana University School of Medicine; Attending, Indiana University Hospital and Wishard Memorial Hospital, Indianapolis, Indiana
Perinatal Evaluation and Management of Premature Birth, Breech Presentation, and Multiple Gestation

James H. Diaz, M.D., MHA
Clinical Associate Professor of Anesthesiology, Tulane University School of Medicine; Director, Pediatric Anesthesia, and Co-Director, Intensive Care Unit, Ochsner Clinic and Alton Ochsner Medical Foundation, New Orleans, Louisiana
Are Anesthetics Teratogens?; The Physiologic Changes of Pregnancy Have Anesthetic Implications for Both Mother and Fetus; Anesthetic Management of the Pregnant Patient Undergoing Nonobstetric Surgery; Perinatal Evaluation and Management of Premature Birth, Breech Presentation, and Multiple Gestation; Anesthetic Management of Premature Neonates, Term Neonates, and Infants; Perioperative Management of Conjoined Twins Undergoing Separation Surgery; Postoperative Critical Care Management of Neonates

v

Robert H. Friesen, M.D.
Associate Clinical Professor of Anesthesia and Pediatrics, University of Colorado School of Medicine; Associate Director of Anesthesiology, Children's Hospital, Denver, Colorado
Neonatal Physiologic Adaptations and Their Anesthetic Implications

Eric B. Furman, M.B., B.Ch. (RAND), D.A. (RAND), FFA (SA)
Clinical Professor of Anesthesia, University of Texas Medical School at San Antonio, San Antonio, Texas; Director, Department of Anesthesia, Cook–Fort Worth Children's Medical Center, Fort Worth, Texas
Perioperative Management of Conjoined Twins Undergoing Separation Surgery

Jay P. Goldsmith, M.D.
Associate Clinical Professor of Pediatrics, Tulane University School of Medicine; Chairman, Department of Pediatrics, and Chief, Section of Neonatology, Ochsner Clinic and Alton Ochsner Medical Foundation, New Orleans, Louisiana
Resuscitation of the Neonate; The Neonatal Effects of Anesthetic Agents and Techniques

Michael R. Harrison, M.D.
Professor of Surgery and Pediatrics, University of California, San Francisco, School of Medicine; Chief of Pediatric Surgery and Co-Director, Fetal Treatment Program, University of California, San Francisco, Medical Center, San Francisco, California
Perioperative Management of the Fetus Undergoing Surgery in Utero

Timothy Huckaby, M.D.
Staff Anesthesiologist, Arnold Palmer Hospital for Children and Women, Orlando, Florida
Perinatal Management of Maternal and Fetal Emergencies

Edward H. Karotkin, M.D.
Associate Professor of Pediatrics, Eastern Virginia Medical School; Director, Neonatal Medicine, Children's Hospital of the King's Daughters, Norfolk, Virginia
Resuscitation of the Neonate

Michael T. Longaker, M.D.
Research Fellow, Fetal Surgery Laboratory, University of California, San Francisco, School of Medicine; Research Fellow, Department of Surgery, University of California, San Francisco, Medical Center, San Francisco, California
Perioperative Management of the Fetus Undergoing Surgery in Utero

Warren N. Otterson, M.D.
Professor and Chairman, Department of Obstetrics and Gynecology, School of Medicine in Shreveport, Louisiana State University Medical Center, Shreveport, Louisiana
Perinatal Management of Maternal and Fetal Emergencies

Jonathan H. Skerman, B.D.Sc., M.Sc.D., D.Sc.
Professor of Clinical Anesthesiology and Obstetrics and Gynecology, School of Medicine in Shreveport, Louisiana State University Medical Center, Shreveport, Louisiana
Perinatal Management of Maternal and Fetal Emergencies

Andrea L. Starrett, M.D.
Assistant Professor, School of Allied Health Professions, Louisiana State University Medical Center; Director, Child Development Center, Ochsner Clinic and Alton Ochsner Medical Foundation, New Orleans, Louisiana
The Neonatal Effects of Anesthetic Agents and Techniques

Elizabeth B. Walker, R.N.C.
Clinical Specialist in Inpatient Obstetrics, University Hospital, Louisiana State University Medical Center, Shreveport, Louisiana
Perinatal Management of Maternal and Fetal Emergencies

Foreword

Anesthesia as an adjunct to the surgical repair of wounds came into use centuries ago when opiates or alcoholic mixtures were given to stupefy patients and so reduced pain and the need for restraints. Today, synthetic opiates, anxiolytics, and tranquilizers are administered to effectively prepare patients for modern anesthetics, which may be volatile gases that are inhaled or local anesthetics that function as regional nerve blocks.

In this new and unique work, *Perinatal Anesthesia and Critical Care*, a variety of authors from different specialties address important issues in perinatal anesthesia, including the placental transfer of local and general anesthetics, the prenatal effects of anesthetics on the fetus, and the postnatal effects of anesthetics on neonates. New techniques and pharmacologic agents employed in the anesthetic and perioperative care of patients undergoing such radical and new surgical procedures as fetal surgery and complex separation of conjoined twins are also described and discussed.

Recent advances in perinatal medicine enable more premature infants to survive the neonatal period. Anesthetic and perioperative care is required for the surgical repair of commonly acquired defects such as retinal detachment from retinopathy or prematurity or obstructive hydrocephalus from intracranial hemorrhage.

In short, both the populations of aging gravidas giving birth prematurely and their premature offspring are growing. Surgical procedures will be required to ensure both the preservation of the pregnancies and the survival of the infants. *Perinatal Anesthesia and Critical Care* will serve as a valuable reference resource for a variety of specialists in perinatal care who treat high-risk gravidas, their fetuses, and newborns.

JOHN C. WEED, M.D., M.S.
Professor Emeritus of Obstetrics and Gynecology,
Department of Obstetrics and Gynecology,
Tulane University School of Medicine;
Chairman Emeritus, Department of Obstetrics and Gynecology,
Ochsner Clinic and Alton Ochsner Medical Foundation,
New Orleans, Louisiana

Preface

Historically, the choice of anesthetic agents and techniques was limited to a few inhaled anesthetics (ether, nitrous oxide) or local anesthetics (cocaine) for use in general or regional anesthesia, respectively. Many early pioneers in anesthesiology used these limited technical and pharmacologic resources to provide safe and skillful anesthesia during the development of daring pediatric surgical procedures now considered commonplace, such as cleft palate repair and ligation of the patent ductus arteriosus. Many times, new anesthesia instruments, endotracheal tubes, and breathing circuits were designed on the spot, fashioned from spare parts and tubes, and used for new procedures in small patients when existing equipment for adults was unsuitable.[1]

With flammable anesthetics unsafe for wartime use, early anesthesiologists on the front lines combined wit with available resources to develop unique combinations of anesthetic agents and techniques for wound management. Some of these combined techniques are still in use today, especially in gravidas and neonates during dissociative anesthesia and neuroleptanesthesia.

Dissociation is the separation of mind from body, in which pain is received but not perceived or experienced. Neuroleptanesthesia, or, more commonly, balanced anesthesia, is the combination of pharmacologic agents and anesthetic techniques to achieve complete analgesia and amnesia. Early anesthesiologists often combined opioids, alcohol, and distraction for dissociation during battlefield amputations. During World War I, topical application, wound infiltration, and even spinal blocks, all performed with cocaine, were often combined with nitrous oxide inhalation for neuroleptanesthesia, then known as anoci-association, for wound debridements and even more extensive operations.[2] Today, modern perinatal anesthesiologists combine intravenous ketamine with epidural anesthesia for dissociation during cesarean section and mix muscle relaxants with narcotics and inhaled anesthetics for neuroleptanesthesia during neonatal tracheoesophageal fistula repair.

In the past, anesthesiologists, unlike their colleagues in surgery, obstetrics, and pediatrics, were slow to embrace rapid subspecialization in medicine, preferring to serve all patients with the same degree of dedication and intensity. This is now changing rapidly. With the evolution of intensive care units and the development of critical care medicine as a specialty, many primary specialists from anesthesiology, surgery, and pediatrics have preferred to limit their clinical practices to perioperative and critical care in operating rooms and specialized postoperative units. Many obstetrician–gynecologists have also preferred to limit their practices to the medical and obstetric management of high-risk gravidas and their fetuses. Such specialists from many backgrounds now base their practices in tertiary care centers and work closely together in the same specialized units. Despite the appearance of a limited focus, perinatal specialists need a broad background to communicate effectively with one another when treating the same patient or, more appropriately, the same two patients, mother and fetus.

Perinatal Anesthesia and Critical Care not only treats the basic principles of maternal–fetal physiologic adaptations and the modern concepts of perioperative management of gravidas and neonates but also introduces new clinical strategies in perinatal critical care, such as surgical palliation of congenital defects in utero and extracorporeal membrane oxygenation for neonatal respiratory failure. New pharmacologic agents for use in gravidas and neonates are discussed and new mechanisms of action for older, existing pharmacologic agents are presented.

As a complete work, *Perinatal Anesthesia and Critical Care* presents a chronology or, more appropriately, a continuum of human development from conception through infancy. Suggestions for anesthetic and critical care accompany the anatomic and functional descriptions of pregnancy and parturition, fetal growth and development, and infant growth and development after preterm or term birth. Comprehensive tables and illustrations summarize anatomic and functional changes, often in a comparative manner juxtaposing weeks of gestation for pregnancy and chronologic ages for neonates. The latest developments in perinatal medicine are also placed chronologically in the text and are presented in such a way that the normal contrasts with the abnormal so as to suggest a logical set of anesthetic implications and corresponding management techniques.

This is not a textbook of pediatric anesthesia and intensive care, nor is it a text of obstetric anesthesia and intensive care. It is instead a complement to numerous existing works in pediatric and obstetric anesthesia and a new and unique companion to a growing subspecialty of both obstetrics and pediatrics, perinatal medicine. *Perinatal Anesthesia and Critical Care* is aimed at the perinatal specialist from any primary field who treats gravidas and neonates in operating rooms and specialized care units and who needs a basic appreciation of those clinical sciences allied to but outside his or her primary specialty.

Controversial new issues in perinatal care, including anesthetic teratogenicity, in utero fetal surgery, extracorporeal membrane oxygenation, and perioperative management of conjoined twins, are not addressed in the many existing works in anesthesiology, neonatology, and maternal–fetal medicine. Thus, *Perinatal Anesthesia and Critical Care* should fill an important niche in the literature of perinatal medicine, answer many current questions, and pose new ones for physicians who treat pregnant women, their fetuses, and neonates. Even physicians who treat patients at maternity or children's hospitals exclusively will find the topics in this text useful in their clinical practices. Frequently, physicians treat only mothers whose babies are swiftly transported elsewhere or babies whose mothers were delivered elsewhere.

It is not enough for perinatal clinicians to limit their basic clinical knowledge to narrow areas of their expertise and subspecialty. Effective communication among a variety of perinatal specialists demands a broad knowledge base, well grounded in the anatomic and functional changes of pregnancy, the pharmacokinetics of placental drug transfer, and the normal and abnormal development of the fetus and the neonate in both gestational and chronologic time. Only by a full understanding and appreciation of perinatal events will the treating physician, whether anesthesiologist, obstetrician, pediatrician, or surgeon, become better prepared to provide comprehensive care to the mother, her fetus, and her neonate.

A simple algorithm depicting a continuum of anesthetic and critical care for the mother, for her fetus, and subsequently for the neonate is presented in Figure 1. As always, planning ahead for what can happen is the key; a logical thought process allows for planning and prevents surprises and unwelcomed outcomes. A continuum of care concept shows an understanding and appreciation of perinatal events and better prepares the perinatal clinician to provide comprehensive care.

A number of anesthesiologists, obstetricians, pediatricians, and surgeons have contributed to *Perinatal Anesthesia and Critical Care* with the hope that new subspecialists within these primary specialties will develop and grasp a unique appreciation for the continuum of care required by the gravida, her fetus, and her newly born infant—whether preterm or term, perfectly formed or malformed.

From its beginning to its end, from conception through infancy, *Perinatal Anesthesia and Critical Care* presents the anatomic and physiologic changes and the pathophysiology of pregnancy, fetal life, parturition, and neonatal life. Logical treatment plans are developed to meet

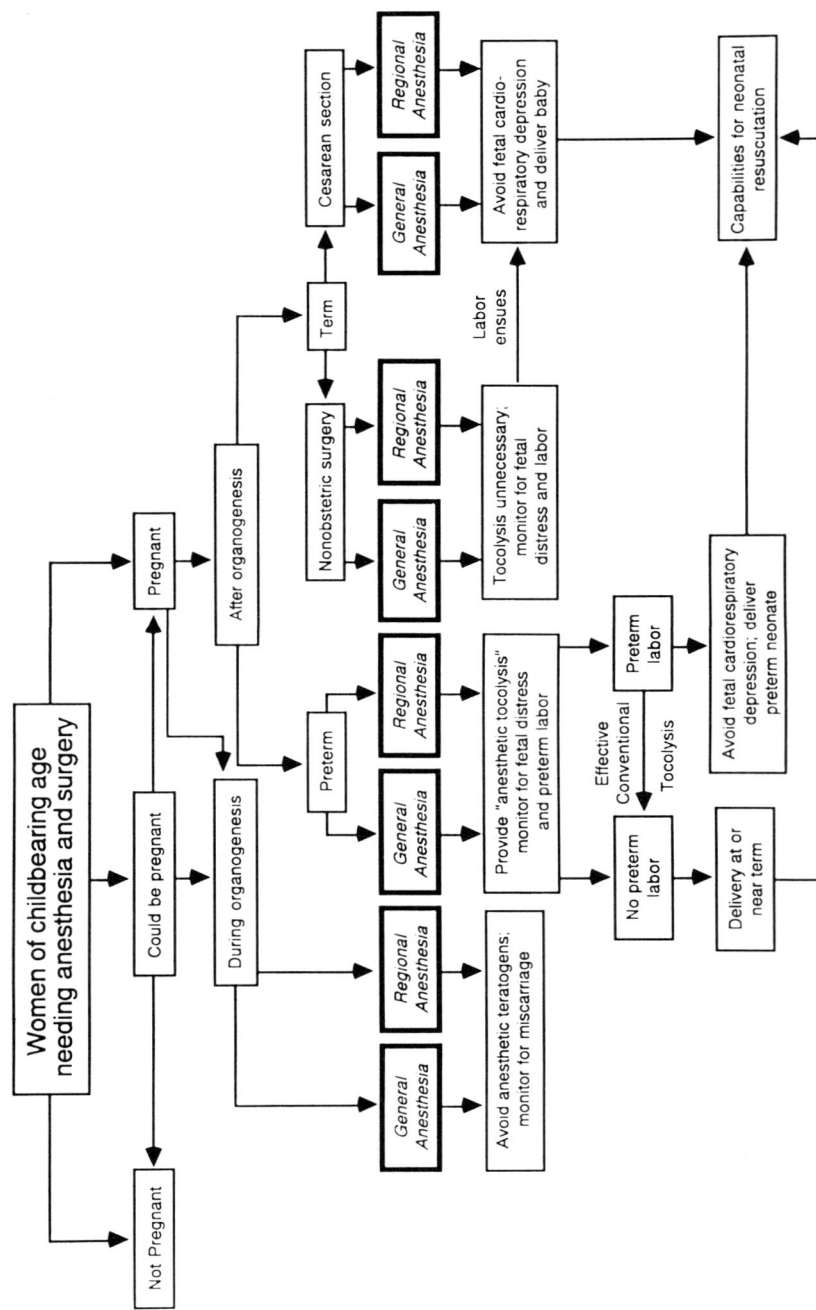

FIGURE 1. Algorithm of a continuum of anesthetic and critical care: mother, fetus, and neonate.

normal and abnormal functional needs of the mother, fetus, and neonate requiring anesthesia and critical care. By itself, or complementing other existing works in perinatal medicine, *Perinatal Anesthesia and Critical Care* bridges the gap in critical care management between fetal and neonatal life. This book's themes stress flexibility, preparedness, and vigilance in ensuring a smooth transition through surgery and the perioperative period for the mother, the fetus, and the neonate.

JAMES H. DIAZ

REFERENCES

1. Ayre P: The T-piece technique. Br J Anaesth 28:250, 1956
2. Forrest RD: Early history of wound treatment. J R Soc Med 75:198, 1982

Contents

1. Are Anesthetics Teratogens?

James H. Diaz, M.D.

INTRODUCTION

Abnormal fetal development may occur in 9% to 10% of the annual 2 million live births in the United States.[1] These developmental abnormalities may be divided into major (e.g., tracheoesophageal fistula) and minor (e.g., supernumerary digit) birth defects that together affect the lives of 15 million Americans.[1-3] Congenital abnormalities are, therefore, not rare and, in 3% to 7% of cases, will require some form of immediate treatment at birth,[2] as in the case of tracheoesophageal fistula. Congenital defects are the leading causes of both hospitalization and surgery in neonates and infants and are second only to accidental injuries as the cause for hospitalizations of children ages 1 to 18 years.[1-3]

According to Wilson,[4] only 2% to 3% of developmental defects are caused by drugs or environmental agents that, if identified by human or

---

Some portions of this chapter have been reproduced or adapted with permission from Diaz JH: Perioperative management of the pregnant patient undergoing nonobstetric surgery. Anesthesiology Review, January/February, 1991.

animal teratogen studies, can be avoided (Table 1–1). Unfortunately, 69% to 73% of congenital abnormalities are of unknown origin (see Table 1–1).[1, 3]

Although nitrous oxide is teratogenic in animals and myelosuppressive in both animals and humans, most other anesthetics do not cause more birth defects or spontaneous abortions in humans than occur naturally in human pregnancies without anesthetic exposures. In fact, the incidence of spontaneous abortion in unexposed human pregnancies is almost equal to the incidence of spontaneous abortion in anesthetic-exposed pregnancies. These facts should be comforting to those who administer a variety of anesthetics to the more than 50,000 pregnant women having surgical procedures each year in the United States.[4]

This chapter describes the pharmacokinetics of drug-induced teratogenesis in humans, identifies periods of human organogenesis most susceptible to teratogenesis (Tables 1–2 and 1–3), evaluates fetomaternal risk factors for teratogenesis, and compares animal and human studies of anesthetic-induced teratogenesis. Later chapters will discuss the physiologic changes of pregnancy (Chapter 2) and the physiologic alterations produced by general and regional anesthetics (Chapters 2 and 4) as they affect pregnancy outcome in humans. The indirect effects of anesthetics on the fetus from maternal cardiorespiratory depression may appear to be more important in determining neonatal outcome than any direct teratogenic potential of anesthetics (see Chapters 2 and 3).

DEFINITIONS

Teratogenicity is the ability of an agent or physical insult to induce a birth defect (morphologic, biochemical, or behavioral) at any stage of gestation that may be detected at birth or later.[2] Teratogens are agents that alter development of somatic cell lines during gestation, causing congenital abnormalities limited to single germ cell layers. Mutagens are toxic agents or physical insults that provoke deoxyribonucleic acid (DNA) alterations among all germ cell layers, causing widespread developmental

Table 1–1. Causes of Congenital Anomalies

Cause	Incidence (%)
Genetic transmission	20
Maternal	
Infections	2–3
Metabolic imbalance	1–2
Drugs or toxins	2–3
Radiation	1
Unknown	69–73

From Goldberg JD, Golbus MS: The value of case reports in human teratology. Am J Obstet Gynecol 154:479–482, 1986. Used with permission.

defects.[2] Mutations have limited etiologies and occur rarely.[2] Teratic changes occur frequently and may be caused by a number of diverse mechanisms including enzyme inhibition, osmolar imbalance, substrate deprivation, and membrane deformities.[2, 5]

A congenital anomaly or malformation is a primary structural defect, recognizable at birth or later, that results from a localized developmental error.[2] In contrast, a congenital deformity is a structural alteration of a previously normal part caused by mechanical forces during fetal development, such as clubfoot caused by intrauterine compression during pregnancies with oligohydramnios.[2, 6] A syndrome is a frequently occurring and easily recognized pattern of congenital anomalies with the same cause.[2, 6] Common drug-induced syndromes include the fetal alcohol syndrome, fetal phenytoin syndrome, aminopterin embryopathy, phencyclidine syndrome, lithium syndrome, and the thalidomide syndrome, which first brought public attention to drug teratogenicity in 1960.[2, 6]

Anomalies that occur together more frequently than expected by chance, do not have a common cause, and therefore do not represent a syndrome are known as *associations*.[7, 8] Common associations include the aniridia-Wilms' tumor association and the VATER (or VATERR) association.[8] The VATER mnemonic describes a nonrandom group of congenital anomalies of various causes consisting of *v*ertebral defects, *a*nal atresia, *t*racheoesophageal fistula, *e*sophageal atresia, and *r*adial or *r*enal dysplasia.[8, 9] Like other associations, the phenotypic expression of each part of the VATER association may not receive the same emphasis, so when one part of the association is detected, other parts should be sought carefully.[9]

THE PHARMACOKINETICS OF TERATOGENS

A 1973 survey by Forfar and Nelson[10] reported that women took an average of almost four drugs during pregnancy, excluding the most commonly prescribed nutritional supplements, vitamins, and iron. Only 20% of women responding to the survey abstained from drug use during pregnancy, excluding nutritional supplements.[9] Almost 50% of patients took medications during the first trimester of pregnancy, and almost one-half of total drug consumption during pregnancy occurred during periods of organogenesis.[1, 2, 9] Multiple drug use is therefore very common during pregnancy, especially during periods of organogenesis in the first trimester, and it complicates large-scale evaluations of drug teratogenesis in humans.[2] Table 1–2 shows the periods of human organogenesis during which teratogens may cause specific developmental anomalies in susceptible fetuses.[2]

In addition to the sheer number of critical drug exposures during

Table 1–2. Human Organogenesis*

Period of Development	Time (wk-mo)	Fetal Length		Cardiac Development	Neural Development	Limb Development	Genitourinary Development
		Somites	Crown–Rump Length (mm)				
PRE-EMBRYONIC	3rd week	1	NA	Heart tubes form	Neural groove forms	Intraembryonic mesoderm forms	Cloacal membrane forms
	4th week	10	NA	Heart tubes fuse	Neural tube closes; brain and optic and otic vesicles appear	Limb buds appear	Nephric ducts bud from nephrogenic cord
	5th week	22–30	NA	Septum primum and endocardial cushions appear	Spinal nerve roots, otic cups, and lens vesicles appear	Joint flexing occurs, hands and feet form	Nephric ducts reach cloaca; ureteric buds reach metanephros; urorectal septum and genital tubercle appear

			Cardiovascular/Hematopoietic	Nervous System	Musculoskeletal	Reproductive
EMBRYONIC	6th week	NA	5–10	Ostium primum closes; aorticopulmonary septation begins; cardiac muscle develops; hepatic hematopoiesis starts	Cerebral hemispheres and cerebellum develop	Chondrification and intramembranous ossification begin	Müllerian ducts and urethral plate appear
	7th week	NA	15–20	Interventricular septum complete	Choroid plexus produces CSF; eyelids develop	Skeletal muscle, fingers, and toes develop	Cloacal membrane breaks down; distinctive testes or ovaries form; nephrons develop and elongate
	8th week	NA	20–30	Fetal heart complete	Cerebral development continues	Endochondrial ossification starts; smooth muscle develops	Müllerian ducts fuse
FETAL	3rd month	NA	30–70	Hematopoiesis begins in bone marrow	Eyelids fuse	Muscular development and further ossification continue	Testes near internal inguinal ring; distinctive external genitalia appear
	4–7 months	NA	70+	Pulmonary alveoli and fetal cardiopulmonary circulation develop	Eyelids separate; pupils open; extensive CNS myelination occurs	Musculoskeletal development continues	Testes enter inguinal canal; vaginal plate canalizes

Modified with permission from Council on Scientific Affairs, American Medical Association: Effects of toxic chemicals on the reproductive system. JAMA 253:3431–3437, 1985. Copyright 1985, American Medical Association.
*CNS = central nervous system; CSF = cerebrospinal fluid; NA = not applicable.

Table 1–3. *Potential Drug-Induced Congenital Malformations Related to Period of Organogenesis and Time That Defect Occurs*

Time (Week of Development)	Potential Congenital Malformation
3rd	Ectopia cordis
	Omphalocele
4th	Omphalocele
	Tracheoesophageal fistula
	Hemivertebrae
5th	Cataracts
	Microphthalmia
	Facial clefts
	Phocomelia
6th	Cleft lip
	Congenital heart defects (septal)
	Aortic arch anomalies
7th	Congenital heart defects (valvular)
	Cleft palate
	Micrognathia
8th	Congenital heart defects (all types)
	Brachycephaly
	Nasal bone ablation
	Digital stunting

Reproduced with permission from Council on Scientific Affairs, American Medical Association: Effects of toxic chemicals on the reproductive system. JAMA 253:3431–3437, 1985. Copyright 1985, American Medical Association.

human pregnancy, a large number of drugs and toxic agents have been implicated in frequent case reports and animal studies as potential teratogens.[9, 10] Shepard[11] lists 1353 drugs and environmental toxins as teratogens in both animals and humans in his *Catalogue of Teratogenic Agents.* Potential drug-induced malformations and their relationships to the periods of organogenesis and timing of insult are listed in Table 1–3.[2]

At present, it is best to consider all drugs as potential teratogens, to prescribe the least amount of drug therapy in pregnant women and in women of childbearing age, and, if necessary, to use the oldest form and lowest dosage of effective drug therapy with effects that have been monitored for generations.[2, 3] Recent studies have shown that the human fetus is not protected by a "placental barrier" from teratogens and toxins.[11] In fact, all drugs and environmental agents of low to moderate lipid solubility and molecular weight can cross from the maternal circulation to the fetal circulation and allow fetal serum concentrations to equal or even exceed maternal serum concentrations.[11]

Besides the myth of the placental barrier, frequent drug exposures, and unsubstantiated reports of teratogenicity, a number of other factors cloud the study of human teratogenesis. Such factors include maternal pharmacokinetics, placental transfer, and fetal pharmacokinetics.[2, 3] Finally, the pattern of drug-induced birth defects varies among infants exposed to the same teratogens, and not all fetuses exposed to potential teratogens in utero will develop birth defects.[2, 3, 5, 9]

Maternal pharmacokinetic factors influencing the likelihood that a teratogen will or will not cause birth defects are determined by the physiochemical changes of pregnancy and include altered drug absorption, limited protein binding, reduced hepatic biotransformation, and enhanced renal elimination of maternal drugs.[3] The maternal physiochemical factors influencing placental transfer of drug teratogens are depicted in Figure 1–1.

Progesterone, a smooth muscle relaxant, will delay gastric emptying and reduce intestinal motility during pregancy, augmenting gastrointestinal absorption of some oral drugs and limiting absorption of others. Maternally administered drugs may often be diluted in an expanded extracellular fluid volume that limits protein binding and permits more placental transfer of free drug than in nonpregnant states. Biliary stasis during pregnancy and accelerated hepatic degradation of progesterone will occupy hepatic enzyme systems and limit hepatic biotransformation of many maternally administered drugs.[11] An increased maternal cardiac output in pregnancy provides more renal blood flow, increasing glomerular filtration and speeding elimination of water-soluble drug metabolites (see Fig. 1–1).[11] Acting together, the increased gastric and intestinal absorption, limited protein binding, and delayed hepatic biodegradation of many maternally administered drugs can increase the likelihood of drug teratogenicity during pregnancy.[11] However, the maternal factors that may permit drug teratogenicity are usually overwhelmed by the more protective effects of teratogen dilution in an expanded maternal plasma volume and rapid renal elimination of active teratogens and their metabolites.[11]

Placental transfer of drug teratogens is related to drug physiochemical characteristics and transplacental differences in serum pH.[11] The physiochemical characteristics of drugs that determine transplacental passage across the chorionic membrane include molecular weight, degree of ionization, lipid solubility, and the affinity for maternal protein binding already discussed. Highly lipid-soluble drugs and drugs that are only slightly ionized at physiologic pH are more easily transferred across the placental membranes than are highly ionized, lipid-insoluble drugs (see Fig. 1–1).[11] Drugs with molecular weights of 1000 or greater are transferred across placental membranes at much slower rates and in lower concentration than are drugs with molecular weights of 500 or less.[11] Finally, the transplacental differences in serum pH can have a clinically significant impact on the fetal distribution and accumulation of drugs with pKa values near physiologic pH.[11] Since fetal plasma pH is 0.1 to 0.2 unit less than maternal plasma pH, basic drugs preferentially

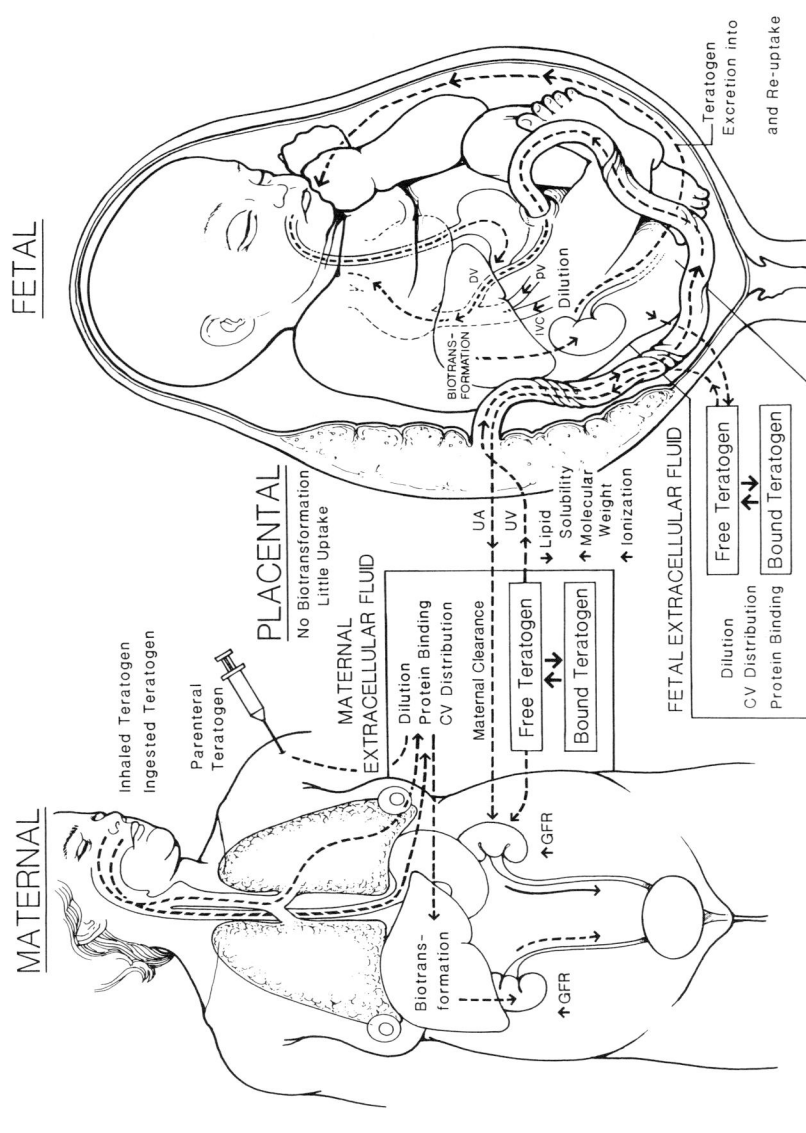

FETAL

Teratogen
Excretion into
and Re-uptake

BIOTRANS-
FORMATION

DV
IVC PV
Dilution

BIOTRANS-
FORMATION

UA
UV

PLACENTAL

No Biotransformation
Little Uptake

↑ Lipid
↑ Solubility
↑ Molecular Weight
↑ Ionization

FETAL EXTRACELLULAR FLUID

Dilution
CV Distribution
Protein Binding

| Free Teratogen |
| Bound Teratogen |

MATERNAL EXTRACELLULAR FLUID

Dilution
Protein Binding
CV Distribution

Maternal Clearance

| Free Teratogen |
| Bound Teratogen |

↑ GFR

MATERNAL

Inhaled Teratogen
Ingested Teratogen

Parenteral
Teratogen

Biotrans-
formation

↑ GFR

↑ GFR

FIGURE 1–1. The pharmacokinetics of placental transfer of drug teratogens. *CV,* cardiovascular; *DV,* ductus venosus; *GFR,* glomerular filtration rate; *IVC,* inferior vena cava; *PV,* portal vein; *UA,* umbilical artery; *UV,* umbilical vein.

accumulate in fetal blood and especially in fetal blood made even more acidotic by stress or asphyxia.[11]

Fetal physiochemical factors promoting drug teratogenicity include limited fetal biotransforming capabilities, prolonged and repeated exposures to teratogens in amniotic fluid, and reliance on maternal renal function for complete drug clearance (see Fig. 1–1).[12] The fetal physiochemical factors influencing fetal distribution are depicted in Figure 1–1.

Effective uteroplacental transfer of drugs and drug metabolites can allow the fetus to rapidly achieve from 50% to 100% of maternal serum drug levels in most cases.[11] As noted, the asphyxiated fetus can develop even higher serum levels of maternally administered drugs than the nonasphyxiated fetus due to ion trapping of basic drugs like local anesthetics, barbiturates, and narcotics in acidotic fetal blood.[11] As pregnancy progresses toward term, drug dilution in fetal extracellular fluid diminishes and fetal protein binding of drugs is limited by low plasma protein levels. Since amniotic fluid bathes the fetus, is absorbed through the skin, and is swallowed, the fetus is often re-exposed to drugs that were previously excreted into amniotic fluid.[11, 12] The fetal kidneys, therefore, cannot completely clear the fetal environment of drug teratogens, making the mother's kidney serve as the final excretory organ for the fetus.[11] Thus, placental transfer and fetal drug handling capabilities provide less fetal protection from drug teratogenicity than do maternal pharmacokinetics (see Fig. 1–1).[12]

In addition to fetomaternal factors and timing of drug exposures in pregnancy, two other main areas of concern remain in describing the pharmacokinetics of drug-induced birth defects: (1) The applicability of animal teratogen experiments to human teratogenesis and (2) human individual differences in susceptibility to drug teratogenesis. These concerns are especially important in studies of anesthetic teratogenicity, since most evidence implicating anesthetics as teratogens has come from intentional animal exposures and human case reports.[9]

In general, the marked variation in species susceptibility to drug-induced teratogenesis makes results obtained in animal testing difficult to apply to the human risks of teratogenesis from the same drugs.[10, 13, 14] The major problems with animal studies of drug teratogenesis are best exemplified by the findings with thalidomide.[13] When tested in rat fetuses, thalidomide did not produce the phocomelia later observed in monkey, rabbit, and human fetuses.[13] On the other hand, most information on human susceptibility to drug teratogenicity comes from retrospective (case reports) and prospective epidemiologic studies that, like animal data, are also conflicting.[13] Prospective drug studies are limited by the small number of teratogen exposures even in large study populations.[13] If no increases in malformations are seen in study populations compared with unexposed control populations, one still cannot be certain that the same drug may not act as a teratogen in smaller, more susceptible populations.[13] Human genetic polymorphisms in susceptibility to teratogens are very common and often place large populations at little risk and only a few selected patients at high risk of drug teratogenicity.[13]

In conclusion, animal teratogen studies yield poor predictive values for human fetuses. Animal studies should continue, but they cannot be relied upon for conclusive evidence of drug teratogenicity in humans. Only clinical observations of pregnancies and offspring will provide conclusive evidence of drug teratogenicity. The limited reliability of animal studies, human case reports, and epidemiologic surveys in predicting human drug teratogenicity has now made therapeutic nihilism the safest and most reasonable approach in most pregnancies. Occasionally, situations arise in which drugs, even known teratogens, must be prescribed in pregnancy (e.g., phenytoin for epilepsy). In these cases, counseling should be based on risk data from the largest epidemiologic studies, and drugs with the widest and longest human exposures should be prescribed.[13]

ARE ANESTHETICS TERATOGENS?

Chronic exposure of pregnant women to trace concentrations of anesthetic gases in unscavenged operating rooms has been poorly correlated with increased incidences of spontaneous abortions and congenital malformations. Several animal studies now show that nitrous oxide (N_2O) is teratogenic in rats, inducing fetal resorptions, visceral and skeletal abnormalities, and soft tissue defects even after short-term exposure to clinical dosages.[15, 16] On the other hand, large-scale prospective studies of N_2O teratogenicity in human pregnancies have had conflicting results.[15, 16] Recent prospective animal studies on the reproductive and teratogenic effects of inhaled anesthetics, intravenous anesthetics, and anesthetics combined with N_2O confirmed consistent animal teratogenesis with N_2O alone and in combinations, but showed no adverse effects from other inhaled or intravenous anesthetics administered without N_2O.[17–19] At present, only N_2O is a consistent animal teratogen among the anesthetic gases. In humans, only N_2O may cause a slight (statistically insignificant) increase in spontaneous abortions in chronically exposed pregnant health care workers.

In 1967, Vaisman[20] reported 354 Russian anesthesiologists, most of them female, with an unusually high incidence of headache, fatigue, irritability, and nausea following prolonged exposure to trace combinations of anesthetic gases in unscavenged operating rooms. Vaisman also noted that 18 of 31 pregnancies in female anesthesiologists ended in spontaneous abortion. Unfortunately, Vaisman's work had no control populations for comparison with the reported study populations. This 1967 study did, however, promote early interest in anesthetic reproductive and teratogenic effects and stimulated a number of large epidemiologic surveys throughout the world. Like the antimetabolite aminopterin, most abortifacients are also powerful teratogens, and early surveys of increased abortion risk in anesthetic-exposed pregnancies suggested high likelihood of anesthetic-induced birth defects as well.

In a 1970 questionnaire study, Askrog and Harvald[21] in Denmark showed that the frequency of abortion increased from 10% to 20% after women started working as anesthestiologists in unscavenged operating rooms. In the United States, Cohen and coauthors[22] later confirmed this increase in spontaneous abortions and reported the highest abortion rate to date (38%) among female anesthesiologists compared with other female physicians. These investigators reported an abortion rate of $17.1 \pm 2.0\%$ in female anesthesiologists compared with $8.9 \pm 1.8\%$ in female pediatricians ($p = 0.01$).[22] They also observed increased abortion rates in nurse anesthetists and operating room nurses and estimated the overall risks of abortion in female operating room workers to be 1.3 to 2 times that of unexposed female health care workers.[22] Knill-Jones and associates[23] also demonstrated an increased abortion rate of 18% among British female anesthesiologists compared with a 14% incidence of spontaneous abortions in pregnancies of retired female anesthesiologists, those no longer working in unscavenged operating rooms.

The true incidence of spontaneous abortion in the general population is unknown, but the estimated incidence in small study groups ranges from 15%[21, 22] to 31%.[24] Abortions occur most often in the first 3 weeks of gestation, often before women realize they are pregnant, and are unusual after 15 weeks unless there is cervical incompetence, intrauterine infection, abdominal trauma, or peritonitis.[24] The observed incidences of spontaneous abortion among trace anesthetic–exposed operating room personnel (18% to 38%) do not appear unduly high when compared with the estimated incidence of spontaneous abortion in the general population (15% to 31%).[22–24] Nevertheless, abortions occur more frequently among female anesthesiologists than in control groups, and working anesthesiologists have more abortions than do retired anesthesiologists.[20–23] Effects of job-related stress and maternal age on pregnancy outcome have not, however, been studied in working or retired female operating room personnel.[20–23] Despite a lack of supporting evidence, some authorities have recommended that pregnant women, particularly those in the first trimester, should adhere to national standards[25] and avoid working in unscavenged operating rooms with levels of halogenated anesthetics greater than 1 ppm and N_2O levels greater than 25 to 60 ppm.[22]

Since most abortifacients are also teratogens, earlier reports of increased abortions among N_2O-exposed personnel prompted epidemiologic surveys on the incidence of congenital anomalies in exposed health care workers. N_2O alone and N_2O combined with some halogenated agents are teratogenic in animals, but the risk of congenital anomalies in children of exposed female health care workers is hard to predict from these animal studies, for the reasons presented earlier. Corbett and associates[26] reported a 5.9 ± 1.4% incidence of major congenital anomalies in children of nurse anesthetists, providing another possible reason for pregnant women to avoid unscavenged operating rooms, especially during the first trimester. However, when compared with the 9% to 10% incidence of all birth defects in the general population, the study by Corbett and associates[26] does not appear to place the pregnant anesthesiologist at any higher risk for congenital anomalies than other pregnant women.[1]

A variety of large retrospective surveys have documented no significant increase in the incidence of congenital abnormalities in offspring of first- and second-trimester surgical patients compared with nonoperated control patients (Table 1–4).[27–30] Fetal loss following surgery in these studies was due to premature labor and delivery triggered by surgical pathology and not by anesthetic techniques or agents.[27–30] Acute surgical illnesses, particularly cervical incompetence and acute appendicitis, are the major determinants of postoperative premature labor and fetal loss in most pregnant surgical patients.[27–29]

Nitrous Oxide

In humans and experimental animals, N_2O inactivates vitamin B_{12}, reduces tissue folate stores, inhibits synthesis and activity of methionine synthetase, and makes less methionine and thymidine available for DNA synthesis.[31, 32] The effects of N_2O on vitamin B_{12}, folate, and methionine synthetase activity in humans are rapid and may be detected after exposure to clinical concentrations of N_2O (50% to 70%) for periods as brief as 1.25 to 2.75 hours.[31–33] Leukopenia and thrombocytopenia from bone marrow depression and megaloblastic anemia from vitamin B_{12} inactivation have been reported after both long-term (12 hours to 3 days) and short-term (5 to 12 hours) exposure to 50% to 70% N_2O.[16, 31–33] Megaloblastic changes in bone marrow and in peripheral blood have also been reported in critically ill patients exposed to the same concentrations of N_2O for periods as brief as 2 hours.[34]

The bone marrow depressant effects of N_2O have been well studied in humans and have linked even short-term exposure to clinical concentrations of N_2O to potential inhibition of DNA synthesis through inhibition of methionine synthetase and its essential cofactor, vitamin B_{12}. A minimum of 5 hours of exposure to 50% or more N_2O is required in uncompromised patients before evidence of bone marrow suppression

Table 1–4. Surveys of Fetal Wastage and Congenital Defects in Liveborn Offspring of Women Undergoing Surgery During the First and Second Trimester

Study Author(s)	Year Published	Obstetric Population	First Trimester			Second Trimester		
			Operations*	Abortions	Congenital Defects	Operations*	Abortions	Congenital Defects
Smith[27]	1963	18,493	10	2	0	45	5	0
Shnider and Webster[28]	1965	9,073	47	3	4	58	5	6
Brodsky et al.[29]	1980	12,929	187	9	3	100	4	3
Crawford and Lewis[30]	1986	548	333	28	11	24	0	3

*Various anesthetics.

becomes demonstrable by morphologic changes in bone marrow aspirates and abnormal deoxyuridine suppression tests.[35, 36] However, less sensitive blood tests of bone marrow activity, such as peripheral blood smears, have failed to confirm morphologic damage to blood elements after longer exposures (24 hours) to N_2O in healthy human volunteers.[37] In all cases in which morphologic changes in marrow aspirates have occurred after N_2O exposure, they have resolved completely within 10 days.[38] As noted, debilitated patients may be susceptible to bone marrow suppression from N_2O even after short exposure.[34]

The teratogenic effects of N_2O in a variety of experimental animals have been attributed to N_2O suppression of DNA synthesis. Recent animal investigations have shown that folinic acid supplements can reduce the incidence of birth defects and protect against the myelosuppressive effects of N_2O in pregnant rats exposed to N_2O for 24 hours or longer.[39, 40] Folinic acid protection against the teratogenic and myelosuppressive effects of N_2O in animals is presumed to result from enhanced DNA synthesis via alternate metabolic pathways in the presence of methionine synthetase inhibition.[40]

Despite considerable animal data, N_2O has not been established as a consistent teratogen in humans, and there are no current indications to pretreat pregnant women with folinic acid before administration of N_2O.[31] Despite its adverse effects on cellular metabolism in humans and animals, short-term clinical exposure to N_2O does not cause an increased incidence of fetal abnormalities or low birth weights in human offspring.[31] As noted, the increased incidence of fetal abnormalities after N_2O inhalation first reported by Corbett and others[26] in 1974 has not been confirmed by several retrospective studies of general anesthetics in pregnancy.[27-29] Additionally, N_2O in clinical concentrations did not influence the success rates for in vitro fertilization and subsequent pregnancy in seven women (60%) undergoing laparoscopy for oocyte retrieval, in vitro fertilization, and subsequent zygote transfer.[40]

Crawford and Lewis[30] examined the hospital records of 463 patients undergoing general anesthetics with N_2O during the first two trimesters of pregnancy and compared outcomes with pregnant patients having similar procedures during regional anesthesia. Outcomes reported over a 14-year period included spontaneous abortions, congenital malformations, and low birth weights. There were no significant differences between the two groups in incidence of abortions or neonatal outcomes. Another epidemiologic survey by Duncan and others[41] studied the entire population of Manitoba, Canada, between 1971 and 1978 and matched a series of 2565 patients having surgery during pregnancy with an equal number of nonoperated control subjects of similar age and residence. The anesthetics, however, were only categorized as none (18%), general (57%), spinal (2%), and local (24%).[30, 41] Thus, one can only assume that

N_2O was administered to the majority of patients undergoing general anesthesia for major surgery in pregnancy. Once again, the incidences of abortions and congenital malformations were the same in the operated and nonoperated groups.[41] Another study by Brodsky and others[29] compared returned questionnaire data from 287 pregnant dental hygienists and pregnant wives of dentists who underwent general anesthesia with data from unexposed and nonoperated control groups (Table 1–4). This study also found no association between N_2O exposure in the dental office or during surgery and congenital malformations in offspring.[29] This study did, however, report a higher incidence of fetal loss in the operated group compared with the nonoperated control group.[29]

Despite excellent data supporting both the myelosuppressive effects of N_2O in humans and in animals and the teratogenetic effects of prolonged exposure to N_2O in animals, the incidence of congenital anomalies among children of women who undergo general anesthesia with N_2O while pregnant is not increased. As noted, there is at present no indication to pretreat pregnant women with folinic acid supplements before N_2O administration.[31] It appears safe to administer N_2O to healthy pregnant women for single operative procedures lasting less than 6 hours.[29, 31] However, pregnant patients compromised by acute critical illness, trauma, or chronic disease may be at greater risk of the myelosuppressive effects of N_2O even after short exposures.[34] Although N_2O diminishes the amount of thymidine available for DNA synthesis by dividing cells, the anesthetic does not affect human oocyte release, subsequent human fertilization, or early embryologic development during in vitro fertilization procedures.[40] Conclusions regarding the relationship of N_2O to spontaneous abortion in operating room personnel have been difficult to develop because of conflicting data. At present, most studies suggest that the underlying disease processes (e.g., cervical incompetence, acute appendicitis) that led to the operation during pregnancy are more significant risk factors for fetal wastage than is the choice of anesthetic or use of N_2O.[24, 31]

Volatile Anesthetics

For more than a decade, Mazze and associates have studied the reproductive and teratogenic potential of both N_2O alone and in combination with other volatile anesthetics or narcotics in rodent models.[42–48] To date, the only consistent teratogenic effects in rodents have been produced with N_2O,[17, 45, 46, 48–50] confirming the original report of N_2O teratogenesis in animals by Fink and coworkers in 1967[49] and a subsequent "rediscovery" of N_2O teratogenesis in animals by Lane and associates in 1980.[50]

Women who undergo general anesthesia during pregnancy often

receive combinations of inhaled agents and multiple parenteral agents. Volatile anesthetics are usually administered in N_2O and oxygen (O_2) as carrier gases. These combinations of inhaled and parenteral anesthetics limit the applicability of human anesthetic teratogenicity studies to animal studies conducted with single volatile agents in O_2. To date, only one large controlled epidemiologic study of reproductive outcome in women undergoing general anesthesia during pregnancy, known as the Collaborative Perinatal Project, has been reported.[51] The project's findings with the commonly administered volatile anesthetics are summarized in comparison with animal studies with the same agents.[51]

Halothane. The frequency of congenital anomalies was not significantly increased among offspring of 25 women receiving halothane anesthetics during the first trimester of pregnancy in the Collaborative Perinatal Project reported by Heinomen and colleagues in 1977.[51] In mice, fetal death, congenital anomalies, and growth retardation were common among offspring of animals repeatedly anesthetized with halothane during pregnancy, but such exposures usually produced maternal deaths from circulatory depression.[42, 52] In direct contrast, no increased maternal toxicity or teratogenic effects were observed in rats or in rabbits after similar exposures.[48, 53] However, behavioral abnormalities have been observed among adult rats born to female rats anesthetized with halothane during pregnancy.[54] In a recent experiment, Mazze and others actually prevented N_2O-induced fetal wastage and teratogenicity in rats by adding halothane (0.27%) to N_2O inhalation.[55] The authors attributed the protective effects of halothane against N_2O-mediated teratogenicity in rats to halothane's ability to maintain uterine blood flow and reverse N_2O-mediated increases in adrenergic tone with reduced uteroplacental perfusion.[55]

Enflurane. No epidemiologic studies of congenital anomalies in offspring of women receiving enflurane anesthetics during pregnancy have been reported to date. Limb and abdominal wall defects have, however, been observed more frequently than expected in offspring of rabbits anesthetized with clinical concentrations of enflurane during pregnancy.[56] In another study,[44] increased incidences of cleft palate, skeletal anomalies, and fetal growth retardation were reported among the offspring of mice repeatedly anesthetized with enflurane during pregnancy. In contrast, no teratogenic effects were observed among mice or rats receiving similar enflurane anesthetics in other studies.[48, 57]

Isoflurane. No epidemiologic studies of congenital anomalies in offspring of women receiving isoflurane anesthetics during pregnancy have been reported to date. In one study, increased incidences of cleft palate, skeletal anomalies, and fetal growth retardation were observed among the offspring of pregnant mice repeatedly exposed to subanesthetic doses of isoflurane.[47] In contrast, other animal studies have shown no teratogenic effects among the offspring of pregnant rats or rabbits receiving repeated anesthetics with clinical doses of isoflurane.[48, 58] Interestingly, one study reported that the addition of isoflurane (0.35% or 0.25 minimum alveolar concentration [MAC] in rats) stopped the majority of congenital anomalies caused by N_2O in rodents.[17] Like the halothane-N_2O study conducted by Mazze and others,[55] this study also suggested that isoflurane's protective effects against N_2O-mediated teratogenicity in rats might be due to maintenance of uterine blood flow, reduced adrenergic tone in the uteroplacental circulation, or prevention of N_2O-inhibition of methionine synthetase activity.[17]

Parenteral Anesthetic Agents and Adjuvants

In the past, reliable studies of parenteral anesthetic agents, especially the barbiturates and narcotics, were not possible in experimental animals because of the direct maternal and indirect fetal cardiovascular toxicity associated with bolus drug administration and resulting circulatory depression.[59-61] The older narcotics (morphine, meperidine, and methadone) caused adverse reproductive and teratogenic effects in experimental animals only at doses high enough to cause maternal cardiorespiratory depression, presumably with intrauterine fetal asphyxia.[60-65] Recently, chronically implanted subcutaneous osmotic infusion pumps have permitted researchers to study the teratogenic effects of parenteral anesthetics without adverse maternal consequences and fetal asphyxia from maternal cardiopulmonary depression.[59, 66]

Narcotics. Fujinaga and associates[19, 59] studied the teratogenic potential of narcotics and narcotic-N_2O combinations in rats, using infusion pumps for safer drug administration. The addition of the narcotic fentanyl does not significantly alter the adverse reproductive and teratogenic effects of N_2O in rodents.[18, 59] Only N_2O alone or in combination with fentanyl has caused significant bone resorptions in rodent fetuses and major visceral and soft tissue malformations in rat offspring.[18]

The chronic use of subcutaneously implanted infusion pumps has now permitted the continuous delivery of high total daily doses of fentanyl, alfentanil, and sufentanil at constant serum levels throughout organogenesis in rats without maternal toxicity.[18, 19, 59, 66] Fentanyl, in doses up to 500 μg/kg/day, delivered by infusion pump for 2 weeks before breeding and throughout pregnancy, was devoid of adverse reproductive and teratogenic effects.[59] No significant adverse reproductive or teratogenic effects were produced by either sufentanil (10, 50, or 100 μg/kg/day) or alfentanil (8 μg/kg/day), administered continuously by infusion pumps from day 5 through day 20 of rodent pregnancy.[19]

In conclusion, the newer narcotic supplements available for use during anesthesia (fentanyl, sufentanil, and alfentanil), when administered in high doses by infusion pumps throughout animal pregnancies, do not cause abortions or congenital anomalies.[18, 19, 59] The subcutaneously implanted infusion pump has facilitated the study of reproductive and teratogenic effects of narcotics in animals by permitting slow, continuous delivery of large doses that would not be tolerated by bolus injection or might otherwise complicate experimental designs.[8, 19, 59, 66] Despite the weaknesses of applying animal data to humans, fentanyl, sufentanil, and alfentanil can be presumed safe for use during human pregnancy.[18, 19, 59, 66] More extensive clinical use of these narcotics during anesthesia in pregnant patients without adverse reproductive or teratogenic effects will, however, be required to confirm the extensive animal data on the safety of narcotic adjuvant use during human pregnancy.

Barbiturates

Thiopental. The frequency of congenital anomalies in offspring of 152 women receiving thiopental during the first trimester of pregnancy was no greater than expected in the Collaborative Perinatal Project.[51] The frequency of congenital anomalies was also not increased among the offspring of mice or rats treated during pregnancy with 1.5 to 3 times the usual human dose of thiopental.[67–70] Human and animal data suggest that the risk of congenital anomalies in children of women receiving thiopental early in pregnancy is not substantially greater than the risk in the general population.[69, 70]

Methohexital. The frequency of congenital anomalies in offspring of 41 women receiving methohexital during the first trimester of pregnancy was no greater than expected in the Collaborative Perinatal Project.[51] No studies of methohexital teratogenicity in experimental animals have been reported.[68, 69]

Thiamylal. The frequency of congenital anomalies in offspring of 21 women receiving thiamylal during the first trimester of pregnancy was no greater than expected in the Collaborative Perinatal Project.[51] However, limb and digital anomalies were observed more frequently than expected among the offspring of mice treated during pregnancy with thiamylal.[68, 69]

Tranquilizers.
Human case reports and numerous prospective studies in experimental animals have associated the use of the benzodiazepines (diazepam and chlordiazepoxide) and the phenothiazines (chlorpromazine) during pregnancy with a significantly increased risk of congenital malformations.[2] Safra and Oakley[71] reported a significant association between cleft lip alone and with cleft palate and prenatal exposure to diazepam. During pregnancy, especially during periods of organogenesis in the first trimester, the use of the benzodiazepines, the phenothiazines, or related drugs, like the butyrophenones (droperidol and haloperidol), is not recommended.[2, 69, 70]

Other Parenteral Anesthetics

Etomidate. No epidemiologic studies have been reported to date of congenital anomalies among offspring of women anesthetized with etomidate during pregnancy. The frequency of congenital anomalies was no greater than expected among offspring of rats treated during pregnancy with etomidate in doses 40 times those used to induce anesthesia in humans.[72]

Ketamine. To date, no epidemiologic studies of congenital anomalies among offspring of women anesthetized with ketamine during pregnancy have been reported.[51, 69] The frequency of congenital anomalies was no greater than expected among offspring of rats treated during pregnancy with ketamine in doses 10 times those used in humans.[73]

Local Anesthetics

Lidocaine. Fujinaga and Mazza[60] have also used infusion pumps to administer clinical doses of lidocaine to rats throughout pregnancy without adverse reproductive or teratogenic effects. The frequency of major or minor congenital anomalies in offspring of 293 women treated with lidocaine as a local anesthetic during the first trimester of pregnancy was no greater than expected in the Collaborative Perinatal Project.[51] However, no epidemiologic studies of congenital anomalies have been conducted in pregnant women treated with lidocaine for cardiac arrhythmias.[69]

Mepivacaine. A twofold increase in the frequency of congenital anomalies was observed among the children of 82 women who received mepivacaine during the first trimester of pregnancy in the Collaborative Perinatal Project.[51] This disturbing increase in the incidence of congenital anomalies associated with mepivacaine use in early pregnancy was not repeated in the offspring of another group of 224 pregnant women treated with mepivacaine throughout pregnancy.[51] No teratologic studies of mepivacaine use in pregnant experimental animals have been reported to date.[69] Findings in the Collaborative Perinatal Project would recommend avoiding mepivacaine use in early pregnancy.[51]

Procaine. The frequency of congenital anomalies in offspring of 1340 women receiving procaine as a local anesthetic during the first trimester of pregnancy was no greater than expected in the Collaborative Perinatal Project.[51] In a case-control study of 266 infants with congenital anomalies, the frequency of maternal treatment with procaine during the first trimester was not greater than expected.[74] No teratologic studies of procaine in experimental animals have been published to date.[69]

Tetracaine. The frequency of congenital anomalies in the children of 23 women treated with tetracaine during the first trimester of pregnancy was no greater than expected in the Collaborative Perinatal Project.[51] No teratologic studies of tetracaine in experimental animals have been reported.[69]

Other Local Anesthetics. The following commonly used local anesthetic agents have not been adequately studied for teratogenic effects: bupivacaine, chloroprocaine, etidocaine, and prilocaine.[69] No epidemiologic studies have been reported among offspring of women receiving these local anesthetics during pregnancy.[69] No teratologic studies of these local anesthetics in pregnant experimental animals have been conducted.[69]

CONCLUSIONS

Currently administered inhaled anesthetics and most local anesthetics are not teratogenic in humans. Among the modern anesthetic gases, only N_2O causes abortions and birth defects in laboratory animals exclusively. Although the myelosuppressive effects of N_2O occur in both animals and humans, these effects have no significant impact on human pregnancy except that they worsen preexisting anemia in women with chronic illnesses, folate deficiency, or dilutional anemia. The local anesthetics (excluding mepivacaine), barbiturates, ketamine, etomidate, and narcotics are not teratogenic in animals and can probably be used safely throughout human pregnancy. The benzodiazepines, notably diazepam and chlordiazepoxide, and the phenothiazines, most notably chlorpromazine, are teratogenic both in animals and in humans and should be avoided as anesthetic adjuvants throughout the first trimester of pregnancy and possibly throughout gestation.[2, 70]

Operating rooms and dental offices should be scavenged of waste anesthetic gases to provide better working conditions for all health care workers and reduce levels of halogenated gases to 1 ppm or less and N_2O to 25 to 60 ppm or less in accordance with National Institute of Occupational Safety and Health standards.[22, 25] Gas scavenging systems should be provided not only on anesthesia machines but also for the operating room or dental office itself. Pregnant health workers should avoid unscavenged operating rooms to reduce their risks of chronic N_2O exposure with its attendant myelosuppressive effects.

Pregnant patients who need surgery may receive most local anesthetics and narcotics as needed. Healthy pregnant patients may receive N_2O for operative procedures lasting less than 6 hours.[30] Pregnant patients compromised by chronic disease, acute critical illness, or trauma should not receive N_2O because of significant myelosuppression even after short exposure. Since elective and semielective operations should be delayed until after delivery and the puerperium, most patients undergo nonobstetric surgery during pregnancy for urgent reasons, most notably for cervical incompetence, acute appendicitis, ovarian torsion, or traumatic injury. Such patients should not receive N_2O during emergency surgery.

In conclusion, anesthetics are often blamed for abortions or birth defects without documentation or evidence. Detailed investigations of the reproductive and teratogenic effects of anesthetics have now been completed in experimental animals and in humans. These studies have identified only N_2O as a consistent abortifacient and teratogen in animals exclusively. As noted, N_2O is myelosuppressive in animals and in humans, but it does not cause significantly more human abortions or birth defects than would occur normally in the general population. The narcotics and a number of local anesthetics are safe for use throughout pregnancy. The benzodiazepines and phenothiazines should not be used as anesthetic adjuvants throughout organogenesis and possibly throughout gestation. Advanced maternal age, environmental exposures, and surgical illnesses appear to have more impact on fetal wastage and deformity than do anesthetics.

References

1. Goldberg JD, Golbus MS: The value of case reports in human teratology. Am J Obstet Gynecol 154:479–482, 1986
2. Council on Scientific Affairs, American Medical Association: Effects of toxic chemicals on the reproductive system. JAMA 253:3431–3437, 1985
3. Persaud TVN, Chudley AE, Skalko RG: Basic Concepts in Teratology. New York: Alan R. Liss, 1985, pp 13–29
4. Wilson JG: Environmental effects in development—teratology. In: Assali NS (ed): Pathophysiology of Gestation, vol 2. New York: Academic Press, 1972, pp 269–353
5. Brodsky JB: Anesthesia and surgery during early pregnancy and fetal outcome. Clin Obstet Gynecol 26:449–457, 1983
6. Pernoll MC, King CR, Prescott GH: Genetics for the clinical obstetrician-gynecologist. In: Wynn RM (ed): Obstetrics and Gynecology Annual, vol 9. New York: Appleton-Century-Crofts, 1980, pp 1–53
7. Smith DW: An approach to clinical dysmorphology. J Pediatr 91:690–692, 1977
8. McKusick VA: On lumpers and splitters, or the morphology of genetic disease. Birth Defects 5:23–32, 1969
9. Jones OW: Reproductive genetics: Basic genetics and patterns of inheritance. In: Creasy RK, Resnik R (eds): Maternal-Fetal Medicine: Principles and Practice. Philadelphia: W.B. Saunders, 1984, pp 3–92
10. Forfar JO, Nelson MM: Epidemiology of drugs taken by pregnant women: Drugs that may affect the fetus adversely. Clin Pharmacol Ther 14:632–642, 1973
11. Shepard T: Catalogue of Teratogenic Agents, 4th ed. Baltimore: Johns Hopkins University Press, 1983
12. Brendel K, Duhamel RC, Shepard TH: Embryotoxic drugs. Biol Res Pregnancy Perinatol 6:1–6, 1985
13. Spielberg SP: Pharmacogenetics and the fetus. N Engl J Med 307:115–116, 1982
14. Blake DA: Requirements and limitations in reproductive and teratogenic risk assessment. In: Niebyl JR (ed): Drug Use in Pregnancy. Philadelphia: Lea & Febiger, 1982, pp 1–8
15. Keeling PA, Rocke DA, Nunn JF, et al: Folinic acid protection against nitrous oxide teratogenicity in the rat. Br J Anaesth 58:528–534, 1986
16. Aldridge LM, Tunstall ME: Nitrous oxide and the fetus. Br J Anaesth 58:1348–1356, 1986
17. Fujinaga M, Baden JM, Yhap EO, et al.: Reproductive and teratogenic effects of nitrous oxide, isoflurane, and their combination in Sprague-Dawley rats. Anesthesiology 67:960–964, 1987
18. Mazze RI, Fujinaga M, Baden JM: Reproductive and teratogenic effects of nitrous oxide, fentanyl, and their combination in Sprague-Dawley rats. Br J Anaesth 59:1291–1297, 1987
19. Fujinaga M, Mazze RI, Jackson EC, et al.: Reproductive and teratogenic effects of sufentanil and alfentanil in Sprague-Dawley rats. Anesth Analg 67:166–169, 1988.
20. Vaisman AI: Usloviia truda v operatisionnykh i ikh vliianie na zdorov'e anesteziologov. Eksp Khir Anest 12:44–49, 1967

21. Askrog V, Harvald B: Teratogen effect of inhalationsanestetika. Nord Med 83:498–500, 1970
22. Cohen EN, Bellville JW, Brown BW Jr: Anesthesia, pregnancy, and miscarriage: A study of operating room nurses and anesthetists. Anesthesiology 35:343–347, 1971
23. Knill-Jones RP, Rodrigues LU, Moir DD, et al.: Anaesthetic practice and pregnancy: Controlled survey of women anaesthetists in the United Kingdom. Lancet 1:1326–1328, 1972
24. Wilcox AJ, Weinberg CR, O'Connor JF, et al.: Incidence of early loss of pregnancy. N Engl J Med 319:189–194, 1988
25. U.S. Department of Health, Education, and Welfare (National Institute for Occupational Safety and Health): Criteria for a recommended standard—occupational exposure to waste anesthetic gases and vapors. Cincinnati: DHEW (NIOSH) Publication No. 77-140, Public Health Service Center for Disease Control, 1977
26. Corbett TH, Cornell RG, Endres JL, et al.: Birth defects among children of nurse-anesthetists. Anesthesiology 41:341–344, 1974
27. Smith BE: Fetal prognosis after anesthesia during gestation. Anesth Analg 42:521–526, 1963
28. Shnider SM, Webster GM: Maternal and fetal hazards of surgery during pregnancy. Am J Obstet Gynecol 138:1165–1167, 1965
29. Brodsky JB, Cohen EN, Brown BW, et al.: Surgery during pregnancy and fetal outcome. Am J Obstet Gynecol 138:1165–1167, 1980
30. Crawford JS, Lewis M: Nitrous oxide in early human pregnancy. Anesthesia 41:900–905, 1986
31. Mazze RI: Nitrous oxide during pregnancy. Anaesthesia 41:897–899, 1986
32. Amess JA, Burman JF, Rees GM, et al.: Megaloblastic haemopoiesis in patients receiving nitrous oxide. Lancet 2:339–342, 1978
33. Skacel PO, Chanarin I, Hewlett A, et al.: Failure to correct nitrous oxide toxicity with folinic acid (letter). Anesthesiology 57:557–558, 1982
34. Amos RJ, Amess JAL, Hinds CJ, et al.: Incidence and pathogenesis of acute megaloblastic bone-marrow change in patients receiving intensive care. Lancet 2:835–838, 1982
35. Kano Y, Sakamoto S, Sakuraya K, et al.: Effect of nitrous oxide on human bone marrow cells and its synergistic effect with methionine and methotrexate on functional folate deficiency. Cancer Res 41:4698–4701, 1981
36. O'Sullivan H, Jennings F, Ward K, et al.: Human bone marrow biochemical function and megaloblastic hematopoiesis after nitrous oxide anesthesia. Anesthesiology 55:645–649, 1981
37. Thompson PL, Lown B: Nitrous oxide as an analgesic in acute myocardial infarction. JAMA 235:924–927, 1976
38. Chanarin I: The effect of nitrous oxide on cobalamins, folate and on related events. CRC Crit Rev Toxicol 10:179–213, 1982
39. Amos RT, Amess JAL, Nancekievill DG, et al.: Prevention of nitrous oxide-induced megaloblastic changes in bone marrow using folinic acid. Br J Anaesth 56:103–107, 1984
40. Rosen MA, Roizen MF, Eger EI II, et al.: The effect of nitrous oxide on in vitro fertilization success rate. Anesthesiology 67:42–44, 1987
41. Duncan PG, Pope WEB, Cohen MM, et al.: Fetal risks of anesthesia and surgery during pregnancy. Anesthesiology 74:790–794, 1986
42. Wharton RS, Wilson AI, Mazze RI, et al.: Fetal morphology in mice exposed to halothane. Anesthesiology 51:532–537, 1979
43. Wharton RS, Sievenpiper TS, Mazze RI: Developmental toxicity of methoxyflurane in mice. Anesth Analg 59:421–425, 1980
44. Wharton RS, Mazze RI, Wilson AI: Reproduction and fetal development in mice chronically exposed to enflurane. Anesthesiology 54:505–510, 1981
45. Mazze RI, Wilson AI, Rice SA, et al.: Reproduction and fetal development in mice chronically exposed to nitrous oxide. Teratology 26:11–16, 1982
46. Mazze RI, Wilson AI, Rice SA, et al.: Reproduction and fetal development in rats exposed to nitrous oxide. Teratology 30:259–265, 1984
47. Mazze RI, Wilson AI, Rice SA, et al.: Fetal development in mice exposed to isoflurane. Teratology 32:339–345, 1985
48. Mazze RI, Fujinaga M, Rice SA, et al.: Reproductive and teratogenic effects of nitrous

oxide, halothane, isoflurane, and enflurane in Sprague-Dawley rats. Anesthesiology 64:339–344, 1986
49. Fink BR, Shepard TH, Blandau RJ: Teratogenic activity of nitrous oxide. Nature 214:146–148, 1967
50. Lane GA, Nahrwold ML, Tait AR, et al.: Anesthetics as teratogens: nitrous oxide is fetotoxic, xenon is not. Science 210:899–901, 1980
51. Heinomen OP, Slone D, Shapiro S: Birth Defects and Drugs in Pregnancy. Littleton, MA: Publishing Sciences Group, 1977
52. Wharton RS, Mazze RI, Baden JM, et al.: Fertility, reproduction, and postnatal survival in mice chronically exposed to halothane. Anesthesiology 48:167–174, 1978
53. Kennedy GL, Smith SH, Keplinger ML, et al.: Reproductive and teratologic studies with halothane. Toxicol Appl Pharmacol 35:467–474, 1976
54. Smith RF, Bowman RE, Katz J: Behavioral effects of exposure to halothane during early pregnancy in the rat: Sensitive period during pregnancy. Anesthesiology 49:319–323, 1978
55. Mazze RI, Fujinaga M, Baden JM: Halothane prevents nitrous oxide teratogenicity in Sprague-Dawley rats; folinic acid does not. Teratology 38:121–127, 1988
56. Ramazzotto LJ, Carlin RD: Ethrane teratogenicity—a preliminary report (abstract). J Dent Res 57(Special Issue A):289, 1978
57. Saito N, Urakawa M, Ito R: Influence of enflurane on fetus and growth after birth in mice and rats. Oyo Yakuri 8:1269–1276, 1974
58. Kennedy GL, Smith SH, Deplinger ML, et al.: Reproductive and teratologic studies with isoflurane. Drug Chem Toxicol 1:75–88, 1977
59. Fujinaga M, Stevenson JM, Mazze RI: Reproductive and teratogenic effects of fentanyl in Sprague-Dawley rats. Teratology 34:54–57, 1986
60. Fujinaga M, Mazze RI: Reproductive and teratogenic effects of lidocaine in Sprague-Dawley rats. Anesthesiology 65:626–632, 1986
61. Harpel HS, Gautieri RF: Morphine-induced fetal malformations. J Pharm Sci 57:1590–1597, 1968
62. Zagon IS, McLaughlin PJ: Effects of chronic morphine administration on pregnant rats and their offspring. Pharmacology 15:302–310, 1977
63. Geber WF, Schramm LC: Congenital malformations of the central nervous system produced by narcotics and analgesics in the hamster. Am J Obstet Gynecol 123:705–713, 1975
64. Hutchings DE, Hunt HF, Towey JP, et al.: Methadone during pregnancy in the rat: Dose level effects on maternal and perinatal mortality and growth in the offspring. J Pharmacol Exp Ther 197:171–179, 1976
65. Jurand A: Teratogenic activity of methadone hydrochloride in mouse and chick embryos. J Embryo Exp Morphol 30:449–458, 1973
66. Theeuwes F, Yum SI: Principles of the design and operation of generic osmotic pumps for the delivery of semisolid or liquid drug formation. Ann Biomed Eng 4(4):343–353, 1976
67. Persaud TVN: Tierexperimentelle Untersuchungen zur Frage der teratogenic Wirkung von Barbituraten. Acta Biol Med Ger 14:89–90, 1985
68. Tanimura T: Effect of administration of thiamylal sodium to pregnant mice upon the development of their offspring. Acta Anat Nippon 40:323–328, 1965
69. Friedman JM: Teratogen update: Anesthetic agents. Teratology 37:69–77, 1988
70. Tanimura T, Owaki Y, Nishmura H: Effect of administration of thiopental sodium to pregnant mice upon the development of their offspring. Okajimas Folia Anat Jpn 43:219–226, 1967
71. Safra MJ, Oakley GP: Association between cleft lip with or without cleft palate and prenatal exposure to diazepam. Lancet 2:478–480, 1975
72. Doenicke VA, Heinrich KF, Boll H, et al.: Teratogene Schäden durch Narkotika. In: Henschel WF, Lehman C (eds): Schädigungen des Anaesthesie-Personals durch Narkose-Gase und Dämpfe. Berlin: Springer-Verlag, 1975, pp 90–106
73. El-Karim AHB, Benny R: Embryotoxic and teratogenic action of ketamine hydrochloride in rats. Ain Shavis Med J 27:459–463, 1976
74. Mellin GW: Drugs in the first trimester of pregnancy and the fetal life of Homo sapiens. Am J Obstet Gynecol 90:1169–1180, 1964

2. The Physiologic Changes of Pregnancy Have Anesthetic Implications for Both Mother and Fetus

James H. Diaz, M.D.

24

INTRODUCTION

Most of the normal anatomic and physiologic alterations of pregnancy, labor, and delivery have significant effects on the fetal and maternal responses to regional and general anesthetics. Many of the physiologic changes of pregnancy are quite beneficial, such as an increased blood volume, which permits better tolerance of acute blood losses of 500 to 1000 ml at delivery. Other physiologic changes, such as aortocaval compression, offer no significant advantages and may pose serious risks of hemodynamic compromise to both the mother and the fetus during anesthetics for labor and delivery. The anatomic and physiologic changes of pregnancy with greatest effects on obstetric anesthetics can be classified by organ systems into cardiovascular, respiratory, gastrointestinal, and renal changes, all of which are summarized in Figure 2–1, *A* and *B*.

CARDIOVASCULAR SYSTEM

Blood Volume

A very rapid expansion of total maternal blood volume occurs during normal pregnancy to approximately 30% to 45% over nonpregnant levels (Fig. 2–2).[1–3] The maximum increase in circulatory volume is usually achieved by 30 to 34 weeks of gestation[4] and is due primarily to an expanded plasma volume of 35% to 45% over nonpregnant levels.[1, 4] Lagging behind plasma volume expansion, red blood cell mass also increases during pregnancy to approximately 20% over nonpregnant levels.[2] A mild dilutional anemia occurs by midpregnancy because plasma volume expansion (40%) occurs earlier and is more pronounced than red blood cell mass expansion (20%).[2] The physiologic, dilutional anemia of pregnancy usually results in hematocrit values near 35% and hemoglobin levels near 12 g/dl at term.[2] Figure 2–2 summarizes the changes in maternal circulatory volume and blood components that occur during normal pregnancy and in the puerperium.

Plasma Volume (*see Fig. 2–2*). Plasma volume expansion during pregnancy begins at 6 to 12 weeks' gestation, is complete by 30 to 34 weeks, and has a measured volume 1200 to 1500 ml higher than in nonpregnant states.[1] The degree of plasma volume expansion during pregnancy is quite variable and can be significantly greater in multiple gestations. The etiology of plasma volume expansion during pregnancy is poorly understood, but its existence explains both the dilutional anemia during gestation and the spontaneous autotransfusion at delivery.[2]

A dilutional reduction in total plasma protein concentration to 4 to 6 g/dl also occurs during pregnancy. The decrease in albumin concentration is relatively greater than the decrease in globulin concentration, with a

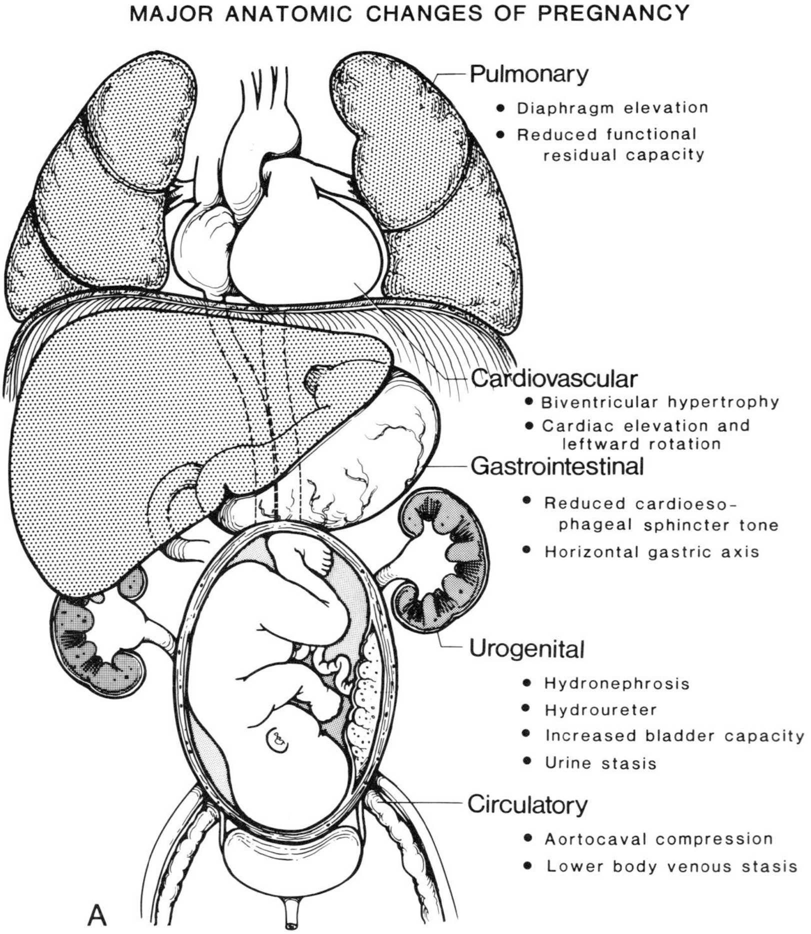

MAJOR ANATOMIC CHANGES OF PREGNANCY

Pulmonary
- Diaphragm elevation
- Reduced functional residual capacity

Cardiovascular
- Biventricular hypertrophy
- Cardiac elevation and leftward rotation

Gastrointestinal
- Reduced cardioesophageal sphincter tone
- Horizontal gastric axis

Urogenital
- Hydronephrosis
- Hydroureter
- Increased bladder capacity
- Urine stasis

Circulatory
- Aortocaval compression
- Lower body venous stasis

A

FIGURE 2–1. *A*, The anatomic changes during pregnancy and their anesthetic implications.

consequent decline in the albumin-globulin ratio from 1.5 to 1.0.[2] Albumin binding of drugs and local anesthetic is, therefore, less in pregnant states than in nonpregnant states.

Red Blood Cell Volume (see Fig. 2–2). As noted, total red blood cell mass begins to increase after plasma volume expansion starts and reaches levels of 250 to 450 ml over nonpregnant red cell mass.[4] This expansion in red cell mass is related to increased hematopoiesis in the bone marrow and the liver and is not due to prolonged erythrocyte life span. Dilutional anemia, increased hematopoiesis, and the associated transfer of approximately 300 mg of maternal iron to the fetus during gestation create an iron deficit of approximately 800 mg by midpregnancy.[4] Since iron stores

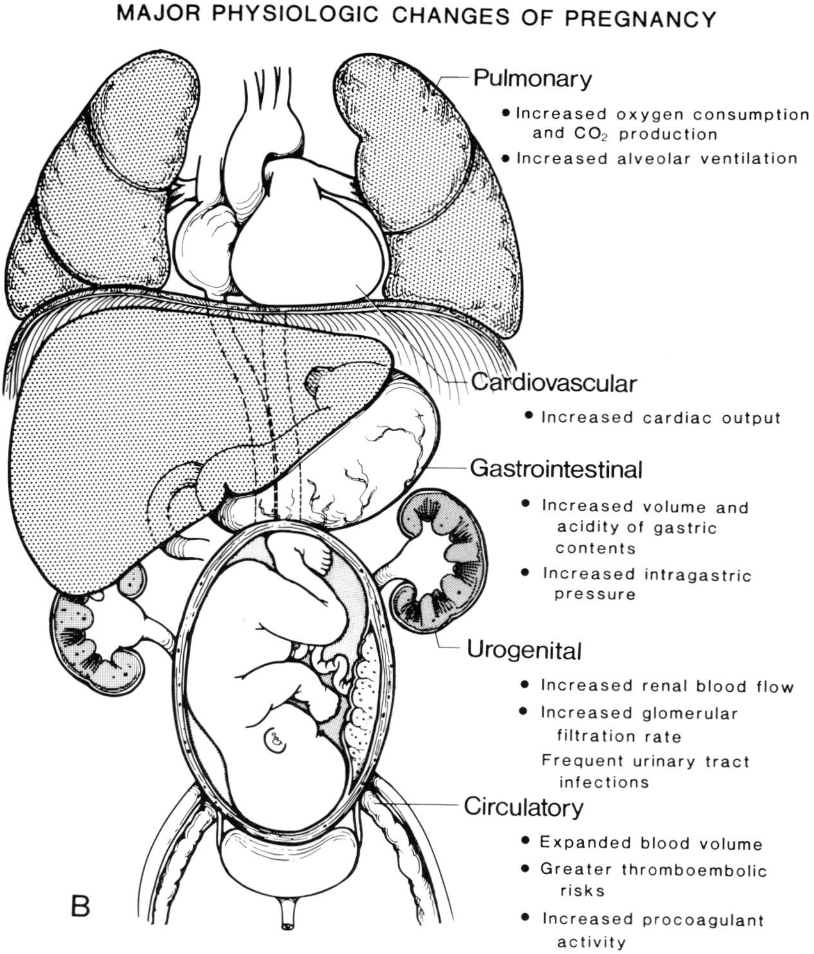

MAJOR PHYSIOLOGIC CHANGES OF PREGNANCY

Pulmonary
- Increased oxygen consumption and CO_2 production
- Increased alveolar ventilation

Cardiovascular
- Increased cardiac output

Gastrointestinal
- Increased volume and acidity of gastric contents
- Increased intragastric pressure

Urogenital
- Increased renal blood flow
- Increased glomerular filtration rate
  Frequent urinary tract infections

Circulatory
- Expanded blood volume
- Greater thromboembolic risks
- Increased procoagulant activity

B

FIGURE 2–1 Continued B, The physiologic changes during pregnancy and their anesthetic implications.

in menstruating, reproductive-age women are lower than comparable iron stores in men, iron deficits during gestation should be treated with supplemental iron and folic acid therapy.[4] Red blood cell 2,3-diphosphoglycerate (2,3-DPG) concentration is also higher during pregnancy than in nonpregnant states and decreases the affinity of maternal hemoglobin for oxygen, enhancing oxygen dissociation from maternal hemoglobin for uteroplacental transfer to the fetus and to fetal hemoglobin.[5]

White Blood Cell Volume (see Fig. 2–2). The total white blood cell count increases considerably during pregnancy from a nonpregnant level of 5000 to 6000 cells/mm³ to 12,000 cells/mm³, a 40% to 50% increase.[3]

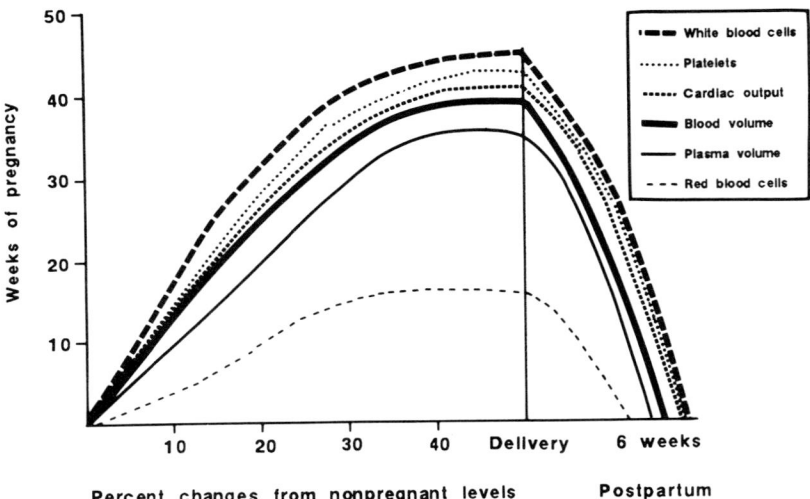

FIGURE 2-2. Circulatory volume changes during pregnancy and the puerperium. (Data from Lund CJ, Donovan JC: Blood volume during pregnancy: Significance of plasma and red cell volumes. Am J Obstet Gynecol 98:393, 1967; Pritchard JA: Changes in blood volume during pregnancy and delivery. Anesthesiology 26:393, 1965; and Efrati P, Presentey B, Margalith M, et al.: Leukocytes of normal pregnant women. Obstet Gynecol 23:249, 1964.)

Heart and Great Vessels

Maternal myocardial hypertrophy during pregnancy has been documented by both histologic and echocardiographic studies and is a normal response to the increased circulatory volume load of pregnancy.[6] Echocardiographic studies during pregnancy have demonstrated biventricular increases in both end-diastolic volume and end-diastolic ventricular wall thickness, indicating increased cardiac muscle mass, wall thickness, and chamber size during pregnancy.[6] At echocardiography, there is also a biventricular increase in posterior wall motion and circumferential fiber shortening during gestation.[6, 7] Such findings may indicate enhanced myocardial contractility related to intracardiac conduction changes.[7] The electrocardiographic changes of pregnancy include left axis deviation as a result of diaphragm elevation with corresponding cardiac elevation and leftward rotation, flattened T waves in lead V_3, insignificant ST interval and Q wave changes, and frequent transient supraventricular tachyarrhythmias that are rarely symptomatic or clinically significant.[4]

Heart Rate. A significant increase in heart rate occurs during pregnancy, with a 32% increase in supine heart rate over nonpregnant heart rates by 36 weeks.[8] Significant changes in heart rate may be associated with sitting, standing, and supine positions during pregnancy, with changes stabilizing, at least for supine and standing positions, by about

32 weeks.[4] Standing and sitting heart rates exceed the supine heart rate throughout pregnancy.[4]

Cardiac Chamber Size and Pressures. Echocardiographic studies have now enabled accurate determination of heart chamber size throughout pregnancy and the puerperium. An expanded maternal blood volume with increased diastolic filling results in larger left and right ventricular end-diastolic dimensions.[7] An increased stroke volume results in no change in left and right ventricular end-systolic dimensions.[7] Changes in cardiac chamber size during pregnancy correspond well with cardiac catheterization data. Early in gestation, right atrial pressure increases slightly as a result of total blood volume expansion.[4] There are also slight decreases in mean pulmonary artery pressure and pulmonary vascular resistance.[4] The onset of contractions causes significant increases in cardiac chamber sizes and pressures, with a 33% increase in stroke volume over preterm levels and a 4- to 6-cm H_2O increase in right atrial pressure with each contraction.[4]

Heart Sounds. Phonocardiographic studies have made possible detailed investigations of changes in heart sounds and murmurs associated with pregnancy. The first heart sound increases in loudness, with an exaggerated split between its mitral and tricuspid components, due to earlier closure of the mitral valve during pregnancy.[9] There are no changes in the aortic and pulmonary components of the second heart sound during the first 30 weeks of pregnancy.[9] Thereafter, the interval between aortic and pulmonary closure sounds varies little with respiration, unlike in the nonpregnant state.[9] Up to 90% of pregnant women develop a loud third heart sound, usually before 20 weeks' gestation.[9] Phonocardiography has identified a fourth heart sound in 16% of pregnant patients.[9] Innocent heart murmurs are very common during pregnancy; 95% of pregnant women develop systolic murmurs best heard along the left sternal border by midpregnancy. Nearly one-half of these early- to mid-systolic murmurs are intensified on inspiration, and approximately 15% are grade 1/4, and 85% are grade 2/4. Grade 1 to 2 systolic murmurs during pregnancy are usually related to systemic vasodilation with augmented cardiac ejection and forward flow biventricularly.[9]

Cardiac Output. A progressive increase in cardiac output occurs during pregnancy, beginning in the first trimester and extending through the second trimester and into the early third trimester.[10] The greatest increases in cardiac output during pregnancy occur during the first trimester, and further increases during the second and third trimesters are variable and slight.[10] The early increases in cardiac output during the first trimester are due to increases in resting heart rate and circulatory volume. Overall, cardiac output increases 30% to 50% during pregnancy, with the greatest increases in cardiac output occurring prior to 20 weeks.[10]

As term approaches, maternal position has a greater effect on cardiac output. Cardiac output is profoundly affected by positional change during the late second and third trimesters. Cardiac output decreases in the supine position by 20 to 24 weeks and is lowest at 38 to 40 weeks.[11] Reductions in cardiac output caused by the supine position at term result from aortocaval compression, with reduced caval venous return and loss of stroke volume (Fig. 2–3).[12, 13] Aortocaval compression results from occlusion of both the inferior vena cava and the abdominal aorta by the gravid uterus in the supine position (see Fig. 2–3).[12, 13] Although the epidural and azygous venous plexi provide alternative routes for venous return to the heart from the lower body during aortocaval compression, such a compensation in venous return is usually inadequate to maintain cardiac output even with heart rate increases of 12 to 15 beats per minute and heightened sympathetic tone. The consequences of increased venous capacitance in the paravertebral venous collaterals caused by aortocaval compression during pregnancy include significant volume reductions in the spinal subarachnoid and epidural spaces; diminished meningeal circulation; increased cerebrospinal fluid opening pressure, especially during contractions; and reduced negative pressure within the epidural space.[14] Peridural venous distensibility during the third trimester may increase by 150%.[14]

The hemodynamic changes that occur during aortocaval compression, also known as the supine hypotensive syndrome, include reduced inferior vena caval venous return, reductions of 30% or more in stroke volume and cardiac output, 10% to 15% increases in heart rate, and 20% to 30% reductions in mean arterial blood pressure (see Fig. 2–3).[13] Caval compression in the supine position is also accompanied by abdominal aortic compression with impaired abdominal, aortic, renal, and uteroplacental blood flow.[12, 13] Consequently, maternal renal function and urinary output are more significantly increased in lateral positions than in supine positions, especially during the third trimester.[12, 13] Figure 2–3 demonstrates the significant aortocaval compression caused by the gravid uterus in the supine position during late pregnancy (see Fig. 2–3, A) and its relief by left uterine displacement, achieved by placing a wedge under the right hip (see Fig. 2–3, B).

Great Vessels. Collagen softening occurs throughout the venous circulation, and all vascular smooth muscle hypertrophies to meet the increased circulatory loads during pregnancy.[15] All vessels carry greater volumes of blood per unit of time throughout gestation. The pulmonary arteries and their branching tributaries make prominent vascular markings on the chest x-ray film by the third trimester. Central venous pressure is reduced in the supine position by the late second trimester, with worsening aortocaval compression.[16]

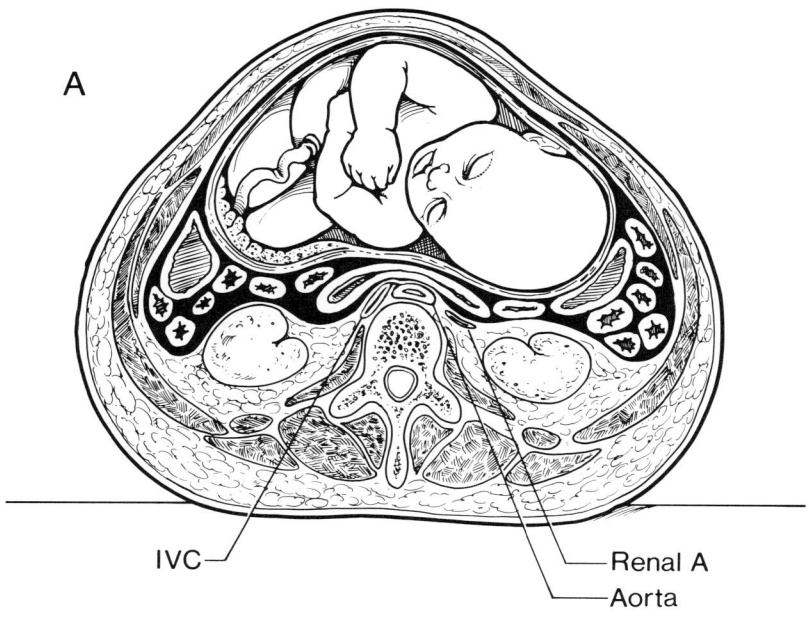

A

IVC — | — Renal A
— Aorta

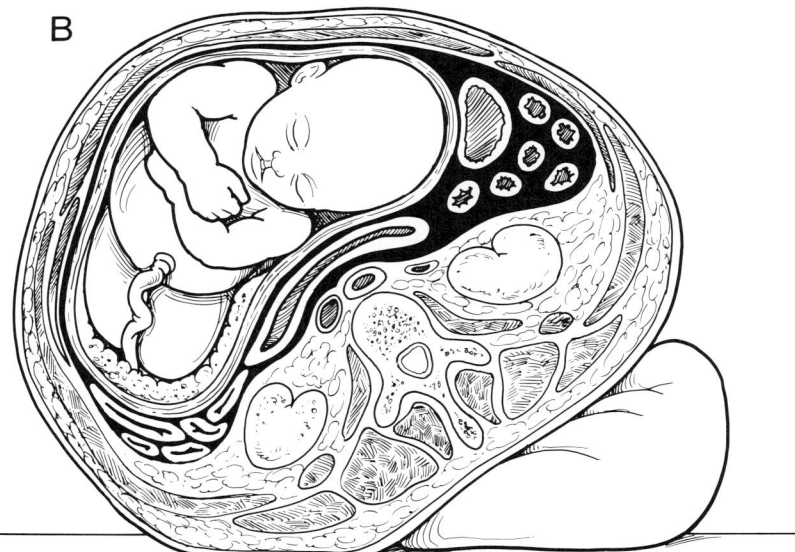

B

FIGURE 2–3. Aortocaval compression during late pregnancy. *A*, Supine position. *B*, Supine position with left uterine displacement to relieve aortocaval compression. (Data from Kerr MG, Scott DM, Samuel E: Studies of the inferior vena cava in late pregnancy. Br Med J 1:532, 1964; and Bleniarz J, Crohogini JJ, Curuchet E, et al.: Aortocaval compression by the uterus in late human pregnancy. Am J Obstet Gynecol 100:203, 1968.)

Peripheral Vasculature

Arterial Vascular Bed. Sitting and standing systolic arterial pressures remain relatively constant throughout pregnancy, at around 110 to 130 mmHg.[4, 8] Sitting or standing diastolic arterial pressures demonstrate a progressive decrease during the first two trimesters of pregnancy; the lowest value, reached by 28 weeks, is 65 to 67 mmHg.[4, 8] During the remainder of the third trimester, there is a progressive return toward nonpregnant diastolic pressures, reaching 72 mmHg by 40 weeks.[4, 8] After 24 weeks, a greater change in systolic pressure occurs in response to positional changes, with systolic pressures decreasing by about 8 mmHg in the supine position.[8] Similar reductions are also observed in diastolic pressures in supine positions.[8] During the last 4 weeks of pregnancy, diastolic pressure increases sharply in the left lateral decubitus position to within 4 mmHg of normal pregnant values.[8]

Regional Blood Flows. The uterus receives 10% to 20% of the cardiac output during pregnancy, with a uterine flow at term of 300 to 800 ml/min.[4] Renal blood flow is also increased during pregnancy, with a maximum increase by term of nearly 50% over nonpregnant levels.[4] Skin and mammary blood flow are also increased during pregnancy. No significant changes in cerebral or hepatic blood flows occur during pregnancy.

Circulatory Times. Circulatory times are often increased during pregnancy, as demonstrated by arm-to-tongue intervals.[17] The shortest circulatory time measured by arm-to-tongue interval, 10.2 seconds, occurs in the third trimester when velocity of blood flow is greatest.[17]

Systemic Vascular Resistance. Total systemic vascular resistance is decreased during pregnancy because of a slight decrease in mean arterial pressure and a marked increase in cardiac output. The low-resistance uteroplacental circulation, in addition to the low vascular resistances offered by the kidneys and the skin, help to reduce systemic vascular resistance by accepting larger proportions of the cardiac output than in nonpregnant states. Acting together, uteroplacental, renal, and skin circulations produce an arteriovenous fistula effect on central circulatory dynamics during gestation by reducing vascular resistances, lowering arterial pressures, and increasing cardiac output.[4]

Autonomic Nervous System. Sympathetic tone is augmented during pregnancy, rendering pregnant women particularly sensitive to the cardiodepressant effects of autonomic blockade. Assali and coworkers[18] concluded that increased autonomic tone in the peripheral arterial circulation during pregnancy results from increased sympathetic nerve transmission rather than from changes in vessel wall neural density. Pharmacologic sympatholysis by either conduction anesthesia or ganglionic blockade may cause a more exaggerated decrease in arterial pressure and cardiac output in pregnant patients than is observed in nonpregnant states.[18] In addition to arterial autonomic imbalance, loss of venomotor tone results in significant venous pooling throughout pregnancy that is often exaggerated in the pelvis and lower extremities by progressive aortocaval compression and is characterized physically by hemorrhoids, varicose veins, pedal edema, and labial varicosities and edema.[4]

Venous Vascular Bed. The venous capacitance circuit becomes engorged during pregnancy. Venous prominence is most apparent in the lower extremities, where hydrostatic forces, expanded blood volume, caval compression, and greater venous distensibility act together to reduce venous return to the heart.[19] Venous stasis in the pelvis and lower extremities is common during the third trimester and may predispose the pregnant patient to thromboembolic phenomena.[19] The exact mechanisms responsible for increases in venous capacitance during pregnancy are unknown; proposed mechanisms include progesterone-mediated relaxation of venous smooth muscle, altered elastic properties of venous walls, and autonomic deficiencies in venomotor tone.[4]

Pulmonary Vascular Bed. Pulmonary blood volume is increased during pregnancy and is responsible for prominent pulmonary vascular markings on chest x-ray films at term.[4] Mean pulmonary artery pressure is decreased throughout pregnancy, as is pulmonary vascular resistance.[20] Pulmonary capillary wedge pressure remains in a low to normal range of 4.5 to 6.5 mmHg throughout pregnancy.[20]

Arterial Blood Gases

Maternal oxygen and carbon dioxide dissociation curves are shifted to the right during pregnancy and enhance oxygen release from maternal hemoglobin to fetal hemoglobin in the uteroplacental circulation. Higher erythrocyte 2,3-DPG concentrations during pregnancy also reduce the affinity of maternal hemoglobin for oxygen and facilitate further dissociation of oxygen from maternal hemoglobin for placental and fetal transfer.[5] A decrease in the partial pressure of carbon dioxide ($PaCO_2$) from a normal nonpregnant level of 39 mmHg to approximately 31 mmHg during pregnancy results from a slight increase in respiratory rate accompanied by a 40% increase in tidal volume.[4] The mechanism for increased respiratory rates during pregnancy is unknown but is believed to be related to the stimulating effects of progesterone on the medullary respiratory centers. The slight decrease in $PaCO_2$ during pregnancy causes slight compensatory increase in pH to 7.44 in pregnant patients as compared with a normal pH of 7.40 in nonpregnant women. The slightly alkalotic pH of pregnancy is compensated for metabolically by increased renal excretion of hydrogen ions.

Coagulation

The platelet count increases progressively toward term from a non-pregnant level of 187,000 to a term level of 316,000.[21] In addition to more platelets during pregnancy, increases in factors VIII, X, XII, and fibrinogen occur as pregnancy progresses toward term.[21] Fibrinogen concentrations may increase from nonpregnant levels of 250 to 300 mg/dl up to 450 mg/dl at term.[21] Systemic fibrinolytic activity as determined by euglobulin lysis time is considerably depressed during pregnancy but returns to normal shortly after delivery.[21] However, localized fibrinolytic activity is maintained throughout pregnancy, and fibrin degradation products are usually increased slightly toward term. The net effect of the procoagulant changes during pregnancy is to provide protection against catastrophic hemorrhage at delivery. Unfortunately, this is achieved at the expense of rendering the pregnant patient more susceptible to thromboembolic phenomena in late pregnancy and in the immediate postpartal period.

Anesthetic Implications

The anesthetic implications of the cardiovascular changes during pregnancy include (1) concomitant increases in cardiac output and in brain anesthetic tensions; (2) exaggerated blood losses at delivery; (3) aortocaval compression and its relief by positional changes during labor; (4) peridural venous distention with concomitant volume loss in the epidural space; (5) the dramatic effects of sympathetic blocks on augmented sympathetic tone and cardiac output; and (6) maternal thromboembolic risks.

The increased cardiac output of pregnancy speeds the delivery of both inhaled and intravenous anesthetics to the brain and is accompanied by rapid onset of general anesthesia and associated circulatory changes. Additionally, aortocaval compression in the supine position may cause significant hypotension from inadequate venous return to the heart and concomitant reductions in maternal cardiac output, uteroplacental blood flow, and fetal perfusion.

The principal causes of decreased uteroplacental perfusion during pregnancy include aortocaval compression; sympathetic blockade from epidural or subarachnoid anesthetics; maternal hemorrhage; and administration of vasodilators, particularly high concentrations of inhaled anesthetics. Supine hypotension from aortocaval compression and sympathetic blockade from regional anesthesia often occur together, reduce maternal cardiac output and fetal perfusion quickly and without warning, and are best prevented by a combination of effective prophylactic measures. Prophylactic measures to decrease hypotension from aortocaval compression and regional anesthesia at term should include the following:

1. Prehydration of the patient for vaginal delivery with 1000 ml of crystalloid solution and for cesarean section with 1500 to 2000 ml of crystalloid solution. Lactated Ringer's solutions or 0.9% normal saline solutions are preferable to glucose-containing crystalloid solutions for acute hydration prior to vaginal or cesarean delivery to prevent maternal hyperglycemia with fetal acidemia and neonatal hypoglycemia. Intravenous fluids may be warmed to body temperature in blood warmers and administered rapidly to parturients with normal cardiac function. Parturients with congenital or acquired heart disease should be volume expanded incrementally during continuous right atrial or pulmonary arterial pressure monitoring.

2. Insertion of a wedge in the form of a pillow or rolled sheet under the right hip to displace the uterus to the left to avoid the occlusive pressure of the uterus on the inferior vena cava and the abdominal aorta also reduces supine hypotension and restores cardiac output. Like a right-sided wedge, left table tilt or mechanical uterine displacement devices also effectively accomplish left uterine displacement to relieve aortocaval compression.

3. Avoidance of major regional anesthetics in parturients with marked supine hypotensive syndromes that do not respond to either left or right uterine displacement and volume loading.

4. Early recognition of significant maternal hypotension (systolic blood pressure less than 100 mmHg), which often follows maternal sympathetic block.

5. Pharmacologic management of maternal hypotension with intravenous ephedrine sulfate (5 to 10 mg), identified by Ralston and associates[22] as the best injectable vasopressor to use for maternal hypotension. A mildly alpha-adrenergic and predominantly beta-adrenergic agonist, ephedrine restores maternal blood pressure rapidly with little change in uterine blood flow. Pure alpha-adrenergic vasopressors, like phenylephrine and methoxamine, may restore maternal blood pressure, but they also constrict uteroplacental vascular beds and limit fetal perfusion pressures.[22] Intravenous ephedrine administration for maternal hypotension has been known to produce significant increases in fetal heart rate and beat-to-beat variability.[23] Such ephedrine-mediated changes in fetal circulatory dynamics, however, have not been associated with fetal depression, hypoxia, or acidosis as evaluated by fetal capillary Po_2 and pH or neonatal Apgar scores.[23] Datta and associates[24] have now clearly demonstrated that the aggressive use of ephedrine to treat maternal hypotension after spinal anesthesia for cesarean section will prevent further decreases in blood pressure, maintain fetal homeostasis during delivery, and reduce the postpartal incidence of nausea and vomiting.

Venous distensibility in the extradural venous circulation at term will decrease the filling capacities of both the subarachnoid and extradural spaces, enhancing the rapid spread of drugs administered there, slowing capillary circulation in the meninges, and often delaying meningeal absorption of intrathecally or extradurally injected drugs, prolonging their duration. The reduced size of the spinal and epidural spaces at term increases the likelihood of high blocks from routinely injected volumes of local anesthetics. Greater vascularity of the epidural space at term will increase the risk of intravascular injections of local anesthetics with toxic reactions. With each uterine contraction, there are significant increases in central venous pressure, cardiac output, mean arterial pressure, intra-amniotic pressure, epidural space pressure, and spinal subarachnoid space pressure. Increases in epidural and subarachnoid pressures during contractions reduce the normal negative pressure within the epidural space and make loss-of-resistance techniques more difficult to use when identifying the epidural space for local anesthetic injections. Hanging-drop techniques to identify the epidural space are often ineffective during labor because of reduced negative pressures within the epidural space.

Blood loss at delivery is normally well tolerated because of an expanded circulating blood volume, which provides automatic compensation for blood losses of up to 500 ml at delivery. Blood losses greater than 1000 ml during vaginal or cesarean delivery may require earlier volume restoration by blood transfusion than in nonpregnant states. Several studies have shown that choice of anesthetic techniques may influence blood loss during either midforceps vaginal delivery or cesarean section, with apparent advantages in reduced hemorrhage associated with epidural anesthesia over general anesthesia.

Blood constituent and procoagulant changes during pregnancy often produce a hypercoagulable state by the third trimester to provide natural protection against massive vaginal hemorrhage at delivery. Thromboembolic phenomena may, however, occur in pregnant patients predisposed to phlebothrombosis by heightened coagulation activity, reduced fibrinolytic activity, lower extremity venous stasis, and increased bed rest. Venous compression stockings, early postpartal ambulation, and aggressive anticoagulant management of lower extremity or pelvic thrombophlebitis will reduce thromboembolic risks near term and in the puerperium.

RESPIRATORY SYSTEM
Oxygen Consumption

During pregnancy, oxygen consumption rises progressively by 10% to 20% and may increase by 100% during labor. On the average, oxygen consumption rises during pregnancy by 32 to 58 ml/min, with a maximum oxygen consumption at rest of between 249 and 331 ml/min.[25, 26] Basal oxygen consumption during pregnancy is therefore 3.65 ml/kg/min.[27] The increase in oxygen consumption during pregnancy is achieved with little change in the partial pressure of oxygen in arterial vessels. Arterial oxygen tension (PaO_2) usually increases to its highest values of 106 to 107 mmHg in early pregnancy, with a fall to 92 to 103 mmHg at term.[28, 29] Increases in oxygen consumption during pregnancy are associated with corresponding increases in CO_2 production. The respiratory quotient increases from approximately 0.76 before pregnancy to 0.83 in late pregnancy.[30] The increase in CO_2 production during pregnancy is therefore proportionally greater than the increase in oxygen consumption. This effect is likely due to an increase in the proportion of carbohydrates to fats metabolized during pregnancy.[30] The pulmonary diffusing capacities of both O_2 and CO_2 decrease sharply during pregnancy.[27]

Alveolar Ventilation

Since oxygen consumption rises, PaO_2 alters little, and arteriovenous oxygen difference decreases, an increase in ventilation must compensate for these changes during pregnancy. The 40% increase in ventilation during pregnancy is, indeed, impressive, exceeding by 100-fold the increase in oxygen consumption. The hyperventilation of pregnancy is achieved by small increases in respiratory rate of 2 breaths per minute, significant increases in tidal volume from 450 ml in nonpregnant states to 600 ml by midpregnancy, and an increase in diaphragmatic over thoracic breathing.[25–27, 31] The increase in minute ventilation from 7.5 to 10.5 L/min during pregnancy is achieved more efficiently by the increases in tidal volume than by the increases in respiratory rate.[32] A pregnant patient therefore breathes more deeply rather than more frequently to compensate for smaller total lung capacity and greater oxygen consumption. The vital capacity does not change during pregnancy. The summation of a reduced expiratory reserve volume and the residual volume yields a reduction in the functional residual capacity of 20%, or approximately 300 ml by midterm. Reductions in functional residual capacity are intensified in the supine position and in obese parturients. Figure 2–4 summarizes the lung volume changes of pregnancy by comparing spirometric performance at term with a nonpregnant state. Lithotomy and Trendelenburg positions will also reduce functional residual capacity during pregnancy.

The partial pressure of arterial carbon dioxide ($PaCO_2$) falls in pregnancy from nonpregnant levels of 35 to 40 mmHg to 30 to 33 mmHg in the first trimester.[33] The $PaCO_2$ falls early in pregnancy, paralleling changes in ventilation. The fall in $PaCO_2$ is even greater at high altitudes where

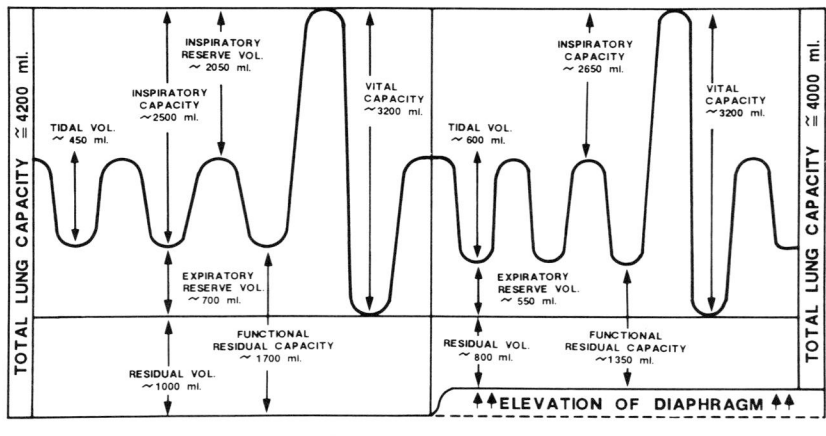

A NONPREGNANT   **B PREGNANT AT TERM**

FIGURE 2–4. Lung volume changes during pregnancy. *A,* Nonpregnant. *B,* Pregnant at term. (Data from Alaily AB, Carrol KB: Pulmonary ventilation in pregnancy. Br J Obstet Gynaecol 85:518, 1978; Pernoll ML, Metcalfe J, Kovach PA, et al.: Ventilation during rest and exercise in pregnancy and postpartum. Respir Physiol 25:295, 1975; and deSwiet M: Maternal pulmonary disorders. In: Creasy RK, Resnik R (eds): Maternal-Fetal Medicine: Principles and Practice. Philadelphia: W.B. Saunders, 1984, pp 781–794.)

pregnant women will hyperventilate further to maintain sea-level PaO_2.[34] The fall in $PaCO_2$ is matched by an equivalent reduction in plasma bicarbonate concentration and buffer base, creating a base excess on arterial blood gas samples. The increase in ventilation and the associated fall in $PaCO_2$ during pregnancy are due to the effect of progesterone.[35] Progesterone will lower the CO_2 response threshold of the medullary respiratory center and act as a primary stimulant to the respiratory center independently of any change in CO_2 sensitivity.[36] In addition, the sensitivity of the medullary respiratory center increases so that an increase in $PaCO_2$ of 1 mmHg increases ventilation by 6 L/min in pregnancy compared with a corresponding 1.5 L/min increase in the nonpregnant state.[36] The respiratory stimulating effect of progesterone has also been used in the treatment of high-altitude pulmonary edema, respiratory failure, and emphysema to improve alveolar ventilation.[37]

Anatomic Changes

Significant anatomic changes in the configuration of the chest wall occur during pregnancy. The subcostal angle increases from 68° to 103° before the enlarging uterus mechanically elevates the hemidiaphragms.[38] The level of the diaphragm rises by about 4 cm, and the transverse diameter of the chest wall increases by 2 cm.[39, 40] Increases in the anteroposterior and transverse diameters of the chest wall during pregnancy account for a 20% decrease in residual volume.[40] Excursion of the hemidiaphragms during ventilation in pregnancy is about 1.5 cm further in either direction than in the nonpregnant state.[39, 40]

Upper Airway Anatomy. Upper airway anatomy may change significantly during pregnancy because of weight gain, edema, and mucosal hypervascularity. A pregnant patient may become obese, developing a short neck and large breasts, which can limit cervical range of motion and restrict accessory muscles of ventilation. Nasal and respiratory tract mucosa become edematous and hyperemic, with more blood vessels that may be traumatized easily and bleed profusely.[41] Nasal congestion and epistaxis are common by midterm and may obstruct the nasal airway, causing voice changes and nasal stuffiness.[42]

Dyspnea in Pregnancy. The degree to which pregnant patients are aware of profound changes in ventilation (breathlessness or dyspnea) varies enormously. About 50% of pregnant women are aware of breathlessness before 20 weeks' gestation.[40] The maximum incidence of breathlessness at rest occurs between 28 and 31 weeks' gestation.[40]

Airway Resistance

Large Airways. Large airway resistance and lung compliance do not change appreciably during pregnancy because of the balancing effects of progesterone and prostaglandins. Prostaglandin F-2-alpha ($PGF_2\alpha$) is a bronchoconstrictor, and prostaglandins E_1 (PGE_1) and E_2 (PGE_2) are bronchodilators; the serum levels of both F and E series prostaglandins increase to similar extents during pregnancy. Progesterone causes bronchodilation, presumably by increasing beta-adrenergic activity.[43, 44] On the other hand, reduced residual volume and respiratory alkalosis may promote a bronchoconstrictor effect on large airways.[45]

Small Airways. Closing volume is increased during pregnancy, with small airway closure beginning during normal tidal volume in 50% of patients.[46] The caliber of small airways less than 2 mm in diameter decreases in pregnancy to the point at which some airways will close during tidal breathing.[47] Small airway closure in pregnancy is intensified by lung disease, advancing maternal age, multiple gestation, obesity, and Trendelenburg and lithotomy positions.

Anesthetic Implications

The most significant anesthetic implications of respiratory changes during pregnancy include upper airway changes, increased oxygen consumption, rapid nitrogen washout, reduced functional residual capacity permitting high alveolar concentrations of anesthetics, and hyperventilation-induced vasoconstriction with reductions in uteroplacental blood flow and fetal perfusion.

Upper airway changes affecting ease of endotracheal intubation, significant increases in oxygen consumption, and reduced ability to store oxygen in the lungs for long periods necessitate 5 to 6 minutes of preoxygenation before elective endotracheal intubation of a pregnant patient at term. Only short periods of apnea should be permitted in pregnant patients. Endotracheal intubation may be difficult in a pregnant patient because of anatomic changes due to weight gain (short neck, large breasts), generalized edema of the nasopharynx and laryngopharynx, and hypervascularity of the respiratory tract mucosa.[41] Even minor trauma inflicted during attempted endotracheal intubation can result in profuse bleeding from the mouth, lips, nose, or pharynx.[41, 42] A selection of smaller endotracheal tubes (6.0 to 7 mm outside diameter), laryngoscopes, and laryngoscope blades should be immediately available in the delivery room.

Cephalad pressure by the expanding uterus results in elevation of the hemidiaphragms with significant reductions in total lung capacity and functional residual capacity by midterm. Any factor that further decreases functional residual capacity, such as obesity, general anesthesia, or positional changes (supine, lithotomy, or Trendelenburg), or that may increase closing volume (advancing age, lung disease) can result in significant airway closure with hypoxemia during tidal breathing and, especially, during sedation or anesthesia. The hyperventilation of pregnancy, particularly during labor, will deliver more inhaled anesthetic to the alveoli. In addition, the decreased functional residual capacity of pregnancy results in less nitrogen dilution of inhaled gases, allowing rapid accumulation of high alveolar concentrations of inhaled anesthetics. Minimum anesthetic concentration (MAC) is decreased during pregnancy (halothane by 25%, isoflurane by 40%), an effect that has been attributed to the sedative effects of elevated levels of progesterone and beta-endorphins.[48, 49] Rapid induction of inhalation anesthesia occurs by midpregnancy from combinations of hyperventilation, small functional residual capacity, rapid nitrogen washout, less dilution of inhaled anesthetics in alveoli, and decreased MACs.

Further hyperventilation during pregnancy, particularly during labor, worsens the preexisting alkalosis of pregnancy and can significantly reduce uteroplacental blood flow and fetal perfusion by promoting vasoconstriction within fetomaternal circulations. Fetal acidosis and hypoxia may result. Respiratory alkalosis, whether produced by spontaneous or controlled hyperventilation, will shift the maternal hemoglobin-oxygen dissociation curve to the left, hindering oxygen unloading from maternal to fetal hemoglobin and aggravating fetal hypoxia during severe maternal alkalosis. The chronic hyperventilation of pregnancy can be worsened by the pain of uterine contractions, which causes exaggerated hypocarbia and respiratory alkalosis, further oxygen debt, and greater cost of breathing. Further hyperventilation during labor and delivery can be reduced or even abolished by providing effective pain relief with conduction anesthesia. Recently, transcutaneous measurements of maternal oxygen tension ($P_{TC}O_2$) have demonstrated dramatic decreases in $P_{TC}O_2$ during contractions in mothers not receiving adequate analgesia.[50] Hyperventilation during painful contractions also reduces $PaCO_2$ to such an extent that respiratory drive is temporarily inadequate when the painful stimulus is absent, leading to hypoventilation between contractions.[51] Narcotic analgesics further depress the ventilatory response to $PaCO_2$, causing even more severe hypoventilation with maternal hypoxia and fetal asphyxia between contractions. In contrast to narcotic analgesia, conduction analgesia by continuous lumbar epidural anesthesia normalizes maternal ventilation and oxygenation during labor and maintains uteroplacental blood flow.

In summary, no beneficial effects accrue from maternal hyperventilation during labor. Regional analgesia for labor and delivery minimizes maternal hyperventilation, improves oxygenation, and decreases oxygen consumption, all of which improve neonatal outcome.[52] The respiratory system adapts quickly and easily to pregnancy, labor, and delivery, because of its ability to increase ventilation more than necessary. With such a reserve in ventilatory capacity, respiratory failure is uncommon in pregnancy. Most chronic respiratory conditions affect older pregnant patients. Respiratory failure may become more common as more patients with cystic fibrosis become pregnant, but the more common causes of respiratory failure in pregnancy are preventable catastrophes, like aspiration of gastric contents or such rare and often unpreventable catastrophes as amniotic fluid embolus and massive pulmonary embolus.

GASTROINTESTINAL SYSTEM

Hepatic Changes

Elevated serum levels of glutamic oxaloacetic acid transaminase, lactic dehydrogenase, alkaline phosphatase, cholesterol, and fibrinogen may occur during pregnancy.[53] Eighty percent of parturients have an abnormal bromosulfathaleine excretion test.[53] Other transaminases, prothrombin, bilirubin, and liver blood flow usually remain unaltered during pregnancy.[54] Abnormal liver function tests do not necessarily indicate hepatic diseases during pregnancy.[54]

Plasma cholinesterase levels decrease significantly as early as the first trimester of pregnancy and remain low until delivery. Average serum cholinesterase activity is reduced by 24% before delivery and by a maximum of 33% at 3 days postpartum, returning slowly to normal activity by 6 weeks postpartum.[55] Dehydration, acidosis, diabetes mellitus, electrolyte disturbances, hypermagnesemia, and the administration of trimethaphan or cholinesterase inhibitors may further depress serum cholinesterase activity during pregnancy and in the puerperium.[56] The etiology of low plasma cholinesterase levels in pregnancy is unknown, but proposed causes include hemodilution of serum cholinesterase levels, hepatic dysfunction with reduced cholinesterase production, hypoalbuminemia, and elevated estrogen levels.

Gastric Changes

Pregnant patients demonstrate significant changes in gastric position, intragastric pressures, cardioesophageal sphincter tone, and gastric acid volume and secretion by midterm. The enlarging uterus causes a progressive shift in the position of the stomach and intestines. By midterm, there is significant cephalad gastric displacement, a shift in the stomach axis from vertical to horizontal, and a changing angle of the cardioesophageal junction. These combined factors result in progressive incompetence of the gastroesophageal sphincter, which allows gastric reflux and the production of acid esophagitis and heartburn in 45% to 70% of pregnant women by midterm.[57]

The gravid uterus mechanically obstructs the duodenum and increases intragastric pressure, especially during labor. With the pylorus displaced upward and backward, gastric emptying is further reduced at the onset of labor. Intragastric pressure increases progressively toward term and may reach levels exceeding 40 cm H_2O during labor and in cases of obesity, multiple gestation, and polyhydramnios.[58]

Progesterone, a placental hormone and muscle relaxant, decreases gastrointestinal motility and reduces gastroesophageal sphincter tone during pregnancy, further promoting gastroesophageal reflux of acid gastric contents. Another hormone, gastrin, also produced by the placenta during pregnancy, acts directly on gastric secretory cells to raise the hydrochloric acid, chloride, and enzyme contents of gastric secretions to above normal levels.[59] Taken together, anatomic and physiologic changes in the gastrointestinal tract make pregnant patients more susceptible to silent regurgitation, active vomiting, and pulmonary aspiration during general anesthesia or impaired consciousness.

Recent studies have identified 60% or more pregnant patients with gastric volumes of 25 ml or more and gastric pH of 2.5 or less.[60] These patients are at considerable risk for pulmonary aspiration of acid gastric contents that can cause severe acid aspiration syndrome with immediate hypoxemia and later respiratory failure. Aspiration of solid gastric contents is associated with atelectasis, lung abscess, and obstructive emphysema.

Gastric hyperacidity, retained gastric contents, intragastric pressure increases, and reduced gastroesophageal sphincter tone are all present by midterm or earlier, regardless of fasting status, and predispose every pregnant woman to a full-stomach status with a significant risk of silent regurgitation and aspiration of gastric contents when obtunded by sedatives or anesthetics. In addition, the regurgitation and aspiration of gastric contents may be further promoted by (1) depolarizing muscle relaxants, which induce muscle fasciculations and cause further increases in gastric pressure; (2) externally applied fundal and abdominal pressure at delivery; and (3) positive-pressure ventilation by face mask, which causes gastric distention during unconsciousness.

Anesthetic Implications

Despite lower levels of serum cholinesterase activity, prolonged respiratory impairment rarely follows appropriate doses of succinylcholine during pregnancy and at term. However, magnesium therapy for preeclampsia or succinylcholine overdoses may cause prolonged neuromuscular blockade in pregnant patients. Blitt and associates[61] recently compared the duration of paralysis following the administration of succinylcholine to 25 patients undergoing cesarean section and to an equal number of nonpregnant women. Although cholinesterase levels were lower in the pregnant women, the time to reach 90% recovery of twitch height was the same in both groups.[61] Careful titration of succinylcholine doses in parturients and frequent monitoring of neuromuscular blockade with a nerve stimulator, particularly in patients receiving magnesium therapy for preeclampsia, are prudent measures during succinylcholine administration in pregnancy.

The dangers of gastric regurgitation and pulmonary aspiration during pregnancy and at term can be reduced by regional anesthesia, which permits consciousness with cough and other airway protective reflexes. However, if general anesthesia is indicated for delivery, the tracheal airway should be isolated quickly by means of a cuffed endotracheal tube. This tube should be inserted at the induction of general anesthesia, immediately following loss of consciousness. Special antiaspiration precautions can be instituted during induction and before airway establishment by endotracheal intubation. Such precautions include:

1. Avoidance of the lithotomy position to prevent further additional increases in intragastric pressure.

2. Forty percent head-up tilt, which also helps to eliminate silent regurgitation. (If time permits, the stomach may be decompressed by means of a nasogastric tube before elective endotracheal intubation, but the tube should be removed before the induction of anesthesia to permit full closure of the cardioesophageal sphincter.)

3. Avoidance of positive pressure ventilation with further gastric distention.

4. Prevention of succinylcholine-induced fasciculations with further increases in intragastric pressure and reduced cardioesophageal sphincter tone by prior injection of small doses of nondepolarizing muscle relaxants during continuous cricoid cartilage pressure (Sellick's maneuver) applied by an assistant to occlude the underlying esophagus before and during endotracheal intubation.

Acidity of gastric juice can be reduced effectively by oral administration of antacid solutions, particularly noncolloidal, clear antacids like sodium citrate, which will pose no additional hazard if aspirated. Gastric acidity may also be reduced by specific histamine (H_2) blockers, such as cimetidine and ranitidine, which may be administered orally or intravenously.[62] Intravenous metoclopramide has also been used to reduce the risk of aspiration pneumonitis and prepare the pregnant patient with a full stomach for general anesthesia. Metoclopramide increases pressure in the lower esophageal sphincter and at the gastric fundus and increases peristaltic contractions in the esophagus, gastric antrum, and small intestine. Taken together, these effects hasten esophageal clearance, promote rapid gastric emptying, and shorten transit time through the small bowel. Narcotics and anticholinergics have an opposite effect on gastroesophageal sphincter tone and prolong gastric emptying time significantly.

A pregnant patient near term should be considered a patient with a full stomach who is at risk for regurgitation and pulmonary aspiration of retained gastric contents. Every effort should be made to reduce intragastric pressure as well as the volume and acidity of gastric contents. Gastric pH can be raised above 3.5 by antacids or H_2 blockers, and gastric volume can be reduced below 25 ml by metoclopramide or nasogastric suction to further reduce the risk of acid aspiration. Regurgitation and aspiration of gastric contents during pregnancy occur when protective airway reflexes are obtunded by sedatives, general anesthetics, or high-level regional blocks. The simplest and most effective antiaspiration measures include the administration of antacids, a head-up position for tracheal intubation, avoidance of lithotomy and fundal pressure, prevention of succinylcholine-induced fasciculations prior to tracheal intubation, avoidance of positive pressure ventilation, and a rapid induction-intubation sequence with effective cricoid pressure applied by an assistant. For maximum effectiveness, oral antacid solutions should be given in volumes of 15 to 30 ml at least 30 minutes before induction of general anesthesia, to allow for adequate mixing and acid buffering. Oral antacid therapy may be repeated after 3 hours to counteract acid rebound phenomena. With large gastric volumes, antacids may not increase pH sufficiently above 3.5 to prevent acid aspiration pneumonitis. Therefore, pregnant patients should always be considered at risk for gastric acid aspiration.

RENAL SYSTEM

Anatomic and Dynamic Changes

The renal calyces, pelves, and ureters above the pelvic brim dilate progressively beginning at the twelfth week of pregnancy, as a result of mechanical compression at the pelvic inlet, initially by the iliac arteries and later by the enlarging uterus. The precise etiology of gestational hydronephrosis is unknown but probably represents a combination of ureteric compression by the iliac arteries, ovarian veins, and gravid uterus, and ureteric smooth muscle relaxation directed by one or more gestational hormones, particularly progesterone. A more pronounced obstructive pattern of hydronephrosis is noted on the right side in 75% of patients studied by intravenous urography during pregnancy.[63] The difference in renal dilatation on the right and left sides has been related to dextrorotation of the enlarging uterus, greater right ureteral compression by the right ovarian vein, and the cushioning effect offered by the sigmoid colon on the left side.[63] Dilatation of the urinary collecting system in pregnancy increases the capacity of the urinary tract by about 200 ml.[64] The urinary bladder easily accommodates this increase in urine capacity with near-term bladder capacity double that of the nonpregnant state.[64] The increases in bladder capacity during pregnancy are associated with a decrease in bladder tone causing urgency, frequency, and incontinence. Urinary stasis within the bladder, ureteral dead spaces, and dilated calyceal systems is common by midpregnancy and contributes to the frequency of urinary tract infections during pregnancy.

Functional Changes

Glomerular Filtration Rate and Renal Plasma Flow. The glomerular filtration rate (GFR) increases significantly during pregnancy, with the highest rates of increase in GFR occurring in the first and early second trimesters, reaching 40% to 50% above nonpregnant levels by 20 weeks.[4] During the remainder of the second trimester and until 28 weeks, the rate of increase in GFR slows, with no more than an additional 10% increase.[4] Changes in GFR during the third trimester are variable; most studies demonstrate relative stability or a slight decrease in GFR. The normal GFR by midpregnancy is between 110 and 150 ml/min.[4] Like GFR, renal plasma flow (RPF) also begins to increase in the first trimester, following a pattern of increase similar to that of GFR, with a maximum increase of 35% to 40% by midpregnancy.[4] Aortocaval compression by the gravid uterus in the supine position may significantly decrease RPF. In the lateral position, near-term values for RPF are 750 ml/min, and in the recumbent position RPF drops to approximately 600 ml/min. In late pregnancy, GFR, RPF, urine output, and urinary sodium and chloride excretion decrease when measured in the supine position. There is a 40% reduction in blood urea nitrogen to 8 to 9 mg/dl and in creatinine to 0.46 mg/dl by midpregnancy, due to increases in GFR and RPF.[65]

Renal Tubular Function. Glycosuria is common in pregnancy, may occur in the presence of normal blood glucose levels, and is probably related to augmented GFR, which results in a filtered load of glucose that exceeds tubular reabsorption capacity. Tubular reabsorption capacity for glucose may actually decrease during pregnancy. Glycosuria of 1 to 10 g/day is not uncommon by midpregnancy and is not usually associated with any pathology, just annoying diuresis.[4]

Amino Acids. Aminoaciduria is also common during pregnancy and may reach urinary levels of 1 to 10 g/day, unassociated with any pathology. Excretion of glycine, histidine, threonine, serine, alanine, lysine, cysteine, taurine, tyrosine, and phenylalanine increases during the first half of pregnancy.[4] It is not known whether the renal threshold or tubular maximum for amino acids is altered by pregnancy.[4]

Uric Acid. Serum uric acid levels are significantly decreased during the first and second trimesters but increase to near-nonpregnant levels by the third trimester.[4] The later increase is attributed in part to increasing production of uric acid by the fetus.[4]

Potassium and Sodium. Urinary potassium excretion during pregnancy parallels nonpregnant potassium balance. There is, however, an increase in the tubular reabsorption of potassium throughout pregnancy, with increased filtered sodium loads of 5000 to 10,000 mEq/day.[4] Increased GFR, increased progesterone production, increased antidiuretic hormone concentration, decreased plasma albumin, and decreased vascular resistance act together to promote sodium excretion in pregnancy. Increased concentrations of aldosterone, estrogens, cortisol, human placental lactogen, and prolactin tend to decrease sodium excretion during pregnancy. Aortocaval compression by the gravid uterus in the supine position decreases sodium excretion by as much as 50% by midterm.[4] Interestingly, sodium plasma concentrations decrease only slightly during pregnancy due to water retention, slight excess of solute, and a balancing effect between hormonal changes and increased GFR.

Renin-Angiotensin-Aldosterone System. All endocrine components of the renin-angiotensin-aldosterone system are elevated during pregnancy because of their increased regulatory roles in circulatory volume and sodium balance. Elevated aldosterone concentrations occur very early in gestation. Renin substrate also increases in concentration until the end of the second trimester; its hepatic production is stimulated by estrogens.[4] Increased concentrations of renin produced by the kidney rapidly convert renin substrate produced by the liver to high levels of angiotensin I and II.[4] Plasma renin activity is significantly increased by 8 weeks' gestation, with a steady increase in activity to 32 weeks, followed by a slight decrease.[4] For unknown reasons, pregnant patients are less sensitive than nonpregnant women to exogenous angiotensin II. It appears that there is little placental transfer of renin, angiotensin, and aldosterone.[4]

Anesthetic Implications

With dilatation of the upper urinary tracts and urinary stasis in the upper and lower tracts, a pregnant patient is at considerable risk of urinary tract infections, especially near term. Urinary retention from motor blockade during conduction anesthesia for labor and delivery may necessitate temporary bladder catheterization that further increases the risks of urinary tract infections. With significant increases in GFR and RPF during gestation, serum levels of creatinine, blood urea nitrogen, and uric acid are significantly reduced to 50% to 70% less than normal nonpregnant values. Elevation in serum levels of creatinine, blood urea nitrogen, and uric acid must take this into account, especially in hypertensive and preeclamptic patients, because laboratory data that at any other time would be within normal limits may indicate significant renal insufficiency during pregnancy.

CONCLUSIONS

Pregnancy is a uniquely altered state of human physiology with a number of normal physiologic changes occurring progressively that would be considered pathologic in nonpregnant states. The greatest maternal risks from pregnancy (sepsis, hemorrhage, and aspiration) have now been well defined, and effective steps to reduce them have been developed. Fetal risks during pregnancy, such as reactive hypoglycemia from maternal hyperglycemia and hypoperfusion acidosis from aortocaval compression, continue to be defined, and new steps to protect the fetus in utero, like left uterine displacement and ephedrine administration, continue to be developed. Only a thorough understanding of the major physiologic changes of pregnancy, particularly the cardiopulmonary, hematologic, gastrointestinal, and renal changes, will enable clinicians to improve prenatal care, better interpret laboratory data, administer safer anesthetics, preserve fetal well-being, and ensure normal neonatal outcome.

References

1. Lund CJ, Donovan JC: Blood volume during pregnancy: Significance of plasma and red cell volumes. Am J Obstet Gynecol 98:393, 1967
2. Pritchard JA: Changes in blood volume during pregnancy and delivery. Anesthesiology 26:393, 1965

3. Efrati P, Presentey B, Margalith M, et al.: Leukocytes of normal pregnant women. Obstet Gynecol 23:249, 1964
4. Brinkman CR III: Maternal cardiovascular and renal disorders: Biologic adaptation to pregnancy. In: Creasy RK, Resnik R (eds): Maternal-Fetal Medicine: Principles and Practice. Philadelphia: W.B. Saunders, 1984, pp 679–794
5. Bille-Brake NE, Rorth M: Red cell 2,3-diphosphoglycerate in pregnancy. Acta Obstet Gynecol Scand 58:19, 1979
6. Laird-Meeter K, Van de Lay G, Bom TH, et al.: Cardiocirculatory adjustments during pregnancy—an echocardiographic study. Clin Cardiol 2:328, 1979
7. Rubler S, Damani PM, Pento ER: Cardiac size and performance during pregnancy estimated with echocardiography. Am J Cardiol 40:534, 1977
8. Wilson M, Morganti A, Zervoudakis J, et al.: Blood pressure, the renin-aldosterone system and sex steroids throughout normal pregnancy. Am J Med 68:97, 1980
9. Cutforth R, Macdonald CD: Heart sounds and murmurs in pregnancy. Am Heart J 71:741, 1966
10. Lees MM, Taylor SH, Scoh DB, et al.: A study of cardiac output at rest throughout pregnancy. J Obstet Gynaecol Br Commonwealth 74:319, 1967
11. Ueland K, Novy MJ, Peterson EN, et al.: Maternal cardiovascular dynamics IV. The influence of gestational age on the maternal cardiovascular response to position and exercise. Am J Obstet Gynecol 104:856, 1969
12. Kerr MG, Scott DM, Samuel E: Studies of the inferior vena cava in late pregnancy. Br Med J 1:532, 1964
13. Bleniarz J, Crohogini JJ, Curuchet E, et al.: Aortocaval compression by the uterus in late human pregnancy. Am J Obstet Gynecol 100:203, 1968
14. Galbert MW, Marx GF: Extradural pressures in the parturient patient. Anesthesiology 40:499, 1974
15. Marazita AJD: The action of hormones on varicose veins in pregnancy. Med Record 159:422, 1946
16. Colditz RB, Josey WE: Central venous pressure in the supine position during normal pregnancy. Obstet Gynecol 36:769, 1970
17. Manchester B, Loube SD: The velocity of blood flow in normal pregnant women. Am Heart J 32:215, 1946
18. Assali NS, Nuwayhid B, Brinkman CR III, et al.: Autonomic control of pelvic circulation: In vivo and in vitro in pregnant and nonpregnant sheep. Am J Obstet Gynecol 141:873, 1981
19. Barwin BN, Roddie IC: Venous distensibility during pregnancy determined by graded venous congestion. Am J Obstet Gynecol 125:921, 1976
20. Bader RA, Bader ME, Rose DJ, et al.: Hemodynamics at rest and during exercise in normal pregnancy as studied by cardiac catheterization. J Clin Invest 34:1524, 1955
21. Hellgren M, Blomback ML: Studies on blood coagulation and fibrinolysis in pregnancy, during delivery, and in the puerperium. Gynecol Obstet Invest 12:141, 1981
22. Ralston DH, Shnider SM, de Lorimier AA: Effects of equipotent ephedrine, metaraminol, mephentermine and methoxamine on uterine blood flow in the pregnant ewe. Anesthesiology 40:354, 1974
23. Wright RG, Shnider SM, Levinson G, et al.: The effect of maternal administration of ephedrine on fetal heart rate and variability. Obstet Gynecol 57:734, 1981
24. Datta S, Alper MH, Ostheimer GW, et al.: Method of ephedrine administration on nausea and hypotension during spinal anesthesia for cesarean section. Anesthesiology 56:68, 1982
25. Alaily AB, Carrol KB: Pulmonary ventilation in pregnancy. Br J Obstet Gynaecol 85:518, 1978
26. Pernoll ML, Metcalfe J, Kovach PA, et al.: Ventilation during rest and exercise in pregnancy and postpartum. Respir Physiol 25:295, 1975
27. deSwiet M: Maternal pulmonary disorders. In: Creasy RK, Resnik R (eds): Maternal-Fetal Medicine: Principles and Practice. Philadelphia: W.B. Saunders, 1984, pp 781–794
28. Lucius H, Gahlenbeck H, Kleine O, et al.: Respiratory functions, buffer system and electrolyte concentrations of blood during human pregnancy. Respir Physiol 9:311, 1970
29. Templeton AA, Kelman GR: Maternal blood-gases ($P_{A}O_{2}$-PaO_{2}), physiological shunt and V_{D}/V_{T} in normal pregnancy. Br J Anaesth 48:1001, 1976

30. Knuttgen HG, Emerson K: Physiological response to pregnancy at rest and during exercise. J Appl Physiol 36:549, 1974.
31. Lehmann V, Fabel H: Lungenfunktionsuntersuchungen an Schwangeren. I. Lungenvolumina. Z Geburtshilfe Perinatol 177:387, 1973
32. Lehmann V, Fabel H: Lungenfunktionsunterschungen an Schwangeren. II. Ventilation, Atemmechanik und Diffusion-Kapazität. Z Geburtshilfe Perinatol 177:397, 1973
33. Kelman GR, Templeton A: Maternal blood gases during human pregnancy. Physiology 244:66, 1975
34. Sobrevilla LA, Carsinelli MT, Carcelen A, et al.: Human fetal and maternal oxygen tension and acid-base status during delivery at high altitude. Am J Obstet Gynecol 111:111, 1971
35. Doring GK, Loeschche HH: Atmung und Säure-Basengleichgewich in der Schwangerschaft. Pflugers Arch 249:437, 1947
36. Skatrud JB, Dempsey JA, Kaiser DG: Ventilatory response to medroxyprogesterone acetate in normal subjects: Time course and mechanism. J Appl Physiol 44:939, 1978
37. Sutton FD, Zwillich CD, Creagh CE, et al.: Progesterone for outpatient treatment of Pickwickian syndrome. Ann Intern Med 83:476, 1975
38. Thompson KJ, Cohen ME: Studies on the circulation in normal pregnancy. II. Vital capacity observations in normal pregnant women. Surg Gynecol Obstet 66:591, 1938
39. Mobius WV: Abruch der Schwangerschaft. Münchener Med Wochenschr 103:1389, 1961
40. Milne JA, Howie AD, Pack AI: Dyspnoea during normal pregnancy. Br J Obstet Gynaecol 84:448, 1978
41. Mackenzie AI: Laryngeal oedema complicating obstetric anaesthesia. Anaesthesia 33:271, 1978
42. Heller PJ, Scheider EP, Marx GF: Pharyngolaryngeal edema as a presenting symptom in pre-eclampsia. Obstet Gynecol 62:523, 1983
43. Hyman AL, Spannhake EW, Kadowitz PJ: Prostaglandins and the lung: State of the art. Am Rev Respir Dis 117:111, 1978
44. Whalen JB, Clancey CJ, Farley DB, et al.: Plasma prostaglandins in pregnancy. Obstet Gynecol 51:52, 1978
45. Newhouse MT, Becklaile MR, Macklem PT, et al.: Effect of alterations in end-tidal CO_2 on flow resistance. J Appl Physiol 19:745, 1964
46. Bevan DR, Holdcroft A, Loh L, et al.: Closing volume and pregnancy. Br Med J 1:13, 1974
47. Garrard CG, Littler WAW, Redman CWL: Closing volume during normal pregnancy. Thorax 33:484, 1978
48. Palahnuik RJ, Shnider SM, Eger EI II: Pregnancy decreases the requirement for inhaled anesthetic agents. Anesthesiology 41:82, 1974
49. Gintzler AR: Endorphin-mediated increases in pain threshold during pregnancy. Science 210:183, 1980
50. Huch A, Huch R: Transcutaneous, noninvasive monitoring of PO_2. Hosp Pract 11:43, 1976
51. Miller FC, Petrie RH, Arce JJ, et al.: Hyperventilation during labor. Am J Obstet Gynecol 120:489, 1974
52. Levinson G, Shnider SM, de Loumer AA, et al.: Effects of maternal hyperventilation on uterine blood flow and fetal oxygenation and acid-base status. Anesthesiology 40:340, 1974
53. Smith BE, Moya F, Shnider SM: The effects of anesthesia on liver function during labor. Anesth Analg 41:24, 1962
54. McNair RD, Jaynes RN: Alterations in liver function during normal pregnancy. Am J Obstet Gynecol 80:500, 1960
55. Shnider SM: Serum cholinesterase activity during pregnancy, labor and puerperium. Anesthesiology 26:335, 1965
56. Weissman DH, Ehrenwerth J: Prolonged neuromuscular blockade in a parturient associated with succinylcholine. Anesth Analg 62:444, 1983
57. Hart DM: Heartburn in pregnancy. J Int Med Res 6:1, 1978
58. Spence AA, Moir DD, Finlay WEI: Observations on intragastric pressure. Anaesthesia 22:249, 1967

59. Attia RR, Eberd AM, Fischer JE: Gastrin: Placental, maternal and plasma cord levels, its possible role in maternal residual gastric acidity (abstract). Anesthesiology 48 (Suppl):547, 1976
60. Roberts RB, Shirley MB: Reducing the risk of acid aspiration during cesarean section. Anesth Analg 53:859, 1974
61. Blitt CD, Petty WC, Alberternst EA, et al.: Correlation of plasma cholinesterase activity and duration of action of succinylcholine during pregnancy. Anesth Analg 56:78, 1977
62. Husemeyer RP, Davenport HT: Prophylaxis for Mendelson's syndrome before elective cesarean section. A comparison of cimetidine and magnesium trisilicate mixture regimens. Br J Obstet Gynaecol 87:565, 1980
63. Schulman A, Herlinger H: Urinary tract dilatation in pregnancy. Br J Radiol 48:638, 1975
64. Youssef AF: Cystometric studies in gynecology and obstetrics. Obstet Gynecol 8:181, 1956
65. Davison JM: The physiology of the renal tract in pregnancy. Clin Obstet Gynecol 28:257, 1985

3. Anesthetic Management of the Pregnant Patient Undergoing Nonobstetric Surgery

James H. Diaz, M.D.

INTRODUCTION AND EPIDEMIOLOGY

More than 50,000 pregnant women undergo nonobstetric surgical procedures in the United States each year.[1] The number of pregnant

Portions of this chapter have been reproduced or adapted with permission from Diaz JH: Perioperative management of the pregnant patient undergoing nonobstetric surgery. Anesthesiology Review, January/February, 1991.

51

patients who undergo nonobstetric surgery is greater than reported because many surgical procedures, particularly gynecologic operations, are performed in patients who are in early gestational states, unaware of their pregnancies. Therefore, truly accurate data on the incidence of surgery during pregnancy do not exist. The incidence of surgery during pregnancy may range from a low of 0.3% to a high of 2.2%.[2, 3]

Maternal mortality associated with nonobstetric surgery during pregnancy was 35% at the turn of the century.[3, 4] Today, maternal mortality associated with nonobstetric surgery during pregnancy continues to be significant and ranges from 5.5% to 34.6%.[3, 4] As discussed in Chapter 2, the surgical diagnosis and the procedure performed during pregnancy have more impact on maternal morbidity and fetal loss than the choice of anesthetics or the effects of anesthetics on perinatal outcome.

Trauma is the most frequent indication for surgery in a pregnant patient. After surgery related to trauma, the acute abdomen is the most common nonobstetric surgical problem in pregnancy, with acute appendicitis ranking first in indications for exploratory laparotomy.[5] An acute abdomen from a perforated appendix or twisted ovarian cyst requires immediate abdominopelvic exploration, increasing the risks of premature labor and delivery with a 33% to 35% fetal mortality.[3–5]

Blunt abdominal trauma during pregnancy is most commonly caused by motor vehicle accidents and is particularly dangerous to the fetus. Placental laceration and abruptio placentae are frequent and often delayed indications of serious blunt injury to the abdomen or pelvis during pregnancy.[6–8] Rothenberger and associates[8] reviewed 103 cases of blunt abdominal trauma during pregnancy and reported that the overall incidence of unsuccessful pregnancy following such trauma was 61%. Of patients admitted to the hospital in shock, 80% had miscarriages.[8]

Uterine rupture may also follow blunt abdominopelvic trauma, especially in women who have had a previous cesarean section.[9] Fetal survival is unlikely following uterine rupture from blunt trauma.[9]

Penetrating trauma to the abdomen or pelvis during pregnancy usually carries a better prognosis for both the mother and fetus than blunt trauma with its increased risks of placental separation and uterine rupture.[9] Fetal mortality from penetrating trauma to the uterus is about 40%.[10] In general, however, penetrating trauma to the uterus is more detrimental to the fetus than to the mother.[9]

Open heart surgery and neurosurgery are rarely indicated during pregnancy but have been performed, with improved outcomes for both the mother and the fetus. In 1958, Leyse and associates[11] first used extracorporeal circulation (ECC) to repair congenital aortic stenosis in a pregnant patient at 18 weeks' gestation. In 1969, Zitnick and associates[12] reviewed 20 cases of open heart surgery during pregnancy, reporting an overall maternal mortality of 5% and a fetal mortality of 33%. In a more recent study of open heart surgery during pregnancy, Becker[13] in 1983 reviewed 55 cases of open heart surgery performed with ECC during pregnancy and found that although maternal mortality had been reduced to 1.8%, fetal mortality had only slightly improved to 21.8% (see Special Anesthetic Techniques later in this chapter).

The real hazards of surgical anesthesia during pregnancy are related to the physiologic changes of pregnancy, the direct effects of anesthetics on fetal well-being, and the possible adverse effects of surgery on the fetus. These hazards are similar to those encountered during obstetric anesthesia, with two important differences. First, the aim of obstetric anesthesia is to permit pain-free labor and delivery without interfering with the course of labor, whereas the aim of surgical anesthesia is to provide maternal and fetal anesthesia during nonobstetric operations without stimulating uterine activity or precipitating premature labor. Second, obstetric anesthetics should provide maternal analgesia without fetal neurologic depression and delayed neonatal breathing, whereas surgical anesthetics are designed to maintain uteroplacental perfusion and prevent premature labor without consideration of fetal sedation or respiratory depression.

INDIRECT EFFECTS OF ANESTHETICS ON FETAL WELL-BEING

Both surgery and anesthesia may interfere indirectly with normal maternal and fetal physiology, harming the fetus even when the anesthetic agents used have no direct embryotoxic or cytotoxic effects. Indirect effects of anesthetic management with the greatest impact on fetal well-being and neonatal outcome include (1) maternal hypoxia with neonatal asphyxia; (2) maternal hypotension with reduced uterine blood flow; (3) improper vasopressor administration with uterine hypoperfusion; (4) maternal hypercarbia with increased circulating maternal catechols, uteroplacental vasoconstriction, and fetal hypoperfusion; and (5) maternal hypocarbia with reduced uterine blood flow.

Since fetal oxygenation is directly dependent on maternal oxygen tension, maternal hypoxia will result in rapid fetal hypoxia and, if uncorrected, fetal asphyxia and death. Maternal oxygen reserve during pregnancy is limited by increased oxygen consumption, reduced hemoglobin concentration, and diminished functional residual capacity. General anesthesia for nonobstetric surgery in pregnant patients should therefore always be preceded by administration of 100% oxygen for denitrogenation in order to reduce the risks of maternal and fetal hypoxia during induction of anesthesia, hypoventilation, and endotracheal intubation. Fetal oxygenation is also directly dependent on maternal oxygen-carrying capacity, hemoglobin content, hemoglobin affinity for oxygen, and uteroplacental perfusion pressure.

Since the uteroplacental circulation is not autoregulated, uterine blood flow is directly determined by uterine vascular resistance and uterine perfusion pressure. Maternal hypotension from a variety of causes, including hemorrhage, sympathetic blockade, or aortocaval compression, will quickly reduce uterine artery blood flow and compromise fetal perfusion. Under normal circumstances, the uteroplacental circulation is maximally dilated so that perfusion pressure rather than uteroplacental vascular resistance is the major determinant of uteroplacental blood flow.[14] Maternal hemorrhage must be controlled during surgery and circulating blood volume restored as indicated by intravenous crystalloid solutions, colloid infusions, and blood transfusions.

Systemic hypotension resulting from sympathetic blockade during spinal or epidural anesthesia in a pregnant surgical patient is best prevented or at least reduced by the intravenous infusion of crystalloid solution prior to the administration of the sympathetic block. Prehydration should be with 1 liter of a dextrose-containing, balanced electrolyte solution such as warmed lactated Ringer's solution.

Starting at 24 to 26 weeks' gestation, compression of the abdominal aorta and the inferior vena cava by the enlarging uterus will significantly reduce central venous return and cardiac output in the supine position. Prevention of aortocaval compression during nonobstetric surgery is best accomplished by positioning the pregnant patient on her side (preferably on the left side). The pregnant surgical patient may remain on her left side whenever supine and during transport to the operating room. Left uterine displacement can be maintained on the operating table by placing a wedge or pillow under the right hip or tilting the operating table to the left. The right pelvis should be elevated at least 15° from the horizontal to prevent aortocaval compression during surgery in the supine position.

Maternal hypotension with intrauterine fetal hypoperfusion and asphyxia may also result from high inspired doses of inhalation anesthetics. Such anesthetic-induced hypotension may be avoided by administering low to moderate inspired concentrations of halogenated anesthetics and supplementing inhaled anesthetics with intravenous narcotic adjuvants to maintain anesthetic depth and limit inspired concentrations of inhaled anesthetics.

Maternal hypotension from any cause requires immediate treatment with circulating volume restoration and careful vasopressor therapy. All vasopressor agents and catecholamines can increase uteroplacental perfusion by direct vasoconstriction, with significant increases in uteroplacental vascular resistance. Pure alpha-adrenergic agonists like methoxamine and phenylephrine cause profound uterine artery vasoconstriction with uterine hypoperfusion and are contraindicated in the management of maternal hypotension. Even mixed agonists like epinephrine and norepinephrine can reduce uterine blood flow, constrict placental vascular beds, and cause fetal hypoperfusion and hypoxia. The systemic absorption of even small amounts of epinephrine commonly used to prolong the effects of local anesthetics during conduction anesthesia may cause vasoconstriction of uterine vessels.[15] On the other hand, ephedrine, another mixed agonist, appears to be the safest vasopressor for use during maternal hypotension because it increases mean arterial pressure, uterine artery pressure, and uterine artery blood flow without a concomitant decrease in uteroplacental perfusion.[16] As a beta-adrenergic agonist, ephedrine increases maternal cardiac output and restores uterine blood flow during maternal hypotension.[16] As a weak alpha-adrenergic agonist, ephedrine, with its mild vasoconstrictive properties, has little impact on uterine vascular resistance.[16] Overall, the increased cardiac output from ephedrine's beta-adrenergic stimulation will maintain uterine artery perfusion pressure and compensate for ephedrine's mild alpha-adrenergic vasoconstriction.[16]

Maternal hypercarbia and hypocarbia may both result in intrauterine fetal asphyxia by interfering with placental perfusion and maternal-fetal oxygen exchange. Hypercarbia from upper airway loss or sedative-induced respiratory depression will increase maternal catecholamine release, promote direct uteroplacental vasoconstriction, and limit uterine blood flow and fetal perfusion pressure. Similarly, maternal hyperventilation with hypocarbia produced by spontaneous tachypnea or rapid mechanical ventilation will also result in uterine artery vasoconstriction, increased uteroplacental vascular resistance, and intrauterine fetal hypoperfusion and hypoxia. The mechanical effects of induced hyperventilation have also been demonstrated to decrease maternal cardiac output and uteroplacental perfusion pressure in pregnant ewes, an effect that was corrected by restoring maternal $PaCO_2$ to normal or above normal levels.[17]

Maternal hypercarbia and hypocarbia with limited uteroplacental circulation often coexist during poorly managed labors or any other painful condition in pregnancy, such as ureterolithiasis and peritonitis. In such conditions, sedative-induced hypoventilation-hypercarbia between pains often alternates with pain-induced hyperventilation-hypocarbia during uterine contractions or other painful paroxysms. Respiratory depression during pregnancy can be avoided by using conduction anesthetics for surgery and for postoperative pain management and by selecting nonsedating agonist-antagonists (nalbuphine, butorphanol) for mild to moderate perioperative pain after organogenesis is complete. Narcotics have been administered to pregnant women for generations without direct fetal effects. On the other hand, the effects of the newer non-narcotic agonists-antagonists have not been studied during early pregnancy, limiting their use to the late second and third trimesters after the risks of drug teratogenicity have passed.

Maternal hyperventilation, whether spontaneous or induced, should be prevented perioperatively by managing pain and anxiety with appropriate nonsedating dosages of analgesics or conduction anesthetics and by avoiding mechanical hyperventilation during general anesthesia. Maternal respiratory alkalosis from any cause will promote uteroplacental vasoconstriction and shift the maternal oxyhemoglobin dissociation curve leftward, making maternal oxygen less available to fetal hemoglobin.

As noted in Chapter 1, the indirect effects of maternal anesthetics, primarily hypoxia, hypotension, hypercarbia, and hypocarbia, pose greater threats to fetal well-being than any teratogenic or cytotoxic potential of anesthetic agents themselves.

DIRECT EFFECTS OF ANESTHETICS ON FETAL WELL-BEING

The embryotoxic and cytotoxic effects of anesthetic agents during periods of organogenesis have been presented in Chapter 1. Other direct effects of anesthetics on the mother and the fetus during nonobstetric surgery include direct effects on uterine tone and on fetal physiology and well-being. Both ketamine and the halogenated anesthetics have significant effects on uterine activity and tone.

In the first trimester, ketamine produces significant increases in intrauterine pressure equal to the effects of ergot preparations. By the third trimester, however, ketamine has little effect on uterine activity and tone. Since the human uterus contains both alpha- and beta-adrenergic receptors, the epinephrine and norepinephrine release stimulated by therapeutic ketamine dosages (≥ 1 mg/kg) during the first trimester may stimulate adrenergic receptors, increasing uterine tone and activity and promoting intrauterine fetal asphyxia.[18] Because uterine adrenergic receptors decrease in number as pregnancy progresses, the sensitivity of uterine muscle to ketamine is significantly decreased by the third trimester.[18]

Unlike ketamine, halogenated agents given in light to moderate dosages of 0.5 to 1.5 minimum alveolar concentration (MAC)* have little effect on uterine blood flow despite reductions of nearly 20% in maternal blood pressure.[19] At low doses (0.5 to 1.0 MAC), halogenated anesthetics promote uterine vasodilation and have limited effects on uteroplacental circulation and fetal well-being.[19] With levels of 2.0 MAC and greater,

---

*MAC is the minimum alveolar concentration of an anesthetic gas that will produce immobility in 50% of patients exposed to a noxious stimulus.

however, halogenated anesthetics cause significant reductions in maternal blood pressure and cardiac output with concomitant reductions in uterine blood flow, fetal perfusion pressure, fetal heart rate, and fetal oxygen saturation.[19]

Animal investigations seem to indicate that equi-MAC concentrations of isoflurane and enflurane may have a more serious detrimental impact on fetal well-being than equi-MAC halothane concentrations, despite similar decreases in maternal blood pressure and cardiac output with all three anesthetics.[20, 21] During administration of low-dose halothane to pregnant ewes, no significant changes occurred in either fetal regional blood flow to vital organs or in fetal cardiac output.[20–22] Fetal oxygenation and acid-base status remained stable, indicating that a fall in fetal peripheral vascular resistance accounts primarily for the decline in fetal blood pressure.[20] In contrast, 2% isoflurane administration to pregnant ewes significantly reduced uteroplacental blood flow and produced progressive fetal acidosis.[21, 22] Deep enflurane anesthesia will cause maternal and fetal bradycardia, decrease uterine blood flow, and promote fetal acidosis in experimental animals.[19]

Other anesthetic drugs may have a variety of insignificant effects on fetal physiology. Atropine has been demonstrated to cross the uteroplacental circulation and to produce fetal tachycardia with loss of beat-to-beat variability.[23] Atropine does not, however, affect uterine activity or jeopardize a normal fetus.[23] Glycopyrrolate, another anticholinergic like atropine, neither crosses the uteroplacental circulation nor influences fetal heart rate or beat-to-beat variability.[19] The intravenous induction of general anesthesia with the ultra-short-acting barbiturate thiopental and the depolarizing muscle relaxant succinylcholine may lower uterine blood flow by 35% without a significant impact on fetal well-being or neonatal outcome.[24] Intravenous dosages of 50, 75, and 100 μg of the synthetic opioid fentanyl have failed to produce significant deleterious changes in any maternal or fetal cardiovascular or acid-base parameter or in uterine blood flow and muscle tone.[25] Evidence to date has also failed to associate maternal cimetidine or ranitidine acid-aspiration prophylaxis with poor fetal outcome or congenital deformities.[26] Cimetidine, however, rapidly crosses the placental circuit and can elevate fetal hepatic transaminases and inhibit fetal oxidative metabolism, indicating that it has effects at the fetal cellular level.[26] Acid-aspiration prophylaxis with the antihistamines cimetidine and ranitidine should be used with caution during organogenesis until more investigations of potential cytotoxic or embryotoxic effects have been conducted.[19, 26]

In addition to barbiturates, narcotics, low-dose volatile anesthetics, and local anesthetics, muscle relaxants are also used frequently with general anesthetics for nonobstetric surgery in pregnant patients. All commonly used muscle relaxants cross the uteroplacental circulation, depending on the dose administered, maternal serum concentration, and drug molecular weight. Clinical dosages of muscle relaxants given during nonobstetric surgery in pregnant patients have no adverse effects on fetal development or neonatal outcome.[19]

In summary, the indirect effects of anesthetic agents and anesthetic techniques appear to have a more significant impact on fetal well-being and neonatal outcome than any direct effects of anesthetic agents on fetal well-being, growth, and development.

TIMING OF SURGERY

Independent of the anesthetics administered, the incidence of fetal loss following nonobstetric surgery during pregnancy in the first and second trimesters appears to be increased.[27, 28] For this reason, all elective surgical procedures should be deferred until at least 6 weeks postpartum, when maternal physiology has returned to normal.[1] Women of childbearing age who are scheduled for elective operations should be questioned carefully during the preanesthetic interview regarding the possibility of pregnancy and tested when appropriate or when uncertain. Elective surgery can be postponed if the patient is found to be pregnant.

Urgent surgical procedures (cardiac surgery, neurosurgery) that must be performed during pregnancy but that can be delayed are best postponed until the late second or early third trimester.[1] For surgery during the first trimester that cannot be postponed, there is no clear evidence that one specific anesthetic agent or technique is safer than another provided maternal blood pressure and ventilation are maintained within normal limits and fetal status is monitored constantly.[1] When applicable, major regional anesthetics (spinal, epidural, caudal) can be employed in the first trimester to reduce teratogenic drug exposures. On the other hand, general anesthetics may prove more advantageous after organogenesis by permitting maximum maternal-fetal oxygenation, avoiding maternal hypotension, and providing uterine relaxation with inhaled anesthetics, thus decreasing the risks of premature labor and delivery.

PREOPERATIVE PREPARATION

Preoperative preparation of pregnant patients undergoing nonobstetric surgery should include personal reassurance to reduce apprehension and anxiety and adequate premedication if time permits. Barbiturate and narcotic premedicants may be prescribed in preference to benzodiazepines, which are teratogenic (see Chapter 1). Anticholinergics may also be used without adverse effects on maternal-fetal physiology.[19] Narcotics or non-narcotic agonists-antagonists should be used to manage preoperative pain, with narcotics preferred early in pregnancy and the non-narcotics reserved for late pregnancy. Vigorous intravenous fluid therapy will help to avert hypovolemia and support uterine blood flow during regional anesthesia such as spinal and epidural blocks. Patients should be transported to the operating room in the left lateral tilt position and should remain tilted to at least 15° to the left during surgery in the supine position to avoid aortocaval compression. Thirty milliliters of 0.3 *M* sodium citrate, a nonparticulate antacid, may be given by mouth within 45 minutes of surgery to increase gastric pH above 2.5. At present, the gastric antihistamines cimetidine and ranitidine and the gastric emptier metoclopramide have unknown teratogenic potential during organogenesis and may elevate fetal hepatic transaminases.[19] Pregnant patients should be well preoxygenated with at least four deep breaths of 100% oxygen prior to the induction of general anesthesia and tracheal intubation. Regional anesthesia, awake endotracheal intubation, and rapid-sequence induction intubation techniques employing cricoid pressure (Sellick's maneuver) will all reduce the risks of silent regurgitation and pulmonary aspiration during nonobstetric surgery in pregnant patients.

A simple preanesthetic checklist (like an airplane pilot's preflight checklist) for nonobstetric surgery during pregnancy is presented in Table 3–1.

INTRAOPERATIVE MANAGEMENT

Appropriate monitoring of a pregnant patient undergoing nonobstetric surgery should include continuous monitoring of maternal-fetal well-being and uterine activity. Specific monitoring should include noninvasive or direct maternal arterial blood pressure measurements, maternal oximetry or blood gas measurements, inspired oxygen analysis, end-tidal CO_2 analysis, maternal electrocardiography, maternal urine output measurement, central venous pressure measurements if indicated in shock, external uterine tocodynamometry to detect the onset of premature uterine contractions, and fetal Doppler echocardiography to monitor fetal heartbeat and beat-to-beat variability. Arterial blood gas monitoring during nonobstetric surgery in pregnant patients will permit maintenance of normal oxygenation and ventilation and, most importantly, allow the anesthesiologist to avoid hypoventilation-hypercarbia or mechanical hyperventilation-hypocarbia.

External fetal heartbeat monitoring becomes possible as early as at 16 to 20 weeks' gestation. Initiation of electronic fetal monitoring allows for the recognition and rapid correction of alterations in fetal heart tones and variability during nonobstetric surgery. If fetal heart rate decreases or increases, inspired oxygen concentrations can be increased and the uterus displaced further laterally and to the left. If surgical manipulations

Table 3–1. *Preanesthetic Checklist: Anesthetics for Nonobstetric Surgery During Pregnancy*

For Any Anesthetic	For Regional Anesthetic	For General Anesthetic
Intravenous Catheter ___ 14–16 gauge IV catheter	*Prehydration* ___ 1000–1500 ml warmed Ringer's lactate solution ___ 500 ml or less in maternal congenital heart disease	*Preoxygenation* ___ 4 min with 100% O_2
Airway Protection ___ Working laryngoscope ___ Assorted blades ___ Endotracheal tubes: Sizes 6.9–7.0 outside diameter ___ Assorted face masks	*Supplemental O_2* ___ Nasal prongs	*Capable Assistant* ___ To apply cricoid pressure ___ To hand entotracheal tube to laryngoscopist
Capability to Ventilate ___ Anesthesia machine ___ Anesthesia ventilator ___ Breathing circuit ___ Sources of O_2 and anesthetic gases	*Additional Monitors* ___ Foley catheter	*Additional Monitors* ___ Foley catheter ___ End-tidal CO_2

Essential Drugs
___ Induction agents: Thiopental Ketamine
___ Anticholinergics: Atropine Glycopyrrolate
___ Muscle relaxants:
  ___ For defasciculation: Curare Atracurium Vecuronium
  ___ For tracheal intubation: Succinylcholine
  ___ For surgical paralysis: Curare Atracurium Vecuronium Pancuronium
___ Vasopressors: Ephedrine, 5 mg/ml dilution		

Monitors ___ Maternal ECG Automated blood pressure Pulse oximetry Uterine tocodynamometry ___ Fetal external echocardiography		
Position ___ Left uterine displacement when supine		

*From Diaz JH: Perioperative management of the pregnant patient undergoing nonobstetric surgery. Anesthesiology Review, January/February, 1991. Used with permission.

60

cause alterations in fetal heart tones, these manipulations can be discontinued to allow a return of fetal heart rate to normal baseline. If uterine activity as monitored by external tocodynamometry increases during abdominopelvic surgery, increasing inspired doses of halothane, enflurane, or isoflurane may be added to balanced anesthetics to provide dose-related uterine relaxation. During the first trimester, thoughtful placement of tocodynamometers and ultrasound transducers over the uterus will be necessary to avoid encroachment on the sterile surgical field. Anesthetic drugs with a history of safe usage over many years and many generations should be selected for pregnant patients undergoing surgery, especially during early pregnancy. Such drugs include thiopental, morphine, meperidine, succinylcholine, curare, and low concentrations of nitrous oxide (N_2O) for short periods. Pregnant patients compromised by acute surgical illnesses, chronic debilitating illnesses, trauma, or shock should not receive N_2O because of significant myelosuppressive effects even after short exposures to clinical concentrations (see Chapter 1).

Maternal hypotension from regional anesthetics or deep general anesthesia should be prevented as much as possible by prehydration with intravenous fluids before administration of regional blocks or induction of general anesthesia. As a regional anesthetic, spinal anesthesia offers the advantage of employing small amounts of local anesthetic but often causes faster and more profound effects on maternal hemodynamic status than does epidural anesthesia. Should maternal hypotension occur at any time despite fluid prehydration, predominantly beta-adrenergic vasopressors, such as ephedrine, should be promptly administered intravenously in preference to purely alpha-adrenergic agonists, like phenylephrine or methoxamine, or predominantly alpha-adrenergic agonists, like norepinephrine and high dosages of epinephrine.[16]

Since the incidence of premature labor following abdominopelvic surgery in pregnancy is approximately 10%, the general anesthetics used should produce profound skeletal muscle relaxation to limit uterine manipulation and provide better surgical exposure and uterine muscle relaxation to limit uterine activity and premature onset of contractions with preterm labor and delivery. Skeletal muscle relaxation for better surgical access and exposure can be achieved with intravenous muscle relaxants, and uterine activity can be reduced during surgery with low inspired dosages of halogenated anesthetics. Supplemental oxygen should be provided during all regional anesthetics, and inspired oxygen concentrations should be no less than 50% during administration of all general anesthetics for nonobstetric surgery during pregnancy.

The intravenous administration of a nondepolarizing muscle relaxant, such as curare, atracurium, or vecuronium, is indicated prior to succinylcholine administration for tracheal intubation to prevent muscle fasciculations with increased oxygen consumption and regurgitation from increased intra-abdominal pressure and reduced cardioesophageal sphincter tone. Small cuffed endotracheal tubes with outside diameters of 6.0 to 7.0 mm should be swiftly inserted into the trachea during cricoid pressure. Regional anesthetics or awake tracheal intubation with topical anesthesia can be employed if difficult tracheal intubation is anticipated. After tracheal placement of the endotracheal tube and cuff inflation, cricoid pressure may be released and positive pressure mechanical ventilation begun. Assisted spontaneous ventilation is not recommended due to further reductions in functional residual capacity with anesthesia and the need to maintain normocarbia during surgery.

During shock, hypovolemic states, or maternal hypotension, ketamine may prove preferable to thiopental as an intravenous induction agent. Ketamine in low doses (1 to 2 mg/kg) has little if any significant effect on uterine tone by the third trimester.[18, 29] However, at higher doses (4 to 5 mg/kg), ketamine can actually increase uterine tone and endanger the fetus, especially during the first trimester.[29, 30] Halogenated agents may be desirable for operations involving the pelvic organs or on the uterus itself because these agents decrease uterine tone and activity and inhibit uterine contractions (see Chapter 5). For these reasons, halogenated agents have been recommended for use during nonobstetric surgery in later pregnancy and during in utero fetal surgery to reduce the significantly increased chances of premature labor following uterine manipulation or incision during pelvic laparotomy[1, 19] (see Chapter 5).

A 17% to 23% reduction in serum cholinesterase activity during pregnancy appears not to clinically prolong the paralyzing effects of succinylcholine unless large doses are administered or the patient is receiving concomitant magnesium sulfate therapy.[1, 19] As noted, nondepolarizing muscle relaxants may be employed safely during general anesthesia in pregnant patients undergoing nonobstetric surgery. However, the rapid intravenous administration of anticholinesterases to reverse the paralysis produced by nondepolarizing muscle relaxants may cause direct acetylcholine release, theoretically increasing uterine tone and stimulating premature labor.[1, 19] Anticholinesterases such as neostigmine and edrophonium should be administered slowly during closure and should be preceded by adequate amounts of an anticholinergic agent such as atropine or, preferably, glycopyrrolate.[19] As noted, atropine crosses the uteroplacental circulation rapidly and has been associated with significant fetal tachycardia and loss of beat-to-beat variability.[23] Narcotic adjuvants like morphine, fentanyl, and sufentanil in clinical dosages do not cause significant deleterious changes in maternal-fetal hemodynamic status and may permit lower inspired dosages of halogenated anesthetics.

POSTOPERATIVE MANAGEMENT

Postoperatively, maternal-fetal monitoring of patients recovering from nonobstetric surgery during pregnancy should be continued to signal premature labor and document fetal well-being by external tocodynamometry and fetal echocardiography. Supplemental oxygen should be provided during emergence, and endotracheal tubes should be removed only when patients resume consciousness with active airway protective reflexes. Maternal blood oxygenation and ventilation should also be monitored, either noninvasively by transcutaneous oximetry and capnometry or invasively by arterial blood gases. Postoperative maternal hypotension should be treated swiftly with intravascular volume restoration, left uterine displacement, and ephedrine administration. Oxygen desaturation may be corrected by administration of higher inspired oxygen concentrations. Pain-induced hyperventilation with hypocarbia can be prevented by continuous conduction analgesia or by adequate postoperative pain control with incremental dosages of narcotics or non-narcotic agonist-antagonists (in the third trimester). Hypoventilation with hypercarbia can be prevented by antagonizing prolonged narcosis with naloxone, reversing residual neuromuscular paralysis with anticholinesterases, and avoiding respiratory depressants with sedatives and anxiolytics.

SPECIAL ANESTHETIC TECHNIQUES
Extracorporeal Circulation

To reduce fetal risks, maternal-fetal monitoring during open heart surgery in pregnancy should include an external uterine tocodynamometer to signal the onset of premature contractions and continuous fetal echocardiography to evaluate the effects of extracorporeal circulation (ECC) on fetal heart rate and variability. Uterine activity during ECC, a time of marginal uterine blood flow, can further compromise uteroplacental perfusion. Thus, monitoring to detect uterine contractions should be employed throughout open heart surgery and ECC and continued postoperatively for at least 72 hours.[13, 31]

Several groups of investigators[32–36] have now used external ultrasonic Doppler transducers to study the changes in fetal heart rate and variability during ECC and have found some significant intraoperative trends. In the absence of hypotension, no change in fetal heart rate was noted during induction of anesthesia or at the onset of ECC with flow rates of 60 ml/kg/min and greater.[34] Uniformly, changes in fetal heart rate and some losses of beat-to-beat variability were associated with significant decreases in cardiopulmonary bypass pump flow.[32–34] Fetal heart rate improved and stabilized in the majority of cases with ECC at flow rates of 60 ml/kg/min and greater.[32-34] Lam and associates[34] described a pregnant patient who, after a short period of cessation of ECC for mitral valve replacement, had low mean perfusion pressures and fetal bradycardia. After administration of ephedrine, mean perfusion pressure increased and fetal heart rate improved.[34]

Circulatory arrest is no longer recommended during ECC for cardiac surgery in pregnancy. Koh and associates[33] noted that fetal heart rate often increased after ECC to 150 to 170 beats/min, returning to normal within 3 hours. All of these studies emphasize the importance of fetal heart rate monitoring during ECC for open heart surgery in pregnant patients.

Deliberate Hypothermia

Moderate hypothermia has been used in pregnant patients during open heart and neurosurgical procedures and as a treatment for closed head injury.[37-39] Although supporting evidence is limited, the effects of moderate hypothermia on the fetus are thought to be benign. Specific complications of induced hypothermia during pregnancy have included fetal-maternal acid-base disturbances, maternal coagulation disorders, and fetal arrhythmias.[40] Hypothermia can cause maternal and fetal bradycardia, maternal ventricular dysrhythmias, and maternal ventricular fibrillation.[13] Hypothermia can also stimulate uterine contractions and promote premature labor.[37] Fetal bradycardia due to hypothermia is difficult to distinguish from fetal bradycardia due to anoxia. Rewarming after induced hypothermia may also stimulate uterine contractions and induce premature labor and preterm delivery.[13]

In summary, deliberate hypothermia has been employed during a number of cardiovascular and neurosurgical procedures in pregnant patients without significant deleterious effects on fetal well-being or neonatal outcome, with the exception of preterm labor and delivery.[37] Careful monitoring for uterine contractions by external tocodynamometry and for fetal heart rate changes by external fetal echocardiography is required during induced hypothermia in pregnant patients.[37]

Deliberate Hypotension

Normally, the maternal vasculature is maximally dilated during pregnancy, making placental perfusion pressure the major determinant of uterine blood flow.[41] Reduced uteroplacental blood flow is therefore always a concern during the institution of deliberate hypotension with vasodilators in pregnant patients. Rapidly acting vasodilators such as hydralazine and sodium nitroprusside are being administered with increasing frequency during pregnancy to control essential and gestational hypertension. Although nitroglycerin has not been widely used in pregnant patients, detrimental effects on uterine blood flow or fetal well-being have not been observed.[42]

The effects of sodium nitroprusside on fetal well-being have, however, been studied more extensively than the effects of other vasodilators employed for deliberate hypotension. Lieb and others[43] showed that sodium nitroprusside decreased uterine blood flow in normotensive and hypertensive ewes. Ellis and associates[44] showed that uterine blood flow, when decreased by phenylephrine, increased somewhat with nitroprusside infusion but not to control levels. Fetal deaths have been reported in several cases of nitroprusside-induced hypotension and in some animal experiments after the administration of sodium nitroprusside for reduction of blood pressure.[45, 46] Nalty and others[47] noted that while low doses ($<$1 μg/kg/min) of sodium nitroprusside caused no fetal deaths, large doses given to gravid ewes resulted uniformly in maternal and fetal deaths. Sodium nitroprusside quickly crosses the placenta of gravid ewes. Because its liver is immature, the ewe fetus is unable to metabolize free cyanide ions cleaved from the nitroprusside molecule during its biotransformation. Metabolic acidosis develops quickly in ewe fetuses during prolonged nitroprusside administration to gravid ewes.[48] Large doses of sodium nitroprusside, however, have now been administered to pregnant human patients perioperatively without fetal compromise or death.[48]

Like sodium nitroprusside, hydralazine has also been studied clinically and experimentally during pregnancy. Positive inotropic and chronotropic properties are responsible for the increased cardiac output and improved uterine blood flow observed during hydralazine-induced hypotension.[49] Hydralazine given intravenously to renovascular hypertensive, pregnant sheep caused a 20% decrease in mean arterial pressure and a significant increase in uterine artery and renal blood flow.[49]

With careful monitoring of maternal blood pressure, uterine activity, fetal heart rate, and maternal acid-base status, deliberate hypotension with a number of vasodilators including nitroglycerin, sodium nitroprusside, and hydralazine can be achieved in pregnant patients without deleterious effects on fetal well-being or neonatal outcome. Cyanide toxicity remains a significant fetal-maternal risk during prolonged sodium nitroprusside-induced hypotension. Cyanide toxicity from sodium nitroprusside therapy can be prevented by administering low doses ($<$1 μg/kg/min) of nitroprusside and discontinuing therapy if any abnormalities in fetal heart tones are detected.[37]

CONCLUSIONS

Anesthetic care of the pregnant surgical patient is unique because the anesthesiologist must monitor two patients simultaneously, provide for good surgical exposure, detect premature labor promptly, and prevent preterm delivery. Intraoperative monitoring during nonobstetric surgery in pregnancy should include external uterine tocodynamometry and continuous fetal echocardiography. The detrimental, indirect effects of anesthetics on maternal-fetal well-being can be reduced and often eliminated by many simple measures, including preoxygenation before anoxic insults like tracheal intubation, prehydration before sympathetic blocks, early vasopressor therapy with ephedrine for maternal hypotension (systolic arterial blood pressure <100 mmHg), left uterine displacement, and maintenance of maternal normocarbia. The few detrimental direct effects of anesthetics on maternal-fetal well-being can be eliminated by the careful selection of anesthetics that maintain uterine artery blood flow and fetal circulatory homeostasis. Perioperative tocolytic therapy for premature labor is discussed in Chapters 5 and 7.

References

1. Brodsky JB: Anesthesia and the pregnant surgical patient. Reg Anaesth 9:119, 1984
2. Brodsky JB, Cohen EN, Brown BW Jr, et al.: Surgery during pregnancy and fetal outcome. Am J Obstet Gynecol 138:1165, 1980
3. Cohen EN, Belville JW, Brown BW: Anesthesia, pregnancy and miscarriage: A study of operating room nurses and anesthetists. Anesthesiology 35:343, 1971
4. Pedersen H, Finster M: Anesthetic risks in the pregnant surgical patient. Anesthesiology 51:439, 1979
5. Kammerer WS: Nonobstetric surgery during pregnancy. Med Clin North Am 63:1157, 1979
6. Marill KI, Rozycki GS, Pedigo RE, et al.: Female reproductive system in trauma. In: Mattox KL, Moore EE, Feliciano DV (eds): Trauma. Norwalk, CT: Appleton & Lange, 1988, pp 553–560
7. Civil ID, Talluci RC, Schwab CW: Placental laceration and fetal death as a result of blunt abdominal trauma. J Trauma 28:708, 1988
8. Rothenberger D, Quattlebaum FW, Perry JF Jr, et al.: Blunt maternal trauma: A view of 103 cases. J Trauma 18:173, 1978
9. Rozycki GS, Champion HR, Drass MJ: Traumatic injuries in the pregnant patient. Hosp Physician April:26, 1989
10. Pierson R, Mihalovits H, Thomas L, et al.: Penetrating abdominal wounds in pregnancy. Ann Emerg Med 15:1232, 1986
11. Leyse R, Ofstun M, Dillard DH, et al.: Congenital aortic stenosis in pregnancy corrected by extracorporeal circulation. JAMA 176:1009, 1961
12. Zitnick RS, Brandenberg RO, Sheldon R, et al.: Pregnancy and open heart surgery. Circulation 39:257, 1969
13. Becker RM: Intracardiac surgery in pregnant women. Ann Thorac Surg 36:453, 1983
14. Greiss FC Jr: Pressure-flow relationship in the gravid uterine vascular bed. Am J Obstet Gynecol 96:41, 1966
15. Wallace KL, Shnider SM, Hicks JS, et al.: Epidural anesthesia in the normotensive pregnant ewe: Effects on uterine blood flow and fetal acid-base status. Anesthesiology 44:481, 1976
16. Ralston DH, Shnider SM, DeLorimier AA: Effects of equipotent ephedrine, metaraminol, mephentermine, and methoxamine on uterine blood flow in the pregnant ewe. Anesthesiology 40:354, 1974
17. Levinson G, Shnider SM, DeLorimier AA, et al.: Effects of maternal hyperventilation on uterine blood flow and fetal oxygenation and acid-base status. Anesthesiology 40:340, 1974
18. Oates JN, Vasey DP, Waldren BA: Effects of ketamine on the pregnant uterus. Br J Anaesth 51:1163, 1979
19. James FM III: Anesthesia for nonobstetric surgery during pregnancy. Clin Obstet Gynecol 30:621, 1987

20. Greiss FC Jr, Still JG, Anderson SG: Effects of local anesthetic agents on uterine vasculatures and myometrium. Am J Obstet Gynecol 124:889, 1976
21. Donchin Y, Amirov B, Sahar A, et al.: Sodium nitroprusside for aneurysm surgery in pregnancy. Br J Anaesth 50:849, 1978
22. Biehl DR, Yarnell R, Wade JG, et al.: The uptake of isoflurane by the fetal lamb in utero. Effect on regional blood flow. Can Anaesth Soc J 30:581, 1983
23. Hellman LM, Johnson HL, Tolles WE, et al.: Some factors affecting the fetal heart rate. Am J Obstet Gynecol 82:1055, 1961
24. Finster M, Poppers PJ: Safety of thiopental used for induction of general anesthesia in elective cesarean section. Anesthesiology 29:190, 1968
25. Kraft JB Jr, Coldrake LA, Boland JC: Placental passage and uterine effects of fentanyl. Anesth Analg 62:894, 1983
26. Williams JG: H_2 receptor antagonists and anesthesia. Can Anaesth Soc J 30:264, 1983
27. Shnider SM, Webster GM: Maternal and fetal hazards of surgery during pregnancy. Am J Obstet Gynecol 92:891, 1965
28. Levine W, Diamond B: Surgical procedures during pregnancy. Am J Obstet Gynecol 81:1046, 1961
29. Marks GF, Hwang HS, Chandra P: Postpartum uterine pressures with different doses of ketamine. Anesthesiology 50:163, 1979
30. Galloon S: Ketamine for obstetric delivery. Anesthesiology 44:522, 1976
31. Cardell R: Intracardiac surgery in pregnant women. Ann Thorac Surg 36:457, 1983
32. Werc A, Lambert HM, Cooly D, et al.: Fetal monitoring and maternal open heart surgery. South Med J 70:1024, 1977
33. Koh KS, Friesen RM, Livingstone RA, et al.: Fetal monitoring during maternal cardiac surgery with cardiopulmonary bypass. Can Med Assoc J 112:1102, 1975
34. Lam MP, Ross SK, Johnson SK, et al.: Fetal heart monitoring during open heart surgery. Br J Obstet Gynaecol 88:669, 1981
35. Trimakas AP, Maxwell DK, Berkay S, et al.: Fetal monitoring during cardiopulmonary bypass for removal of a left atrial myxoma during pregnancy. Johns Hopkins Med J 144:156, 1979
36. Levy DL, Warrener RA, Burgess GE: Fetal response to cardiopulmonary bypass. Obstet Gynecol 56:112, 1980
37. Conroy JM, Bayley MK, Hollen MF, et al.: Anesthesia for open heart surgery in the pregnant patient. South Med J 82:492, 1989
38. Rowbotham GF, Bell K, Akenhead J, et al.: A serious head injury in a pregnant woman treated by hypothermia. Lancet 1:1016, 1957
39. Boatman KK, Bradford VA: Excision of an internal carotid aneurysm during pregnancy employing hypothermia and a vascular shunt. Ann Surg 148:271, 1958
40. Wrights B, Ream A: Uses of hypothermia in cardiovascular surgery. In: Ream A, Fogdall R (eds): Acute Cardiovascular Management, Anesthesia and Intensive Care. Philadelphia: J.B. Lippincott, 1982, pp 830–851
41. Eilen B, Keiser IH, Becker RM, et al.: Aortic valve replacement in the third trimester of pregnancy. Case report and review of the literature. Obstet Gynecol 57:119, 1981
42. Snyder SW, Wheeler AS, James FM: The use of nitroglycerin to control severe hypertension of pregnancy during cesarean section. Anesthesiology 51:563, 1979
43. Lieb S, Zugaib M, Nuwayhio B, et al.: Nitroprusside-induced hemodynamic alterations in normotensive and hypertensive pregnant sheep. Am J Obstet Gynecol 139:925, 1981
44. Ellis S, Wheeler A, James F, et al.: Fetal-maternal effects of sodium nitroprusside used to counteract hypertension in gravid ewes. Am J Obstet Gynecol 143:766, 1982
45. Shoemaker C, Meyer M: Sodium nitroprusside for control of severe hypertensive disease in pregnancy. Am J Obstet Gynecol 149:171, 1984
46. Goodwin R: Fetal and maternal effects of sodium nitroprusside. Am J Obstet Gynecol 146:350, 1983
47. Nalty J, Cefalo R, Lewis P: Fetal toxicity of nitroprusside in the pregnant ewe. Am J Obstet Gynecol 139:708, 1981
48. Rigg D, McDonough A: Use of sodium nitroprusside for deliberate hypotension during pregnancy. Br J Anaesth 53:985, 1981
49. Brinkman CR, Woods JR: Effects of cardiovascular drugs during pregnancy. Cardiovasc Med 1:231, 1976

4. Maternal and Fetal Effects of Anesthesia

B. Wycke Baker, M.D.

INTRODUCTION

On April 7, 1853, the British physician John Snow administered chloroform to Queen Victoria for the delivery of Prince Leopold.[1] Since that historic beginning, obstetric anesthesia has evolved into a well-recognized branch of anesthesiology and critical care medicine. Clinical experience and laboratory investigation have improved our understanding of anesthetic effects on the parturient, fetus, and neonate. Recent advances in animal research enable important maternal and fetal physiologic data, including uterine blood flow and fetal hemodynamic and blood gas status, to be monitored directly and continuously during laboratory investigations. Information obtained from such investigations, while enhancing our knowledge of the maternal and fetal effects of anesthetics, must be interpreted and applied cautiously. Animal data often have provocative implications but limited relevance when applied to human clinical practice. This chapter reviews the physiologic impact—

68

on the parturient, the uteroplacental circulation, and the fetus—of obstetric anesthetics.

MATERNAL EFFECTS

Anesthetic Requirements

Clinical experience has shown that anesthetic requirements during pregnancy are less than in the nonpregnant state. Several animal studies with inhaled and local anesthetics confirm these clinical observations. To evaluate the effect of pregnancy on the requirements for inhaled anesthetics during surgery, Palahniuk and associates[2] determined the minimum alveolar concentrations (MAC) of halothane, methoxyflurane, and isoflurane in both pregnant and nonpregnant ewes. Significantly greater reductions in MAC were found in the pregnant ewes than in the nonpregnant ewes. MAC was reduced by 25% for halothane, 32% for methoxyflurane, and 40% for isoflurane in the pregnant ewes undergoing a noxious, surgical stimulus. To evaluate the effect of pregnancy on the requirements for local anesthetics, Datta and coworkers[3] measured the time to onset of conduction block in in vitro vagus nerve preparations exposed to bupivacaine. Investigators measured the conduction velocity and the time required for 50% depression of the action potential in A, B, and C fibers of vagus nerves excised from pregnant and nonpregnant rabbits. Conduction velocity was significantly slower and onset of nerve block was faster in all nerve fibers from pregnant rabbits when compared with similar nerve fibers from nonpregnant rabbits.

What are the reasons for the decreased anesthetic requirements during pregnancy? Several possible explanations exist, including the following:

1. Physiologic changes. Significant cardiovascular and respiratory changes occur during pregnancy, which may reduce anesthetic requirements (see Chapter 2). Increases in cardiac output hasten disposition and onset of action of intravenous anesthetics during pregnancy. Increases in alveolar ventilation and decreases in functional residual capacity during pregnancy permit rapid equilibration between inspired and alveolar concentrations of inhaled anesthetics, accelerating induction and establishment of general anesthesia.

2. Anatomic changes. Increased blood volume during pregnancy and inferior caval compression by the enlarging uterus lead to progressive engorgement of epidural veins. As a result, the diameter and size of the epidural and subarachnoid spaces are reduced, and the level of sensorimotor blockade during epidural and spinal anesthesia spreads higher in pregnant women.

3. Hormonal changes. Increasing blood and cerebrospinal fluid levels of progesterone and rising blood levels of beta-endorphin may also

decrease anesthetic requirements during pregnancy.[4, 5] Large doses of progesterone exert potent anesthetic effects in animals and produce mild sedative effects in humans.[6, 7] The intrathecal administration of beta-endorphin produces intense analgesic effects in humans.[8] In addition, pain tolerance increases during pregnancy in experimental animals.[9] These increases in pain tolerance may be reversed with narcotic antagonists, suggesting that endogenous opioids such as beta-endorphin enhance analgesia during pregnancy.

Although these changes may influence the maternal response to anesthesia, they do not completely explain the decreased anesthetic requirements in each stage of pregnancy. Fagraeus and associates[10] reported that exaggerated spread of local anesthetic agents in the epidural space occurs even during the first trimester of pregnancy, before significant anatomic changes occur. Many physiologic changes of pregnancy are present by the first trimester, but the blood volume shifts that reduce the size of the epidural and subarachnoid spaces are not thought to be significant until the third trimester. Other, as yet unrecognized, changes occurring in earlier stages of gestation may unite with well-recognized later changes in reducing anesthetic requirements throughout pregnancy.

The clinician must be alert to the exaggerated effects of anesthetics throughout gestation. Pregnant patients may experience more rapid loss of consciousness and protective airway reflexes at lower inspired concentrations of inhaled and intravenous anesthetics than nonpregnant patients. Compared with nonpregnant patients, pregnant patients also demonstrate wider dermatomal spread and exaggerated hemodynamic effects during regional anesthesia. Consequences of high spinal or epidural blocks can be serious and may include pulmonary aspiration, upper airway obstruction, unconsciousness, profound hypotension, and cardiorespiratory arrest. To manage an obstetric anesthetic safely, the anesthesiologist should reduce and carefully titrate the dosages of both inhaled and injected anesthetic agents to match the pregnant patient's analgesic needs and reduced anesthetic requirements.

Effects on Uterine Muscle

Many studies focus on the indirect effects of anesthetic techniques used in obstetrics on the parturient and the fetus. For example, clinical research continues to evaluate the effects of epidural analgesia on (1) duration of the second stage of labor and voluntary maternal expulsive forces during vaginal delivery, (2) incidence of fetal malpresentation, and (3) need for operative delivery.

While the anesthetic techniques used in obstetrics may exert clinically notable indirect effects, many intravenous, inhaled, and local anesthetics also produce important *direct* effects on uterine resting tone, uterine contraction, and blood loss at the time of delivery.

McGaughey and associates[11] reported increases in the resting tone of isolated uterine muscle strips exposed to local anesthetic solutions in vitro. In a series of studies in pregnant ewes, Greiss and associates[12] also observed increases in uterine tone when local anesthetic agents were injected directly into uterine arteries of experimental animals. Although the increase in uterine tone in these studies occurred after exposure to higher concentrations of local anesthetics than those present during regional anesthesia, paracervical block, excessive doses, or accidental intravascular injection of local anesthetics may also be associated with significant increases in uterine resting tone with reduced uteroplacental perfusion.

Likewise, ketamine can also increase uterine resting tone and muscular activity. Such effects vary with the ketamine dose and the stage of gestation. For example, Galloon[13] administered ketamine in intravenous dosages of 0.275 mg/kg to 2.2 mg/kg during second trimester hysterotomies and measured immediate changes in intrauterine pressure. He observed dose-related increases in basal uterine tone, with peak effects occurring within 2 to 4 minutes. Oats and associates[14] reported similar findings when ketamine, 2 mg/kg, was administered intravenously during second trimester therapeutic abortions. However, when these investigators repeated their study in pregnant patients having cesarean sections at term, significant increases in intrauterine pressure did not occur. Marx and associates[15] evaluated the effects of various dosages of ketamine on intrauterine pressures immediately after delivery. They detected no changes in uterine tone but reported a brief increase in uterine contractile activity postpartum.

A number of investigations describe the direct effects of inhaled anesthetic agents on uterine tone and activity. Nitrous oxide does not affect uterine tone significantly.[16] However, the halogenated vapors (halothane, enflurane, and isoflurane) all reduce uterine resting tone, uterine muscle tension, and spontaneous uterine activity.[17–19] Clinical and laboratory studies indicate that the magnitude of uterine relaxation during inhalation anesthesia is dose-related and is similar for each inhaled agent at an equipotent dose. The direct effects of the halogenated agents on uterine tone often find important clinical application during obstetric maneuvers that require intense uterine relaxation, such as internal podalic version, complete breech extraction, evacuation of retained placenta, nonobstetric surgery during pregnancy, and fetal surgery in utero (see Chapter 3).

The uterine relaxant properties of halogenated anesthetics may be useful and even therapeutic in some instances, as in preventing premature labor after uterine manipulation or incision (see Chapter 5). On the other hand, the uterine relaxant properties of the halogenated agents may increase blood loss at delivery. Increasing inspired concentrations of halothane (to 0.7%), enflurane (to 1.5%), and isoflurane (to 0.75%) have been evaluated for uterine relaxing effects.[20-24] In most studies, significant increases in obstetric blood loss did not occur during general anesthesia with the limited, sub-MAC concentrations of the agents studied. In addition, Marx and associates[25] noted that low concentrations of halogenated agents do not suppress the uterine response to oxytocin stimulation during the postpartum period.

Effects on Uterine Blood Flow

Uteroplacental perfusion is the primary determinant of gas and nutrient exchange across the placenta between the mother and fetus. At term, maximum blood flow to the uterus approaches 1000 ml/min, or 10% to 15% of the maternal cardiac output. The determinants of uterine blood flow can be seen in the following equation:

$$UBF = \frac{UAP - UVP}{UVR}$$

where UBF = uterine blood flow
        UAP = uterine arterial pressure
        UVP = uterine venous pressure
        UVR = uterine vascular resistance

Maternal arterial pressure is the principal flow-limiting factor in this equation and explains why episodes of maternal hypotension may seriously decrease uterine blood flow (UBF). A well-known cause of decreased UBF is uterine contraction during labor. Aortocaval compression may also decrease UBF by two mechanisms: reduced uterine arterial pressure and increased uterine venous pressure. Although uterine vascular resistance (UVR) is usually low during pregnancy, endogenous and exogenous catecholamines and vasopressors—especially alpha-adrenergic agonists—may markedly increase UVR, and thus decrease UBF.[26-28] Unlike the cerebral or coronary circulations, the uteroplacental circulation is not autoregulated. There is also no linear relationship between UBF and respiratory gas tensions, as in the cerebral circulation.[29] Mechanical hyperventilation, however, does cause significant reductions in maternal cardiac output and blood pressure, thereby compromising UBF. In addition, periods of maternal hypoxia or maternal hypercarbia or both may be associated with decreases in UBF, possibly due to the release of endogenous catecholamines that increase uteroplacental vascular resistance.

Anesthetic drugs administered during pregnancy may also affect the determinants of UBF. The ultra-short-acting barbiturate induction agents typically decrease blood pressure and cardiac output by direct cardiac depression and peripheral vasodilation. A series of experiments in pregnant ewes indicate that thiopental, thiamylal, and methohexital all produce brief decreases in maternal blood pressure accompanied by parallel and concomitant decreases in UBF.[30] Because ketamine usually stimulates the cardiovascular system by increasing sympathetic tone, ketamine was initially expected to produce major alterations in UBF. In fact, the effects of ketamine on UBF depend on the dosage (as indicated earlier), the animal species studied, and the presence or absence of active labor. Several animal studies report that intravenously administered ketamine, 2 to 5 mg/kg, may cause decreases in UBF associated with fetal acidosis.[31, 32] Small doses of ketamine up to 1 mg/kg vary in their effects on UBF—which may increase, decrease, or remain constant. Ketamine, in reduced dosages of less than 2 mg/kg administered intravenously, appears to be safe for use during pregnancy without detrimental effects on the uteroplacental circulation or fetal status.

Several investigators have examined the effects of halothane, enflurane, and isoflurane on UBF in pregnant ewes. Each of the halogenated anesthetics can depress the myocardium and produce varying degrees of peripheral vasodilation. As a result, these agents might be expected to reduce UBF. However, during light to moderately deep planes of anesthesia—1.0 to 1.5 MAC halothane or isoflurane, and 0.4% to 1% enflurane—UBF did not alter; uterine vasodilation occurred despite slight reductions in maternal blood pressure.[33] Deeper planes of anesthesia (2.0 MAC) that caused significant decreases in maternal cardiac output and blood pressure also decreased uterine blood flow; fetal hypoxia and acidosis ensued. In these studies, the investigators established stable planes of anesthesia in the absence of surgical stimulation. However, painful or physiologically stressful procedures, such as airway manipulation or surgery in the absence of adequate anesthesia, can also compromise UBF through endogenous catecholamine release. Shnider and associates[34] demonstrated that decreases in UBF and increases in plasma norepinephrine and blood pressure that occurred with noxious stimulation during nitrous oxide–oxygen anesthesia in pregnant sheep did not occur when anesthesia was supplemented with 0.5% halothane or 1% enflurane. Likewise, in the absence of maternal hypotension, regional anesthesia for labor and delivery may also improve uteroplacental perfusion, especially in preeclamptic parturients.[35, 36]

UTEROPLACENTAL PHYSIOLOGY AND PHARMACODYNAMICS

Prior to discussing the effects of anesthesia on the fetus, we should review the unique characteristics of uteroplacental physiology and the

Table 4–1. *Maternal Arterial and Umbilical Blood Gas Tensions*

	pH	P_{O_2}	P_{CO_2}
Uterine artery	7.40	100 mmHg	30 mmHg
Umbilical vein	>7.25	>30 mmHg	<40 mmHg
Umbilical artery	>7.20	>15 mmHg	<50 mmHg

factors governing drug transfer across the placenta. Approaching the placenta, maternal blood is carried through successive divisions of the uterine arteries, terminating at the spiral arteries. The spiral arteries eject oxygenated maternal blood directly into the intervillous space. On the fetal side of the placenta, umbilical blood flow at term is about 500 ml/min or approximately 45% of fetal cardiac output. The two umbilical arteries convey deoxygenated fetal blood to the capillaries that traverse the fetal villi. Exchange of substances occurs between maternal and fetal blood as the fetal villi protrude into the intervillous space. Table 4–1 shows the resulting blood gas tensions. A 70-mmHg gradient exists between the maternal uterine arterial P_{O_2} and the fetal umbilical venous P_{O_2}.

There are several reasons why the placenta is less efficient than the lung as an organ for gas exchange:

1. Diffusion barriers. Maternal and fetal blood are separated by four tissue layers: syncytiotrophoblast, cytotrophoblast, villous connective stroma, and fetal capillary endothelium. Therefore, the average diffusion distance across the placenta is 2.5 μ. This contrasts with the average 0.5-μ distance from alveolus to pulmonary capillary.

2. Anatomic shunts. Neither all of the maternal nor all of the fetal blood directed to the placenta is available for exchange. About 16% of UBF is diverted to the myometrium and the endometrium and never reaches the intervillous space. Likewise, about 6% of total umbilical blood flow is diverted to the fetal chorion. In making an analogy between the placental and pulmonary circulations, it is clear that very large right-to-left shunts exist on both sides of the placenta.

3. Physiologic shunts. The afferent and efferent limbs of the fetal capillary loops are in close apposition as they course along the fetal villi. As a result, a 10% to 15% shunt allows oxygen to diffuse from efferent to afferent limbs, thereby reducing the P_{O_2} within the efferent limb. This diffusion shunt combines with the anatomic shunts to further reduce the efficiency of the placenta.

Despite these barriers to efficient gas exchange, the fetus is adapted to exist at low oxygen tensions. Hemoglobin F binds oxygen more avidly than hemoglobin A (P_{50}* of 19 mmHg versus 26.7 mmHg, respectively).

---

*Partial pressure of arterial oxygen at which hemoglobin is 50% saturated with oxygen.

The fetus is also relatively polycythemic (hematocrit >45%); so, in the fetus, the total blood oxygen content is higher than it would be in an adult at similar oxygen tensions. In addition, the fetal circulation is configured so that blood with the greatest oxygen content perfuses the cerebral circulation.

The transfer of a substance across the placenta depends on its physicochemical characteristics (Table 4–2). In general, low molecular weight (less than 500 daltons), low protein binding, low degree of ionization, and high lipid solubility all favor placental transfer. Fick's diffusion equation describes the relationship between the determinants of placental transfer:

$$Q/t = K\frac{A\,(C_m - C_f)}{D}$$

where Q/t = rate of transfer of substance
  K = constant for substance
  A = surface area for diffusion
  C_m = maternal concentration
  C_f = fetal concentration
  D = diffusion distance

The extent to which a substance undergoes maternal or placental metabolism affects its availability for placental transfer. Likewise, pH gradients between the mother and fetus influence transfer and, in cases of fetal acidosis, may result in fetal ion trapping, with accumulation on the fetal side of the placenta. Uniform placental transfer does not occur for all substances because of the irregular geometry and non-homogeneous blood flow within the intervillous space as well as varying degrees of active versus passive mechanisms of transport across the placenta.

Many anesthetic agents used in obstetrics possess physicochemical properties that favor placental transfer, namely, low molecular weight and high lipid solubility. The depth and duration of maternal and therefore fetal anesthetic exposure are also important factors in uteroplacental pharmacodynamics. In most clinical studies, maternal and umbilical blood is sampled to calculate, for example, the umbilical venous-to-

Table 4–2. Physicochemical Factors Governing Placental Transfer

Molecular weight
Protein binding
Degree of ionization
Lipid solubility

maternal arterial concentration ratio as an index of drug transfer across the placenta. However, unless equilibrium exists—where maternal arterial, umbilical venous, and umbilical arterial concentrations are equal—this ratio provides an incomplete assessment of the total transfer of drug from mother to fetus.

Among the anesthetic induction agents, the thiobarbiturates and ketamine have been evaluated most extensively. Following a maternal intravenous bolus of 4 mg/kg, thiopental crosses the placenta rapidly and can be measured in umbilical venous blood within 30 seconds.[37] Umbilical venous blood concentrations of thiopental peak by 1 minute, and umbilical arterial blood concentrations peak within 2 to 3 minutes. Thereafter, umbilical blood concentrations of thiopental decline and are one-half of peak levels 10 minutes after administration. Larger doses (up to 8 mg/kg) result in high fetal blood concentrations, more than twice those with the 4-mg/kg dose, and may cause perinatal depression. Ketamine also crosses the placenta rapidly, and high doses (2 mg/kg or higher) are associated with neonatal depression, low Apgar scores, and hypertonicity, especially neonatal chest wall rigidity.[38, 39]

Although fetal exposure to intravenous anesthetic agents cannot be avoided, neonatal depression does not occur when limited doses are used because the fetal circulation modifies their distribution significantly. Maternal and fetal shunting and nonhomogeneous blood flow within the uteroplacental circulation reduce the efficiency of drug transfer across the placenta. Umbilical venous blood flowing from the placenta to the right atrium must first pass through the ductus venosus or perfuse the liver directly. Some extraction of drug may occur in the liver, even before reaching the central fetal circulation. Progressive dilution with venous blood in the right atrium also reduces drug concentration. These factors combine to limit fetal cerebral drug exposure.

The depolarizing and nondepolarizing muscle relaxants do not cross the placenta to the same extent as the intravenous anesthetic agents. For example, placental transfer of succinylcholine is hindered by its high degree of ionization. The nondepolarizing relaxants, vecuronium and atracurium, are larger molecules and are low in lipid solubility. Insignificant amounts of these agents cross the placenta when standard doses are used.

The inhaled anesthetics are small, lipid-soluble molecules and therefore cross the placenta easily. Maternal alveolar concentration and duration of exposure directly influence placental transfer of these agents. For example, after 15 minutes of maternal administration of nitrous oxide, the fetal/maternal ratio is 0.8 to 0.9.[40, 41] In clinical studies, maternal administration of 0.65% halothane or 1% enflurane resulted in umbilical vein/maternal artery ratios of 0.35 and 0.60, respectively.[22, 42]

FETAL EFFECTS

Direct Effects of Anesthetics on the Nonstressed Fetus

Interpretation of the following animal and clinical studies requires an understanding of the differences between direct and indirect effects. In clinical studies, information about the fetal effects of anesthesia is evaluated indirectly at the time of delivery and in the early neonatal period using umbilical blood gas tensions, Apgar scores, and neonatal neurobehavioral assessments. Animal studies are more elegant by design and provide more direct hemodynamic data because these variables may be measured continuously in the laboratory during anesthetic interventions. Using both of these approaches, the fetal/neonatal effects of the induction agents and the inhaled anesthetics have been studied.

Levinson and associates[31] investigated the maternal and fetal hemodynamic and acid-base effects of intravenous ketamine (5-mg/kg bolus) in 10 pregnant ewes. Maternal blood pressure and uterine blood flow increased within 2 minutes and there were no adverse effects on fetal hemodynamic or acid-base status. Morgan and associates[43] compared thiopental (3 mg/kg) and methohexital (1 mg/kg) as induction agents for cesarean section in 127 patients. They observed no clinical or biochemical differences between the two groups of mothers and neonates in evaluating Apgar scores, maternal arterial blood gases, and umbilical arterial blood gases. Peltz and Sinclair[44] compared thiopental (3 mg/kg) and ketamine (1 mg/kg) in 100 patients undergoing anesthesia for cesarean section. They found no difference in the incidence of neonatal depression with either thiopental or ketamine. Houlton and associates[45] compared etomidate (0.3 mg/kg) and thiopental (3.5 mg/kg) in 48 healthy patients at term scheduled for elective cesarean section. Neonates whose mothers were induced with etomidate achieved sustained respirations within an average of 13 seconds, whereas the thiopental group required an average of 27 seconds. The base excess gradients between maternal arterial and umbilical arterial and venous blood were narrower in the etomidate group. From this they concluded that etomidate may be beneficial when the fetus is at risk for asphyxiation. Suresh and associates[46] compared the hemodynamics, acid-base status, and side effects of etomidate (0.3 mg/kg) with thiopental (4 mg/kg) at induction of anesthesia for cesarean section. In contrast to the findings of Houlton and associates, no differences in acid-base status were observed between groups.

Gregory and associates[47] determined that MAC (calculated from arterial anesthetic concentrations) for halothane in fetal sheep is 0.33%, which is one-fourth that of the neonatal lamb (1.15%) and one-half that of the pregnant ewe (0.69%). Biehl and associates[48] evaluated the effects of halothane on the normal fetal lamb in utero. They administered 1.5%

halothane to 6 pregnant ewes for 90 minutes. After 8 minutes of maternal halothane administration, the investigators observed a 27% decrease in fetal arterial blood pressure but no significant changes in calculated fetal cardiac output or fetal acid-base status. When the investigators repeated this experiment with 2% isoflurane, they observed no significant changes in fetal hemodynamic or acid-base status until 48 minutes of maternal anesthesia.[49] At that point, significant decreases in fetal pH, base excess, and fetal cardiac index occurred. They concluded that although the normal fetus is likely to tolerate brief exposure to isoflurane, the stressed fetus might develop acidosis and myocardial depression earlier during maternal isoflurane anesthesia.

A few human studies have looked at the effects of the inhaled agents on the fetus. Coleman and Downing[23] evaluated enflurane (0.5% to 0.8%) with 50% nitrous oxide–oxygen as a volatile agent for cesarean section. Comparing blood gas tensions, acid-base status, and Apgar scores with a cohort group, they observed no pharmacologic or biochemical depression. Warren and associates[50] compared the effects of 50% nitrous oxide–oxygen with 0.5% halothane, 1% enflurane, and 0.75% isoflurane for cesarean delivery in 42 healthy parturients. No significant differences in blood gas tension, acid-base balance, blood lactate levels, or Apgar and neurobehavioral scores were observed between groups.

What can we conclude from the studies so far about anesthesia and the nonstressed fetus? It should be clear that brief exposure to limited amounts of these anesthetics results in minimal, if any, deleterious effects. At present, no major differences exist between either the intravenous or inhaled anesthetics.

Direct Effects of Anesthetics on the Stressed Fetus

When the fetus experiences hypoxic stress, adaptive hemodynamic responses are activated. The release of endogenous catecholamines increases systemic vascular resistance and results in fetal hypertension. Fetal cardiac output is redistributed to increase blood flow to vital organs. The fetus possesses the ability to autoregulate cerebral blood flow and to increase regional blood flow within the brain. Autoregulation is lost when oxyhemoglobin saturation decreases below 50%. In addition, when oxygen supply declines acutely, the fetus can preferentially decrease cerebral metabolic activity, within limits, so that cerebral metabolic rate of oxygen consumption ($CMRO_2$) decreases proportionately.

Compromised uteroplacental blood flow and fetal distress require aggressive obstetric management, typically involving rapid anesthetic intervention. In the absence of maternal hypotension, brief exposure of the healthy fetus to regional or general anesthesia produces minimal, if any, deleterious effects. However, the clinical response of the asphyxiated human fetus is largely unknown. Several studies on pregnant ewes have attempted to determine the effects of intrauterine exposure to general anesthesia during experimentally induced fetal hypoxia and acidosis.

Using umbilical cord occlusion to produce fetal asphyxia in pregnant ewes, Pickering and associates[51] evaluated the effects of high-dose and low-dose thiopental and ketamine. Each animal received either thiopental (6 mg/kg or 10 mg/kg) or ketamine (2 mg/kg or 4 mg/kg). The lower doses of each agent resulted in better hemodynamic profiles, and low-dose ketamine caused the least reduction in fetal cerebral blood flow. Leicht and associates[52] compared equivalent doses of thiopental and ketamine for rapid-sequence induction during fetal asphyxia produced by uterine artery occlusion in pregnant ewes. Their preliminary data suggest no clear difference between ketamine and thiopental in the presence of fetal asphyxia.

Palahniuk and associates[53] produced fetal acidosis with partial umbilical cord occlusion before and after 15 minutes of halothane/oxygen anesthesia (4% halothane/oxygen induction, 1% halothane/oxygen maintenance) in pregnant ewes. Fetal blood pressure, cerebral blood flow, arterial pH, and oxygen delivery all decreased during maternal halothane anesthesia. Yarnell and associates[54] produced fetal asphyxia by partial umbilical cord occlusion and then administered 1.5% halothane/oxygen to tracheostomized pregnant ewes for 15 minutes. They observed no significant changes in cardiac output, organ blood flow, or acid-base status, and concluded that *low* levels of halothane anesthesia do not cause further deterioration in the asphyxiated fetus if the duration of fetal exposure is less than 15 minutes.

As opposed to partial umbilical cord occlusion, two studies produced a controlled state of fetal asphyxia by incremental occlusion of the uterine artery. Cheek and associates[55] evaluated the effects of 15 minutes exposure to 1% halothane/oxygen anesthesia in pregnant ewes with this preparation. They found that halothane did not alter the normal fetal responses to asphyxia, such as increased cerebral blood flow and decreased $CMRO_2$. Using the same preparation, Baker and associates[56] investigated the effects of 15 minutes of exposure to 1% isoflurane/oxygen anesthesia. Isoflurane appeared to exacerbate preexisting fetal acidosis, but it preserved the normal pattern of redistribution of fetal cardiac output and maintained a favorable balance between cerebral oxygen supply and demand.

Given these findings, no agent or combination of agents appears to offer distinct advantages in the anesthetic management of fetal distress. Furthermore, as work continues in this area, it is likely that decisions regarding the choice of anesthetic technique during fetal distress must be modified by maternal considerations. The dual nature of obstetric anesthesia management requires that both maternal and fetal/neonatal concerns be balanced.

CONCLUSIONS

Recent progress in obstetric anesthesiology has enhanced our understanding of the physiologic effects of anesthetics on the mother and fetus. Using results from both laboratory and clinical studies, regional and general anesthetic techniques have been refined to optimize maternal, fetal, and neonatal safety. As obstetric anesthesia advances, it is likely that work will continue in many areas, for example, the changes in maternal anesthetic requirements during pregnancy, anesthetic considerations for preterm delivery, and anesthetic management during fetal distress. Experience with intrauterine fetal anesthesia and surgery for correctable lesions before delivery will further improve our knowledge. Likewise, innovations in techniques of maternal and fetal monitoring—such as noninvasive determination of uterine blood flow and continuous intrapartum monitoring of fetal oxygen saturation and pH—will amplify our understanding of the impact of anesthetic interventions on the mother, the uteroplacental circulation, and the fetus.

References

1. Snow J: On Chloroform and Other Anaesthetics. Philadelphia: Lea & Febiger, 1940, p 342
2. Palahniuk RJ, Shnider SM, Eger EI: Pregnancy decreases the requirement for inhaled anesthetic agents. Anesthesiology 41:82, 1974
3. Datta S, Lambert DH, Gregus J, et al.: Differential sensitivities of mammalian nerve fibers during pregnancy. Anesth Analg 62:1070, 1983
4. Yannone ME, McCurcy JR, Goldfein A: Plasma progesterone levels in normal pregnancy, labor, and the puerperium. II. Clinical data. Am J Obstet Gynecol 101:1058, 1968
5. Csontos K, Rust M, Holt V, et al.: Elevated plasma beta-endorphin levels in pregnant women and their neonates. Life Sci 25:835, 1979
6. Selye H: Studies concerning the anesthetic action of steroid hormones. J Pharmacol Exp Ther 73:127, 1941
7. Merryman W: Progesterone "anesthesia" in human subjects. J Clin Endocrinol Metab 14:1567, 1954
8. Oyama T, Akitoma M, Takeo T, et al.: Beta-endorphin in obstetric anesthesia. Am J Obstet Gynecol 137:613, 1980
9. Gintzler AR: Endorphin-mediated increases in pain tolerance during pregnancy. Science 210:193, 1980
10. Fagraeus L, Urban B, Bromage P: Spread of epidural analgesia in early pregnancy. Anesthesiology 58:184, 1983
11. McGaughey HS, Corey EL, Eastwood D, et al.: Effects of synthetic anesthetics on the spontaneous motility of human uterine muscles in vitro. Obstet Gynecol 19:233, 1962
12. Greiss FC, Still JG, Anderson SG: Effects of local anesthetic agents on the uterine vasculatures and myometrium. Am J Obstet Gynecol 124:889, 1976
13. Galloon S: Ketamine for obstetric delivery. Anesthesiology 44:522, 1976
14. Oats JN, Vasey DP, Waldron BA: Effects of ketamine on the pregnant uterus. Br J Anaesth 51:1163, 1979

15. Marx GF, Hwang HS, Chandra P: Post-partum uterine pressures with different doses of ketamine. Anesthesiology 50:163, 1979
16. Munson ES, Maier WR, Caton D: Effects of halothane, cyclopropane, and nitrous oxide on isolated human uterine muscle. J Obstet Gynaecol Br Commonwealth 76:27, 1969
17. Naftalin NJ, Phear WPC, Goldberg AH: Halothane and isometric contractions of isolated pregnant rat myometrium. Anesthesiology 42:458, 1975
18. Munson ES, Embro WJ: Enflurane, isoflurane, and halothane and isolated human uterine muscle. Anesthesiology 46:11, 1977
19. Naftalin NJ, McKay DM, Phear WPC, et al.: The effects of halothane on pregnant and nonpregnant human myometrium. Anesthesiology 46:15, 1977
20. Moir DD: Anaesthesia for cesarean section: An evaluation of a method using low concentrations of halothane and 50 per cent of oxygen. Br J Anaesth 42:136, 1970
21. Galbert MW, Gardner AE: Use of halothane in a balanced technique for cesarean section. Anesth Analg 51:701, 1972
22. Latto IP, Waldron BA: Anaesthesia for cesarean section. Br J Anaesth 49:371, 1977
23. Coleman AJ, Downing JW: Enflurane anesthesia for cesarean section. Anesthesiology 43:354, 1975
24. Abboud TK, Kim SH, Henriksen EH, et al.: Comparative maternal and neonatal effects of halothane and enflurane for cesarean section. Acta Anaesth Scand 29:663, 1985
25. Marx GF, Kim YI, Lin CC, et al.: Post-partum uterine pressures under halothane or enflurane anesthesia. Obstet Gynecol 51:695, 1978
26. Eng M, Berges PU, Ueland K, et al.: The effects of methoxamine and ephedrine in normotensive pregnant primates. Anesthesiology 35:354, 1971
27. Adamsons K, Mueller-Heubach E, Myers RE: Production of fetal asphyxia in the rhesus monkey by administration of catecholamines to the mother. Am J Obstet Gynecol 109:248, 1971
28. Ralston DH, Shnider SM, deLorimier AA: Effects of equipotent ephedrine, metaraminol, mephentermine, and methoxamine on uterine blood flow in the pregnant ewe. Anesthesiology 40:354, 1974
29. Levinson G, Shnider SM, deLorimier AA, et al.: Effects of maternal hyperventilation on uterine blood flow and fetal oxygenation and acid-base status. Anesthesiology 40:340, 1974
30. Cosmi EV: Drugs, anesthetics and the fetus. In: Scarpelli EM, Cosmi EV (eds): Reviews in Perinatal Medicine, vol 1. Baltimore: University Park Press, 1976, p 191
31. Levinson G, Shnider SM, Gildea JE, et al.: Maternal and fetal cardiovascular and acid-base changes during ketamine anaesthesia in pregnant ewes. Br J Anaesth 45:1111, 1973
32. Craft JB, Coaldrake LA, Yonekura JL, et al.: Ketamine, catecholamines, and uterine tone in pregnant ewes. Am J Obstet Gynecol 146:429, 1983
33. Palahniuk RJ, Shnider SM: Maternal and fetal cardiovascular and acid-base changes during halothane and isoflurane anesthesia in the pregnant ewe. Anesthesiology 41:462, 1974
34. Shnider SM, Wright RG, Levinson G, et al.: Plasma norepinephrine and uterine blood flow changes during endotracheal intubation and general anesthesia in the pregnant ewe. In: Abstracts of Scientific Papers, Annual Meeting, American Society of Anesthesiologists, Chicago, 1978, p 115
35. Hollmen A, Jouppila R, Jouppila P, et al.: Effect of extradural analgesia using bupivacaine and 2-chloroprocaine on intervillous blood flow during normal labour. Br J Anaesth 54:837, 1982
36. Jouppila P, Jouppila R, Hollmen A, et al.: Effect of segmental epidural analgesia to improve intervillous blood flow during labor in severe preeclampsia. Obstet Gynecol 59:158, 1982
37. Kosaka Y, Takahashi T, Mark LC: Intravenous thiobarbiturate anesthesia for cesarean section. Anesthesiology 31:489, 1969
38. Little B, Chang T, Chucot L, et al.: Study of ketamine as an obstetric agent. Am J Obstet Gynecol 113:247, 1972
39. Janeczko GF, El-Etr AA, Younes S: Low-dose ketamine anesthesia for obstetrical delivery. Anesth Analg 53:284, 1974

40. Stenger VG, Blechner JN, Prystowsky H: A study of prolongation of obstetric anesthesia. Am J Obstet Gynecol 103:901, 1969
41. Marx GF, Joshi CW, Orkin LR: Placental transmission of nitrous oxide. Anesthesiology 32:429, 1970
42. Dick W, Knoche E, Traub E: Clinical investigations concerning the use of Ethrane for cesarean section. J Perinat Med 7:125, 1979
43. Morgan M, Holdcroft A, Whitwam JG: Comparison of thiopentone and methohexitone as induction agents for cesarean section. Anaesth Intens Care 8:431, 1980
44. Peltz B, Sinclair DM: Induction agents for cesarean section. Anesthesia 28:37, 1973
45. Houlton PC, Downing JW, Buley BM, et al.: Anaesthetic induction for caesarean section with etomidate compared with thiopentone. S Afr Med J 54:773, 1978
46. Suresh MS, Solanki DR, Andrews JJ, et al.: Comparison of etomidate with thiopental for induction of anesthesia at cesarean section. Anesthesiology 65:A400, 1986
47. Gregory GA, Wade JG, Biehl DR, et al.: Fetal anesthetic requirement (MAC) for halothane. Anesth Analg 62:9, 1983
48. Biehl DR, Tweed WA, Cote J: Effect of halothane on cardiac output and regional blood flow in the fetal lamb in utero. Anesth Analg 62:489, 1983
49. Biehl DR, Yarnell R, Wade JG: The uptake of isoflurane by the fetal lamb in utero: Effect on regional blood flow. Can Anaesth Soc J 30:581, 1983
50. Warren TM, Datta S, Ostheimer GW, et al.: Comparison of the maternal and neonatal effects of halothane, enflurane, and isoflurane for cesarean delivery. Anesth Analg 62:516, 1983
51. Pickering BG, Palahniuk RJ, Cote J: Cerebral vascular responses to ketamine and thiopentone during foetal acidosis. Can Anaesth Soc J 29:463, 1982
52. Leicht CH, Baker BW, Rosen MA, et al.: The effect of ketamine or sodium thiopental rapid sequence induction on the asphyxiated fetal lamb. Anesthesiology 65:A387, 1986
53. Palahniuk RJ, Doig GA, Johnson GN: Maternal halothane anesthesia reduces cerebral blood flow in the acidotic sheep fetus. Anesth Analg 59:35, 1980
54. Yarnell R, Biehl DR, Tweed WA: The effect of halothane anesthesia on the asphyxiated foetal lamb in utero. Can Anaesth Soc J 30:474, 1983
55. Cheek DBC, Hughes SC, Dailey PA, et al.: Effect of halothane on regional cerebral metabolic oxygen consumption in the fetal lamb in utero. Anesthesiology 67:361, 1987
56. Baker BW, Hughes SC, Schnider SM, et al.: Maternal anesthesia and the stressed fetus: Effects of isoflurane on the asphyxiated fetal lamb. Anesthesiology 72:65, 1990

5. Perioperative Management of the Fetus Undergoing Surgery in Utero

Michael T. Longaker, M.D., N. Scott Adzick, M.D., and Michael R. Harrison, M.D.

Prenatal diagnosis has undergone an explosion of growth in the past decade. The primary impetus for this rapid expansion has come from the widespread usage of prenatal ultrasonography. After the first reports of in utero ultrasonographic diagnosis of congenital anomalies in the early 1970s, increasingly sophisticated equipment and experience in interpretation have led to the accurate diagnosis before birth of a growing number of surgical lesions. These developments have tremendous implications for any clinician involved in the care of newborns.

83

Table 5–1. Surgical Conditions That May Require Induced Preterm Delivery
and Early Correction Ex Utero

Obstructive hydronephrosis
Obstructive hydrocephalus
Amniotic band malformation complex
Gastroschisis or ruptured omphalocele
Intestinal ischemia/necrosis secondary to volvulus, meconium ileus, and similar conditions
Sacrococcygeal teratoma
Hydrops fetalis
Intrauterine growth retardation

Routine obstetric sonography has changed the surgical management of many congenital anomalies. Most correctable malformations that can be diagnosed in utero are best managed by appropriate medical and surgical therapy after maternal transport and planned delivery at term. Prenatal diagnosis may also influence the timing (Table 5–1) or the mode (Table 5–2) of delivery and in some cases may lead to elective termination of pregnancy (Table 5–3). In rare cases, various forms of in utero therapy may be possible currently or in the future (Table 5–4).

The perinatal management of these patients involves professionals from many different medical disciplines, including obstetricians, sonographers, neonatologists, geneticists, pediatric surgeons, pediatricians, and anesthesiologists. It is essential that the affected family be managed using a team approach and that information and experience be exchanged freely.

Prenatal detection and serial sonographic study of fetuses with anatomic lesions now make it possible to define the natural history of these abnormalities, determine the pathophysiologic features that affect clinical outcome, and formulate management based on prognosis. Prenatal diagnosis has defined a "hidden mortality" for some lesions, such as congenital diaphragmatic hernia, bilateral hydronephrosis, sacrococcygeal teratoma, and cystic hygroma. These lesions, when first evaluated and treated postnatally, demonstrate a favorable selection bias. The most severely affected fetuses often die in utero or immediately after birth, before an accurate diagnosis has been made. Consequently, such a

Table 5–2. Conditions That May Require Cesarean Delivery

Conjoined twins
Giant omphalocele
Large hydrocephalus
Large sacrococcygeal teratoma
Large cystic hygroma
Large or ruptured meningomyelocele
Malformations requiring preterm delivery in the presence of inadequate labor or fetal distress

Table 5–3. *Malformations Usually Managed by Elective Termination*

Anencephaly, porencephaly, encephalocele, and giant hydrocephalus
Severe anomalies associated with chromosomal abnormalities (trisomy 13, trisomy 18,
  and similar conditions)
Renal agenesis or bilateral polycystic kidney disease
Inherited chromosomal, metabolic, and hematologic abnormalities (hemoglobinopathies,
  Tay-Sachs disease, and similar conditions)

condition detected prenatally might have a worse prognosis than the same condition first diagnosed after delivery.[1]

In recent years, there have been attempts to treat prenatally diagnosed fetal medical conditions in utero. The earliest and most successful examples involve the treatment of fetal deficiencies. Fetal anemia secondary to isoimmunization-induced hemolysis can be treated by intraperitoneal or intravascular transfusion of red blood cells.[2] Fetal arrhythmias can be treated by administering appropriate medications to the mother, and various vitamin deficiencies have been treated by maternal vitamin ingestion. Medications can also be injected into the amniotic fluid, where they are swallowed and absorbed by the fetus. An example of this is the treatment of congenital hypothyroidism with intra-amniotic thyroid hormone. In the near future, it may be possible to treat hematopoietic stem cell and hepatic enzyme deficiencies by stem cell and hepatocyte transplantation in utero.[3]

Certain prenatally diagnosed anatomic malformations have been treated with tube decompression in utero. Despite the experimental nature of these procedures, extensive experience has been accumulated. Examples of these conditions include hydrothorax, hydrocephalus, and obstructive uropathy. Relatively extensive experience worldwide with drainage of hydrocephalus in utero has been generally disappointing,[4] and our current approach to fetal ventriculomegaly remains conservative.[5]

A number of congenital anomalies that are potentially lethal or

Table 5–4. *Defects That May Require In Utero Treatment*

Malformation	Effect on Development	In Utero Treatment
Urethral obstruction	Hydronephrosis, lung hypoplasia → renal, respiratory failure	Vesicostomy
Congenital diaphragmatic hernia	Pulmonary hypoplasia → respiratory failure	Thoraco-amniotic shunt
Fetal chylothorax	Pulmonary hypoplasia → respiratory failure	Thoraco-amniotic shunt
Sacrococcygeal teratoma	Massive arteriovenous shunting → placentomegaly, hydrops fetalis	Excision

disabling and cannot or may not best be treated by catheter drainage frequently are diagnosed prenatally. The possibility of open fetal intervention, although a formidable undertaking, may be the only solution for many fetuses. However, this approach is justifiable only if (1) the natural history and pathophysiology of the disease are well understood, (2) if correction in utero is shown to be efficacious in animal models, and (3) if maternal risk is proven to be acceptably low. Over the past 10 years, we have investigated the rationale and feasibility of in utero repair for a number of fetal anomalies, including congenital hydronephrosis, congenital diaphragmatic hernia, sacrococcygeal teratoma, cystic adenomatoid malformation, chylothorax, cleft lip and palate, and simple types of congenital heart disease.

DEVELOPMENT OF TECHNIQUES FOR OPEN FETAL SURGERY

A number of techniques for open fetal surgery have been developed in lower animal models, primarily sheep and rabbits. These animals are ideal for fetal research because they are associated with a relatively low risk of premature onset of labor associated with hysterotomy. Higher animals, like primates, have longer periods of gestation and, like humans, are susceptible to premature labor and delivery following pelvic surgery. It was therefore imperative to develop safe anesthetic and operative techniques in nonhuman primates not associated with premature labor and fetal wastage prior to attempting human open fetal intervention. Our experience with open fetal surgery in more than 200 nonhuman primates[6, 7] led to the development of a satisfactory system for maternal and fetal monitoring and a regimen for the control of premature labor. In addition, techniques were developed for hysterotomy and uterine closure,[8] as well as for exteriorization of the fetal urinary tract,[9] diaphragmatic hernia repair,[10] and pulmonary resection.[11] Maternal mortality and morbidity were minimal in the nonhuman primate models, and future fertility after midgestation hysterotomy appeared not to be affected.[7] Clinical application was first successful in the management of fetal bilateral hydronephrosis, and we will review our experience in this area in detail.

CONGENITAL HYDRONEPHROSIS

Although obstetric ultrasonography frequently detects fetal urologic obstruction, fetuses with bilateral hydronephrosis frequently present with a spectrum of pathophysiology and severity that requires an individualized approach to evaluation and management. Optimal clinical management of both patients, mother and fetus, requires a thorough understanding of the natural history, pathophysiology, and sequelae of obstructive uropathy in the developing fetus. The pathophysiologic rationale for early decompression of the obstructed urinary tract is straightforward: unrelieved obstruction causes progressive damage to the developing kidneys and lungs, which compromises survival at birth. [12, 13] The challenge in management is how to select from the large number of fetuses with dilated urinary tracts those few for whom intervention is appropriate, that is, those with obstruction severe enough to compromise renal and pulmonary function at birth but not so severe that the damage is irreversible. [13]

The theoretical basis for decompression of bilateral fetal hydronephrosis in utero has been established by numerous experimental studies. [14-17] These studies demonstrate that potentially fatal pulmonary hypoplasia caused by oligohydramnios resulting from obstructive uropathy may be ameliorated by decompression in utero. In utero decompression, in addition, may arrest dysplastic morphogenesis of the kidney and preserve renal function, depending on the timing and the duration of the obstruction.

Two major variables complicate the surgical management of a fetus with severe congenital bilateral hydronephrosis: accuracy in predicting outcome and efficacy of decompression in utero. Better selection of patients for prenatal intervention can now be performed based on an improved understanding of the natural history and pathophysiology of the disease as well as qualitative and quantitative tests of fetal renal function.

Diagnostic Methods

Ultrasonography. In many cases, ultrasonography is the only study needed for fetal urologic evaluation. [18] The findings of bilateral renal agenesis, severe renal hypoplasia, or bilateral multicystic dysplasia are uniformly fatal, and the family may be counseled and allowed to choose expectant management or termination of the pregnancy. In cases of unilateral obstruction with normal amniotic fluid production, the patient may be observed by serial ultrasound with no further diagnostic evaluation. In cases of urologic abnormality with associated life-threatening anomalies, evaluation of the urinary tract may assume secondary importance.

In cases of bilateral dilatation with oligohydramnios or decreasing amniotic fluid volume on serial ultrasound examinations, the fetus should undergo a complete prognostic evaluation to determine residual renal function and the potential for normal renal and pulmonary function at birth. [19] The initial step in the assessment of fetal renal function is determination of the quantity of amniotic fluid. Because most amniotic fluid in middle and late pregnancy is a product of fetal urination, the presence of a normal amount of amniotic fluid usually implies the presence of at least one functioning kidney. Amniotic fluid volume status is predictive only in its extremes, with severe oligohydramnios early in gestation suggesting poor renal function, and normal volumes late in gestation suggesting adequate renal function.

By 15 weeks' gestation, the fetal bladder can be easily visualized ultrasonographically to cyclically increase in size and then empty. With distal urinary tract obstruction, however, we have observed that urine reaccumulation and bladder distention after bladder aspiration and bladder distention by furosemide-stimulated urine production are both unreliable diagnostic evaluations of renal function. Similarly, the ultrasonographic evaluation of the fetal kidneys in lower tract obstruction is unreliable as the sole predictor of renal function.[20] Ultrasonographers at our institution previously correlated the sonographic appearance of 49 fetal kidneys with their postmortem histopathology.[20] They concluded that the presence of renal cortical cysts was highly predictive of renal dysplasia (sensitivity 44% and specificity 100%), but the absence of cysts did not preclude the presence of renal dysplasia. The presence of increased renal echogenicity had a sensitivity of 73% and a specificity of 80%, and the presence of hydronephrosis was least predictive (sensitivity 41% and specificity 73%) of renal dysplasia.

In summary, it is clear that ultrasound can accurately delineate the gross anatomy of the dilated urinary tract and provide some qualitative information about renal function. However, in the majority of cases, it cannot determine accurately the degree of irreversible dysfunction or dysplasia or give accurate prognostic information.

Analysis of Fetal Urine. Analysis of fetal urine represents a more direct and quantitative method of evaluating fetal renal function. Fetal urine, which is produced by the thirteenth gestational week, is an ultrafiltrate of fetal serum made hypotonic by selective tubular reabsorption of sodium and chloride in excess of free water. The composition of fetal urine remains constant throughout gestation until just before term. Thus, changes in fetal urine composition might reflect changes in renal function. Total urine output is a combination of glomerular filtration and tubular reabsorption and secretion.

To evaluate the prognostic value of these factors in predicting which fetuses have the potential for normal renal and pulmonary function at birth, we reviewed the management of 40 fetuses with bilateral hydronephrosis and oligohydramnios.[21] Early in our experience, the fetal urinary tract was exteriorized by percutaneous placement of a balloon-tipped catheter into the dilated fetal bladder under ultrasound guidance; more recently, single fetal bladder aspirations have been performed. Based on these results, six prognostic criteria to identify fetuses with "good function" and "poor function" were generated (Table 5–5). The development of prognostic criteria that predict the potential for recovery has greatly simplified counseling of families and selection of appropriate fetal management. The prognostic criteria summarized in Table 5–5 are based on sonographic findings and fetal urine values of urine obtained by needle aspiration of the fetal bladder; they have proven reliable predictors of both neonatal outcome and long-term survival after urinary tract decompression in utero.

Clinical Management

Using the methods described previously, we have derived guidelines for the evaluation and management of the fetus with congenital hydro-nephrosis (Fig. 5–1). Initial evaluation should include ultrasonography to confirm the diagnosis, delineate the anatomy of the obstruction, define the status of the amniotic fluid, and rule out associated life-threatening anomalies. If no associated anomaly is detected and the amniotic fluid is normal, the pregnancy should be followed by serial ultrasonography. If amniotic fluid remains adequate, the mother should receive routine obstetric care, and the fetus can be treated postnatally. If amniotic fluid decreases and oligohydramnios develops, a prognostic evaluation should be performed, including (1) amniotic fluid status at presentation; (2) sonographic appearance of the renal parenchyma; and (3) fetal bladder aspiraton to determine urine Na, Cl, and osmolarity. Although we have only preliminary clinical experience with fetal creatinine clearance, laboratory data suggest that fetal creatinine clearance studies will allow an additional simple, quantitative estimate of fetal renal function.[14]

Prenatal intervention should be reserved for fetuses with adequate renal function for postnatal survival and pulmonary immaturity preclud-ing early delivery. Alternatives for decompression include placement of a percutaneous catheter or fetal surgery. Vesicoamniotic shunts have been placed successfully in more than 80 human fetuses worldwide, but because of the high incidence of catheter clogging and displacement and

Table 5–5. *Prognostic Criteria in the Fetus with Bilateral Obstructive Uropathy*

Predicted Function	Amniotic Fluid Volume Status at the Time of Initial Presentation	Sonographic Appearance of Kidneys	Fetal Urine			
			Sodium (mEq/ml)	Chloride (mEq/ml)	Osmolarity (mosm)	Output (ml/hour)
Poor	Moderately to severely decreased	Echogenic to cystic	>100	>90	>210	<2
Good	Normal to moderately decreased	Normal to echogenic	<100	<90	<210	>2

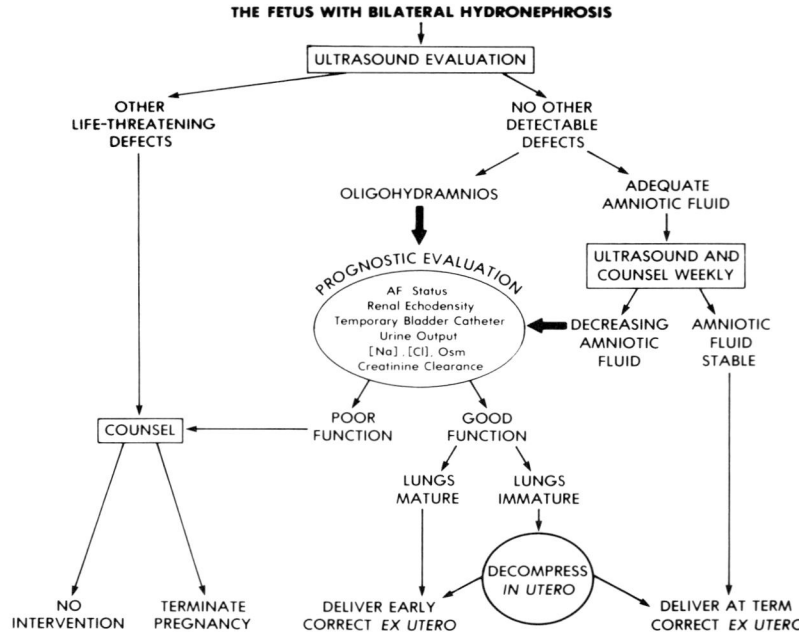

FIGURE 5–1. Management algorithm for fetal bilateral hydronephrosis.

the associated risk of chorioamnionitis, vesicoamniotic shunts are unsatisfactory for long-term fetal urinary tract decompression.[4] We currently favor surgical decompression by bladder marsupialization or bilateral ureterostomies for appropriate fetuses with obstructive uropathy.

OPEN FETAL SURGERY IN HUMANS

Reported experience in human fetal surgery is limited. In the 1960s, fetal exchange transfusions were attempted by direct cannulation of fetal blood vessels exposed through a hysterotomy and partial delivery of a fetal part, usually the lower extremity. Halothane in oxygen was used for inhalation anesthesia. In addition to the uterine relaxation produced by halothane, perioperative tocolytic management for early fetal operations included preoperative isoxsuprine hydrochloride, a betamimetic, and postoperative tocolysis, when indicated, by intravenous alcohol. Asensio[22] reviewed early experiences with fetal operations prior to 1970 and reported that 10 of 15 cases (67%) culminated in premature labor and delivery within 8 days of operation. These and other unreported cases of early fetal loss made fetal surgery so discouraging that all efforts were discontinued for more than a decade and have only recently been resumed.

Prerequisites for Open Fetal Surgery

By the late 1970s, prenatal diagnosis of an increasing number of potentially correctable fetal disorders again raised the possibility of fetal surgical intervention. We identified a few fetal disorders that might require in utero surgery[12, 23] and began to study their pathophysiology experimentally.[9, 24] We also observed an increasing number of human cases that might be appropriate for prenatal intervention.[18] However, we decided early in our studies that we would not attempt open fetal surgery until we had: (1) established the pathophysiology of the fetal disorder in animals; (2) defined the natural history of the untreated condition in human fetuses and learned to select fetuses that required intervention; and (3) proved in a nonhuman primate model that the surgical procedure was feasible and safe for both fetus and mother.[6, 7, 25] This last step was the most difficult, but by the early 1980s, we had enough experience in primates to begin to apply the techniques developed in the laboratory to a few highly selected human cases.

Indications for Fetal Surgery

The indications for prenatal surgical intervention are narrow. Open fetal surgery is indicated only for a select group of fetuses with disorders diagnosed in the late first or early second trimester; with associated oligohydramnios and favorable fetal urine electrolytes and osmolarity; and with normal renal parenchyma observed on ultrasound examination. Open fetal surgery to decompress the urinary tract is preferable to catheter decompression early in gestation, to provide reliable long-term decompression, restore amniotic fluid dynamics, and permit further pulmonary and renal growth and development.

From 1978 to 1988, more than 200 cases of fetal hydronephrosis were referred to the Fetal Treatment Program at the University of California, San Francisco (UCSF) Medical Center. Five patients were found to be suitable for open intervention. One fetus had bilateral ureterostomies and the subsequent four had marsupialization of the bladder at 18 to 24 weeks' gestation.

Operative Technique

Prior to offering fetal surgery to our patients, the efficacy of the proposed fetal procedure was established in sheep, and the feasibility and safety of open fetal surgery were established in primates.[6, 7, 13, 16, 17, 24, 25] The tocolytic, anesthetic, and surgical techniques used were all developed and tested extensively in monkeys. Briefly, maternal tocolytic preparation begins with a 100-mg indomethacin suppository preoperatively. Inspired halothane in oxygen is used for uterine relaxation and fetal and maternal anesthesia intraoperatively. Ritodrine, magnesium sulfate, and/or indomethacin are used postoperatively for tocolysis. Maternal intraoperative monitoring includes automated blood pressure measurement, continuous electrocardiogram, and transcutaneous pulse oximetry (Fig. 5–2).

The uterus is exposed by a low transverse abdominal incision, and intraoperative sonography confirms the fetal position and the placental location.[26] The uterus is opened with either cautery or a newly developed resorbable stapling device, and the lower part of the fetal body is delivered through the hysterotomy.[26] A transcutaneous oximeter placed around the fetal thigh allows continuous monitoring of fetal oxygen saturation and heart rate. The distended and thick-walled bladder is opened and marsupialized to the fetal skin with interrupted sutures (Fig. 5–3).[26] Fetal heart rate has proven to be a very sensitive monitor of fetal condition: any episodes of fetal bradycardia are easily reversed by changing the fetal position to minimize compression of the umbilical cord. The fetal surgical procedure takes 15 minutes or less; the monitoring devices are then removed and the fetus returned to the uterine cavity. Amniotic fluid volume is restored with warm Ringer's lactate containing oxacillin. The uterus is closed with two layers of running polydioxanone (PDS)[26] sutures, making certain to include the amniotic membranes as well as the myometrium in the inner layer. After uterine

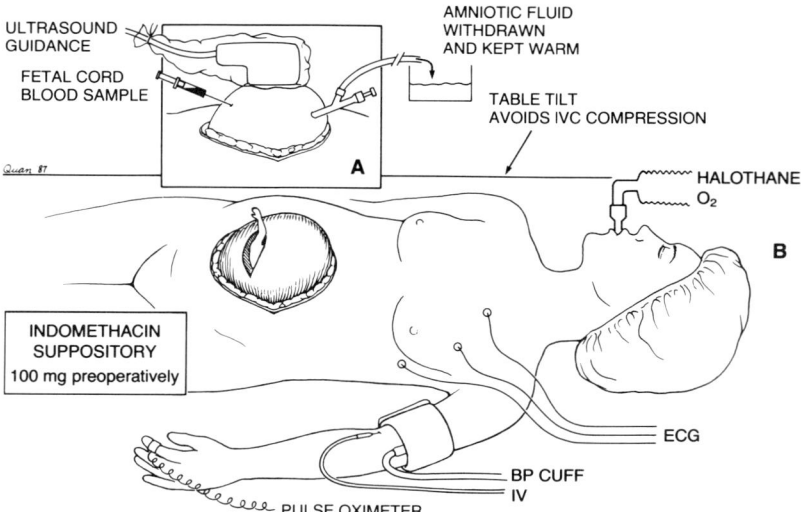

FIGURE 5–2. Maternal monitoring and positioning for open fetal surgery. *(A)* After uterine exposure, fetal umbilical cord blood is sampled and amniotic fluid is withdrawn during ultrasound guidance. *(B)* Hysterotomy permits fetal delivery for open fetal surgery. (IVC = inferior vena cava.)

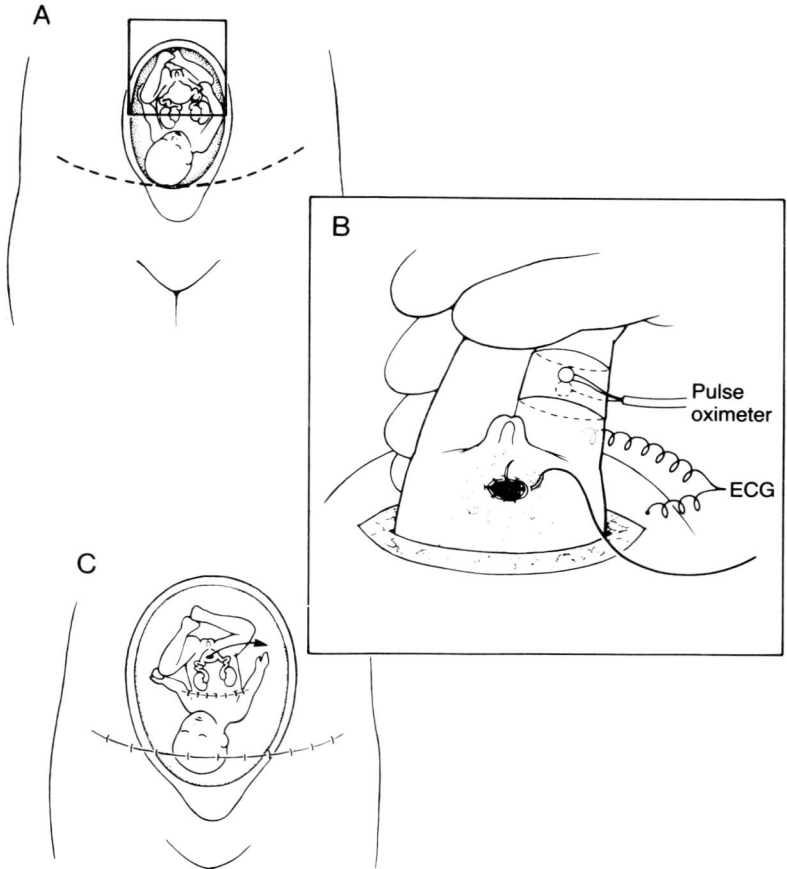

FIGURE 5–3. Example of open fetal surgery for hydronephrosis. *(A)* Bilateral hydrone-phrosis, megalocystis, and oligohydramnios. Guided by intraoperative sonography, a hysterotomy is placed to avoid the placenta and expose the lower body of the fetus without disturbing the umbilical circulation. *(B)* Fetal heart rate and oxygen saturation are monitored by transcutaneous pulse oximetry while a cutaneous vesicostomy is constructed. *(C)* Amniotic fluid volume is restored by fetal urine.

closure, intraoperative sonography can determine fetal heart rate and confirm bladder decompression. Maternal epidural morphine is used postoperatively for analgesia, and perioperative antibiotics are continued for 3 days. Ritodrine hydrochloride or magnesium sulfate is given intravenously for 3 days and then orally to control uterine activity and prevent preterm labor. Mother and fetus usually leave the hospital within 7 to 10 days, are followed weekly thereafter by ultrasonography, and undergo cesarean delivery weeks later.

Postoperative Management

Premature labor remains a constant threat throughout the postoperative course. Tocolytic therapy is started during the procedure with ritodrine and/or indomethacin. Postoperatively, uterine contractions and fetal heart rate are monitored continuously for several days, and tocolytic therapy with betamimetics, magnesium sulfate, and prostaglandin inhibitors is adjusted accordingly. Once the initial period of uterine contractions has subsided, usually within 5 days, oral betamimetics are continued throughout the remainder of the pregnancy. Perioperative antibiotics, generally a cephalosporin, are continued for 3 to 5 days postoperatively. The patient is kept at bedrest for at least 3 days following surgery and then begins a gradual progressive ambulation program. In most patients, a postoperative adynamic ileus is seen for 24 to 48 hours, and oral intake resumes with the return of bowel function. Generally, the patient is discharged on only tocolytic therapy within 10 days of the procedure.

Tocolytic management after open fetal surgery is often exceedingly difficult. Available drugs and combinations of drugs have not always been effective. The management of preterm labor is still the major unsolved problem limiting fetal intervention.

MATERNAL OUTCOME

Between 1981 and April 1988, five women underwent open fetal surgery for congenital hydronephrosis at the Fetal Treatment Program at the UCSF Medical Center. All operations were performed by one of the authors (MRH). All patients received inhalation anesthesia with halothane in oxygen and were monitored intraoperatively by the methods described previously. There was no perioperative maternal mortality, with all of the procedures being technically successful and resulting in a viable fetus postoperatively. Obviously, maternal safety has the highest priority in open fetal surgery, and because our series is small, each mother generally underwent two hysterotomies: the first at the time of the fetal repair and the second at the time of delivery. We have not had any maternal wound complications.

The length of stay postoperatively varied from 7 to 14 days, with an average of 9.4 days. The patients, in general, were ambulatory within 3 days following the procedure, and we have not encountered any problems with persistent postoperative paralytic ileus.

Operative blood loss ranged from 300 to 900 ml, and one patient required blood transfusion. Our hysterotomy technique continues to evolve in an effort to minimize potential blood loss. We have found manual compression of the uterus to be the best way of controlling uterine bleeding. Bleeding from the fetus has not been a problem.

As outlined earlier, our techniques for fetal surgery have continued to improve. The duration of both fetal surgery and total surgery time have decreased. We believe the critical time is the fetal exposure; therefore, for bladder obstruction vesicostomy, we return the fetus to the uterus within 17 minutes (average).

Tocolytic therapy begins with indomethacin preoperatively and halothane intraoperatively. An intravenous tocolytic (ritodrine or $MgSO_4$) is started during the procedure and continued postoperatively. All five patients developed uterine irritability in the immediate postoperative period and were successfully weaned from intravenous tocolysis. They were maintained on oral ritodrine or terbutaline tocolytic therapy until abdominal delivery. All five patients developed premature labor at an average of 9 weeks postoperatively (range 5 to 12 weeks), despite oral tocolytic therapy.

Fortunately, in this early experience, there were no intraoperative complications. In retrospect, postoperative complications that occurred were avoidable. A single leak of amniotic fluid represented a technical error that prompted us to change the method of hysterotomy closure, and it has not recurred in subsequent cases. A mild case of pseudomembranous enterocolitis was secondary to excessively long perioperative antibiotic usage, and it promptly responded to oral vancomycin treatment.

One of the concerns following fetal surgery is the mother's ability to have subsequent pregnancies. In follow-up of our five patients, two have had subsequent pregnancies (three children total), and all deliveries were by repeat cesarean section with a good outcome.

We believe that the paucity of complications in the first five patients with open fetal procedures performed for congenital hydronephrosis is a direct result of our extensive preparation in experimental animal fetuses, which should be a requisite for anyone considering these inherently dangerous procedures.

CONCLUSIONS

From our experience in animals and in our initial clinical experience with open fetal surgery, we have drawn the following conclusions: (1) The anesthetic regimen developed in the nonhuman primate model can successfully be employed in humans, with an acceptable perioperative risk. (2) The uterine irritability induced by hysterotomy can be successfully suppressed perioperatively with intravenous and oral tocolytic agents. (3) Premature labor remains a serious and frequent complication of fetal surgery, requiring early delivery in each of our cases. Despite this, enough tocolytic control was achieved so that fetal lung maturity was adequate in most cases; the morbidity associated with management of preterm labor after fetal surgery will likely be reduced with further experience. (4) Both clinical and experimental evidence suggests that a midgestation hysterotomy, closed with absorbable sutures, has no adverse effect on future fertility.

References

1. Harrison MR, Golbus MS, Filly RA: The Unborn Patient. Orlando FL: Grune & Stratton, 1984
2. Liley AW: Intrauterine transfusion of the foetus in haemolytic disease. Br Med J 2:1107, 1963
3. Flake AW, Harrison MR, Adzick NS, et al: Transplantation of fetal hematopoietic stem cells in utero: The creation of hematopoietic chimers. Science 233:776, 1986
4. Manning FA, Harrison MR, Rodeck C, et al.: Catheter shunts for fetal hydronephrosis and hydrocephalus. N Engl J Med 315:336, 1986
5. Glick PL, Harrison MR, Nakayama DK, et al.: Management of ventriculomegaly in the fetus. J Pediatr 105:97, 1984
6. Harrison MR, Anderson J, Rosen M, et al.: Fetal surgery in the primate. I. Anesthetic, surgical, and tocolytic management to maximize fetal-neonatal survival. J Pediatr Surg 17:115, 1982
7. Adzick NS, Harrison MR, Anderson JV, et al.: Fetal surgery in the primate. III. Maternal outcome after fetal surgery. J Pediatr Surg 21:477, 1986
8. Adzick NS, Harrison MR, Flake AW, et al.: Automatic uterine stapling device in fetal surgery: Experience in a primate model. Surg Forum 36:476, 1985
9. Harrison MR, Nakayama DK, Noall R, et al.: Correction of congenital hydronephrosis in utero. II. Decompression reverses the effects of obstruction on the fetal lung and urinary tract. J Pediatr Surg 17:965, 1982
10. Harrison MR, Ross NA, deLorimier AA: Correction of congenital diaphragmatic hernia in utero. III. Development of a successful surgical technique using abdominoplasty to avoid compromise of umbilical blood flow. J Pediatr Surg 16:934, 1981
11. Adzick NS, Harrison MR, Hu LM, et al.: Compensatory lung growth after pneumonectomy in fetal lambs: A morphometric study. Surg Forum 37:309, 1986
12. Harrison MR, Golbus MS, Filly RA: Management of the fetus with a urinary tract malformation. JAMA 246:635, 1981
13. Harrison MR, Ross NA, Noall R, et al.: Correction of congenital hydronephrosis in utero. I. The model: Fetal urethral obstruction produces hydronephrosis and pulmonary hypoplasia in fetal lambs. J Pediatr Surg 18:247, 1983
14. Adzick NS, Harrison MR, Flake AW, et al.: Development of a fetal renal function test using endogenous creatinine clearance. J Pediatr Surg 20:602, 1985
15. Adzick NS, Harrison MR, Flake AW, et al.: Fetal urinary tract obstruction: Experimental pathophysiology. Semin Perinatol 9:79, 1985
16. Glick PL, Harrison MR, Noall R, et al.: Correction of congenital hydronephrosis in utero. III. Early mid-trimester urethral obstruction produces renal dysplasia. J Pediatr Surg 18:681, 1983
17. Glick PL, Harrison MR, Adzick NS, et al.: Correction of congenital hydronephrosis in utero. IV. In utero decompression prevents renal dysplasia. J Pediatr Surg 19:649, 1984
18. Harrison MR, Golbus MS, Filly RA, et al.: Management of the fetus with congenital hydronephrosis. J Pediatr Surg 17:728, 1982
19. Glick PL, Harrison MR, Adzick NS, et al.: Management of the fetus with congenital hydronephrosis. II. Prognostic criteria and selection for treatment. J Pediatr Surg 20:376, 1985
20. Mahoney BS, Filly RA, Callen PW, et al.: Sonographic evaluation of fetal renal dysplasia. Radiology 152:143, 1984
21. Crombleholme TM, Harrison MR, Golbus MS, et al.: Fetal intervention in obstructive uropathy: Prognostic indicators and efficacy of intervention. Am J Obstet Gynecol 162:1239, 1990
22. Asensio SH: Surgical treatment of erythroblastosis fetalis. In: Adamson K Jr (ed): Diagnosis and Treatment of Fetal Disorders. New York: Springer-Verlag, 1969, pp 264–271

23. Harrison MR, Filly RA, Golbus MS, et al.: Management of the fetus with a correctable congenital defect. JAMA 246:774, 1981
24. Harrison MR, Bressack MA, Churg AM, et al.: Correction of congenital diaphragmatic hernia in utero. II. Simulated correction permits fetal lung growth with survival at birth. Surgery 88:260, 1980
25. Nakayama DK, Harrison MR, Seron-Ferre M: Fetal surgery in the primate. II. Uterine electromyographic response to operative procedures and pharmacologic agents. J Pediatr Surg 19:333, 1984
26. Crombleholme TM, Harrison MR, Anderson RL, et al.: Early experience with open fetal surgery for congenital hydronephrosis. J Pediatr Surg 23:1114, 1988

6. Perinatal Management of Maternal and Fetal Emergencies

Jonathan H. Skerman, B.D.Sc., M.Sc.D., D.Sc.,
Timothy Huckaby, M.D.,
Elizabeth B. Walker, R.N.C.,
and Warren N. Otterson, M.D.

Airway Complications
Malignant Hyperthermia
Pseudocholinesterase Deficiency
Aspiration Pneumonitis

CONCLUSIONS

INTRODUCTION

Although maternal mortality rates have decreased over the past 50 years, pregnancy is still not without risks, and many events can occur that place both the mother and unborn fetus in jeopardy. An event or circumstance that results in immediate risk of serious irreversible injury or death can be considered a maternal/fetal emergency requiring immediate intervention.

Because of the total dependency of the fetus on the mother, many maternal injuries result in fetal emergencies. Emergency care must always begin with the basics of initial management and resuscitation, including establishing control of the airway, providing ventilation, controlling bleeding, and initiating cardiovascular resuscitation when indicated.

In the pregnant patient, fetal evaluation and treatment must not be overlooked in the urgency to provide rapid care to the mother. The maternal and fetal emergencies discussed in this chapter include maternal/fetal trauma, maternal medical emergencies, umbilical cord accidents, and emergencies secondary to the administration of anesthesia.

TRAUMA

Motor Vehicle Accidents and Blunt Trauma

In addition to the medical risks incurred by pregnancy, the modern woman lives in a world where the possibility of traumatic injury to herself and her unborn child is constantly increasing. The parturient no longer stays at home. Because of changing social attitudes and economic roles many women now work outside the home or have other obligations that require travel. With increased mechanization, high-speed travel, and increasing crime rates, the risk of traumatic injury is always present. In addition to possible external dangers, physiologic changes that occur during pregnancy may result in fatigability, hyperventilation, fainting, ligamentous laxity, unsteady gait, and a protuberant abdomen, all of which increase the parturient's vulnerability to injury.

It has been estimated that 6% to 7% of all pregnant patients will experience some type of accidental injury. Not only is minor injury perhaps more common during pregnancy than at any other time in adult life, but traumatic injury is the major cause of nonobstetric maternal deaths in women under the age of 35 (36 deaths per 100,000 pregnancies). Bryant and Wheeler[1] suggest that trauma is the greatest threat to young parturients, since other complications of pregnancy (hemorrhage, pregnancy-induced hypertension, emboli, and infection) result in only 15 maternal deaths per 100,000 pregnancies.

Among the causes of trauma, the motor vehicle has become the greatest threat. In a review of maternal deaths in California, motor vehicle accidents accounted for 13.9% of all maternal deaths.[2] Other causes included assaults (beatings, knifings, shootings), falls, and burns.

The most common maternal injuries include blunt traumatic injuries, fractures, penetrating injuries, and burns. Depending on the extent of the parturient's injury and current health status, there is always the possibility of coexisting fetal distress or demise. Fetal injuries can include direct fetal trauma, abruptio placentae, premature labor, and posttraumatic abortion. With severe trauma, multiple maternal and fetal injuries are often sustained. Several studies have provided important information concerning the etiology of injury, extent of injury, and outcome following blunt trauma during pregnancy. Griswold and Collier[3] reported that motor vehicle accidents accounted for 50% of nonpenetrating abdominal injuries. They observed spleen, kidney, liver, and intestinal injuries in 15% to 20% of accidents, and severe abdominal wall, mesenteric, pancreatic, diaphragmatic, and retroperitoneal hemorrhages in less than 5% of cases. Elliott[4] specifically reported on 39 automotive accidents during pregnancy. Eight parturients sustained severe multiple injuries and died; the primary cause of death was uncontrollable hemorrhage. Bleeding sites included retroperitoneal hemorrhage in five of the eight, and placental separation and intraperitoneal bleeding in three. Elliott further suggested that the increased vascularity associated with pregnancy may have accounted for the large number of deaths secondary to hemorrhage. Of the nonfatal cases, 4 sustained retroperitoneal hemorrhage, 2 had intraperitoneal hemorrhage, 1 had retroplacental hemorrhage, 27 sustained orthopedic injuries, and 44 sustained multiple injuries.

Crosby and Costiloe[5] in 1971 followed 441 pregnant patients who had been involved in automotive accidents. Of the accidents reported, 233 (53%) resulted in minor damage to the automobile and only three patients were injured. Of the other 47%, 15 deaths occurred (3.4%) and 26 (5.8%) nonfatal major injuries were sustained. Causes of death among the 15 fatalities were divided into head injuries (among those who sustained upper body trauma) and internal hemorrhage (among those who sustained lower body trauma). Of the seven who died secondary to head injury, three also had accompanying orthopedic injuries. Among the 26 injured survivors, 5 had pelvic fractures, 2 had rupture of either the liver or spleen, and 19 had lesser injuries including extremity fractures, serious lacerations, and contusions. Crosby and Costiloe[5] noted that the total injury rate was independent of the seating position; however, drivers had the lowest mortality rates. In addition, Crosby and Costiloe[5] noted a significant reduction in ejection from the vehicle among parturients wearing seat belts and therefore recommended that belt restraints should be worn during pregnancy.

Pelvic fracture is the most common traumatic fracture reported to result from motor vehicle accidents involving pregnant women.[6] Although many types of fractures can occur as a result of blunt trauma, fractures of the extremities may not affect the pregnancy. However, pelvic fractures not only produce pain and alteration of the birth canal but may also result in retroperitoneal hemorrhage and fetal injury. The most common site of a pelvic fracture is in the anterior half of the pelvic ring through the horizontal rami of the pubis. Fracture at one location is usually accompanied by a fracture at another site on the ring. Again, with the increased vascularity associated with pregnancy, retroperitoneal hemorrhage following pelvic fracture may be severe and is considered the most serious complication of this injury. Other complications include premature labor, placental abruption, urethral injury, bladder rupture, and pelvic outlet encroachment. Eastman[7] predicts that 5% to 10% of parturients will require a cesarean section secondary to pelvic deformity. Others point out that if gross pelvic deformities are absent, even with recent pelvic fractures, labor and delivery are usually not attended by serious complications.[8]

Blunt trauma may also damage the placenta and uterus. Crosby and Costiloe[5] prospectively followed 211 women injured in severe automotive accidents and noted that there were 12 (5.7% incidence) cases of abruptio placentae. However, among victims involved in minor collisions after the first trimester, they reported no occurrence of placental separation following blunt abdominal trauma. Others agree that premature separation of the placenta occurs in a clinically recognizable degree in less than 6% of the victims of severe collisions.[9] When it does occur, bleeding into the decidua may be self-limiting without any external bleeding. With larger separations there is fetal distress and usually external bleeding. The severity of clinical symptoms and the fetal outcome depend on the surface area of the placental separation. When 25% or less of the placenta is separated, the parturient has uterine tenderness and irritability and possibly some vaginal spotting or bleeding. When greater than 50% of the placenta is separated, there is severe fetal distress, maternal shock, uterine tetany, marked uterine tenderness, and often vaginal bleeding. Disseminated intravascular coagulation (DIC) may also occur or may even have already developed.

In addition to placental abruption, uterine rupture and transection have been reported. Previous uterine surgery may place a parturient at greater risk of uterine rupture as a result of blunt trauma. In a study on acute deceleration and impact injuries with pregnant baboons, Crosby[10] reported intrauterine pressures tenfold higher than pressures recorded during normal labor.

Blunt trauma to the abdomen can produce severe fetal injury, especially in advanced pregnancy, since the fetal head is usually flexed and low in the pelvis and there is decreased buffering action of the amniotic fluid. Fetal fractures, which are the most common injuries, include skull fractures and fractures of the clavicle, femur, tibia, humerus, fingers, and pelvis. Skull fracture, however, is the most common fracture, and dislocation of the fetal cervical spine has been reported. This usually occurs from flexion of the mother's body over the lap belt compressing the fetal skull between the belt and the sacral promontory. If the fetus is not delivered soon after the traumatic event, fetal injury may often go unrecognized. Abdominal ultrasound and roentgenologic examination are necessary to assess fetal injuries from blunt maternal trauma.

Fetal injury may not necessarily result in fetal death; the leading cause of fetal death after any trauma is maternal death. Another primary cause of fetal demise following blunt trauma is extensive separation of the placenta with fetal mortality ranging from 30% to 68%, depending on the degree of placental separation.[8, 10] With a separation of greater than 50%, the fetus usually dies.[5, 6] Fetal distress and death may occur secondary to maternal shock. Uterine perfusion is compromised when maternal blood pressure decreases to 20% below normal baseline. Uterine blood flow can also be reduced by vasoconstriction from high maternal levels of catecholamines released in response to acute stress and by some vasoactive drugs administered to treat maternal hypotension (Chapter 3).

Maternal trauma has been reported to result in both premature labor and spontaneous abortion. The frequency with which this occurs is difficult to estimate because of the difficulty of establishing a causal relationship to trauma and posttraumatic fetal events. An abortion may have already been in progress when the injury occurred. It has been well established with severe maternal and fetal injuries that premature labor and delivery will almost certainly result. Unlike premature labor, abortion following trauma is uncommon but has been reported. At least 50% of all spontaneous abortions are due to abnormalities in development of the embryo or placenta.

Penetrating Injuries

Penetrating injuries sustained during pregnancy are less common and usually result from stabbings or gunshot wounds. Since the enlarged uterus is the most prominent organ in the abdomen, it becomes a major target for penetrating abdominal trauma. Dyer and Barclay[9] state that penetrating abdominal wounds during pregnancy invariably involve the uterus.

Fetal survival following an abdominal stab wound with surgical uterine repair has been reported; however, the outcome is frequently poor because of extensive fetal, placental, or umbilical cord damage. Abdominal gunshot wounds are more common than stab wounds and have a higher maternal and fetal mortality.[9, 11] Maternal mortality rates have been reported to be 9% while fetal mortality rates range from 55% to 75%. Again, the outcome varies as to the point of entry and/or exit of the projectile or weapon.[9, 11]

Traumatic injury frequently involves multiple organ system damage, and thus a complete discussion of treatment is beyond the limitations of this chapter. Certain guidelines, however, are essential for successful management of maternal trauma. Keeping in mind the physiologic changes of pregnancy and their impact on a parturient in shock, the clinician should institute three treatment priorities: establish an airway, ensure ventilation, and stop the bleeding (Chapter 2).

Establishing an airway in a nontraumatized pregnant patient may be very difficult because of laryngeal and airway edema (Chapter 2). With the increased vascularity associated with the hormonal changes of pregnancy, facial and/or neck trauma will result in profuse bleeding and extensive edema that may cause life-threatening airway occlusion (Chapter 2). In addition, all traumatized pregnant patients must be considered to have full stomachs with increased risks of gastric regurgitation and pulmonary aspiration. Nasal airways may cause profuse bleeding and should be avoided. Tracheal intubation should be performed by the most experienced person available, using smaller endotracheal tubes (sizes 7.0, 6.5, and 6.0) to compensate for the diminished laryngeal opening. Total loss of airway patency and/or ventilatory failure in the parturient are acute emergencies. In the second and third trimesters of pregnancy, the functional residual capacity of the lungs is decreased while oxygen consumption is increased (Chapter 2). With cessation of ventilation, hypoxia occurs rapidly with serious consequences for the mother and fetus (Chapter 2). If an airway cannot be established immediately, a cricothyroidotomy may be necessary to provide oxygen while other attempts to establish a satisfactory airway proceed. Once alveolar ventilation is reestablished, maternal hyperventilation should be avoided as it may result in fetal acidosis (Chapters 2 and 3).

Profuse bleeding often accompanies trauma during pregnancy and may be concealed and difficult to estimate. Since blood volume is increased, clinical symptoms may not develop until 30% to 35% of the blood volume is lost.[11] When the systolic blood pressure falls 20% below normal, uterine perfusion may be significantly reduced, and a systolic blood pressure below 80 mmHg is representative of severe maternal shock.[11] Aggressive intervention is needed to prevent fetal and maternal demise. Large-bore intravenous lines should be established and glucose-free balanced salt solutions infused rapidly. Intravenous ephedrine, 5 to 15 mg, will help to restore cardiac output without producing uteroplacental vasoconstriction. As pregnancy nears term, the gravid uterus compresses the vena cava and aorta when the patient is in the supine position, causing a reduction in venous return, cardiac output, and blood pressure (Chapter 2). A wedge should be placed under the right hip to displace the uterus laterally to the left, which will minimize aortocaval compression (Chapters 2 and 3).

Burns

Although the likelihood of sustaining an extensive thermal injury during pregnancy is low, a clear management scheme is needed to provide optimal medical care for both the fetus and mother.

Treatment of the burned parturient is especially difficult since the attending physicians must treat both the mother and the fetus, each of whom may have different medical needs after the injury. Medical treatment of both patients may require compromises that balance the needs of each.

In essence, the goal of treatment for the burned parturient is survival with the best cosmetic and functional recovery possible. In the absence of an inhalation injury, the determinants of survival are the extent and depth (magnitude) of the thermal injury.[12] Topical antimicrobial agents, nutritional support, infection control, and the use of judicious surgical debridement are frequently required to optimize chances of maternal survival after extensive burns.[13] Even after thermal injury that is not life-threatening, surgical treatment and drug therapy are frequently necessary to prevent functional and cosmetic burn deformities, control pain, and prevent infection.

In contrast to the needs of the mother, the fetus is best served by avoiding medication and anesthetics, especially during the first trimester because of the possibility of associated increased risk of birth defects (Chapter 1).[14] The prevention of maternal hypoxia or hypotension is critical to minimize fetal wastage since hypoxia or hypotension, or both, can cause fetal distress and initiate premature labor.[15] Therefore, since extensive surface burns, even in the absence of an inhalation injury, are frequently associated with an increased rate of arteriovenous shunting and hypoxia, prompt institution of supplemental oxygen (O_2) therapy will benefit both fetus and mother. If an inhalation injury has occurred, mechanical ventilatory support should be instituted as early as possible.

Adequate fluid resuscitation should maintain normal maternal intravascular volume and uteroplacental blood flow with normal maternal blood pressures and urine output of 30 to 50 ml/hour.[16]

Fetal survival appears to be related primarily to the gestational age at the time of injury and to maternal survival. During the third trimester, fetal survival depends less on maternal survival and more on gestational age. Thus, it is important to have a good estimate of fetal gestational age for optimal fetal management. Fetuses delivered before 24 weeks' gestation generally will not survive, whereas fetuses delivered after 32 weeks will do well with modern neonatal intensive care, provided they are not born hypoxic or with birth trauma. Most difficult to manage are fetuses between 24 and 32 weeks of gestation when extrauterine survival is difficult to predict. Thus, when preterm labor occurs at this time, pharmacologic inhibition of labor (tocolysis) should be considered during treatment of underlying causes of maternal stress such as hypoxia or hypotension, or as a temporary method of arresting labor while maternal homeostasis is restored (Chapter 7). The administration of beta-mimetic tocolytic agents such as ritodrine or terbutaline to a woman with a thermal injury is not without risk. These agents may cause dangerous myocardial ischemia, pulmonary edema, hyperglycemia, and hypokalemia. Tocolytic therapy using parenteral magnesium sulfate might be better tolerated because magnesium has fewer cardiovascular and metabolic effects than the other agents.[17] Thus, the fetal management scheme begins with an estimate of gestational age based on menstrual history and sonography. Regardless of the gestational age of the fetus, if premature labor occurs, treatable causes of maternal stress should be sought. If the fetus is less than 32 weeks' gestation, tocolysis should be considered in an attempt to improve fetal survival. Beyond 32 weeks' gestational age, it is best to avoid tocolytic therapy because fetal outcome is usually good. Spontaneous vaginal delivery is preferred, but the route and timing of delivery are based on obstetric considerations. Serial fetal sonography and electronic fetal heart rate monitoring often permit timely interventions and prevent intrauterine fetal death by identifying the fetal distress early.

If the mother is burned during the first trimester, fetal wastage appears to be high. In contrast, if the injury occurs during the second trimester, fetal survival appears to be excellent if the mother survives the injury. With burn injuries in the third trimester, the gestational age appears to be the most important variable in fetal survival.

Formulation of a management plan for mother and fetus during the acute phase of the burn injury is difficult, since the effects of various topically and systemically administered drugs on the fetus are largely unknown. In essence, give priority to maintaining normal circulatory volume and avoiding maternal hypoxia to reduce the risk of uteroplacental insufficiency and fetal distress. Topical povidone-iodine cleansing of the burn wound should be avoided since large amounts of iodine may be absorbed through the burn wounds.[18] Diuretics and most antihypertensive drugs can reduce uteroplacental blood flow. The topical agent silver sulfadiazine should be used only in patients with extensive burn injuries or on localized areas of third-degree burns because of the association of absorption of the sulfonamide portion of this agent with kernicterus.[14] Systemic antibiotics are indicated for burn wound sepsis, pneumonia, or urinary tract infection. The choice of antimicrobial drugs is based on blood, urine, and wound cultures. The prompt use of antibiotics in well-documented episodes of infection will benefit the mother by increasing the chance of maternal survival and benefit the fetus by reducing fetal distress and premature birth. Fortunately, most antibiotics are tolerated by the fetus. However, tetracycline should not be used, and chloramphenicol, streptomycin, kanamycin, and sulfonamide should also be avoided. Lastly, the patient is positioned in bed with the right side elevated to prevent uterine compression of the inferior vena cava (Chapter 2).

When surgical treatment is necessary, local or regional anesthesia is preferred whenever possible. If an anesthetic is required, the avoidance of maternal hypotension and hypoxia is more important than the particular agents used.[19] Because of the danger of hyperkalemia after succinylcholine administration, this depolarizing agent should not be used.[20] Instead a nondepolarizing muscle relaxant such as vecuronium or atracurium is preferred.[20] Glomerular filtration rates may be increased or decreased markedly in the pregnant patient with burns, and anesthetic agents that rely primarily on urinary excretion for cessation of action should be administered sparingly.[21]

Pruritus and local wound discomfort are common complaints after the burns have healed. These complaints are best treated with a combination of an antihistamine, topical moisturizers, and compressive garments. Optimal care of burns in pregnant women can best be achieved by a team approach that combines the specialized skills of the obstetrician, burn surgeon, and anesthesiologist.

MATERNAL MEDICAL EMERGENCIES
Cardiac Disease

Pregnancy and labor result in increased cardiac demand, which may lead to cardiac failure in an already compromised heart, producing both a maternal and a fetal emergency. The incidence of heart disease during pregnancy decreased from 3.6% during the 1940s to 1.6% during the 1960s.[22] Although rheumatic heart disease still accounts for the majority of heart disease among parturients, the incidence of pregnant women with congenital heart disease increased from about 14% during the 1940s to about 35% during the 1960s.[23] Rheumatic heart disease consists of mitral stenosis (70% to 90%), mitral regurgitation (6% to 12%), aortic regurgitation (2% to 5%), and aortic stenosis (1%).[23] Mortality ranges from less than 1% in asymptomatic patients to 17% in parturients with mitral stenosis and atrial fibrillation.[24] Congenital lesions include primary pulmonary hypertension, intracardiac shunts (ventricular septal defect, atrial septal defect, tetralogy of Fallot, Eisenmenger's syndrome), valvular dysfunction, and coarctation of the aorta. Congenital lesions tend to have a higher incidence of both maternal and fetal mortality than acquired rheumatic lesions.

CARDIOVASCULAR CHANGES DURING PREGNANCY (see Chapter 2)

When the uterus enlarges as pregnancy advances, displacement of the diaphragm results in a superior and anterior displacement of the heart with left rotation. The apical pulse shifts laterally to the midclavicular line, left axis deviation occurs on the electrocardiogram (ECG), and a larger cardiac silhouette can be seen on chest radiograph. In addition to the left axis deviation, other ECG abnormalities that have been reported include Q waves in leads III and AVF and ST segment depression.[25]

During labor, stroke volume increases and pain and apprehension can further increase cardiac output to 30% to 40% over prelabor values. With each uterine contraction, central blood volume and cardiac output can increase by an additional 10% to 25%. In the immediate postpartum period, central blood volume increases even further and stroke volume increases by as much as 60% to 80% above prelabor values as aortocaval obstruction is relieved.[25] The normal heart tolerates these stresses well, but a diseased heart may fail with serious sequelae.

CARDIAC LESIONS: RHEUMATIC HEART DISEASE

Rheumatic heart disease results from a diffuse inflammatory reaction confined to heart valves following group A beta-hemolytic streptococcal bacteremia. Progressive and permanent damage to the heart valves may occur. The disease preferentially affects children 6 to 15 years of age, causing symptoms that do not appear until later in life. Although the incidence of rheumatic heart disease during pregnancy has decreased, it still accounts for 15% of all cardiac disease among parturients.[26] Major complications include left or right ventricular failure (8.5%), atrial dysrhythmias (6.5%), systemic or pulmonary embolism (1.6%), and infective endocarditis (0.4%).[23]

MITRAL STENOSIS

Mitral stenosis is the most common valvular lesion following rheumatic endocarditis. Symptoms may not appear for 15 years, with right ventricular failure developing 5 to 10 years after the onset of symptoms.[27]

When the mitral orifice area decreases, left ventricular filling is impaired. Left atrial volume and pressure, pulmonary venous pressure, and pulmonary artery wedge pressure increase progressively. Cardiac output falls, and increased extravascular lung water decreases pulmonary compliance, causing progressive dyspnea on exertion. With time, elevated pulmonary vascular resistance produces pulmonary artery fibrosis, right ventricular hypertrophy, cor pulmonale, and then congestive heart failure. Because of the increased cardiac demands during pregnancy and labor, moderate mitral stenosis may become functionally severe.[28] Pregnant patients with mitral stenosis have a 25% incidence of pulmonary edema.[23]

The initial symptoms of mitral stenosis include fatigue and dyspnea on exertion. These often progress to paroxysmal nocturnal dyspnea, orthopnea, dyspnea at rest, and hemoptysis. Severe stenosis may be accompanied by atrial fibrillation, pulmonary embolism, or pulmonary infarction with rapid decompensation.[23]

Physical examination demonstrates a presystolic or mid-diastolic murmur with an opening snap at the left upper sternal border. If the murmur is faint, it may only be heard when the patient lies on her left side. An ECG may show a broadened P wave in lead V_1, indicating left atrial enlargement, or right axis deviation with severe disease. Atrial fibrillation occurs in about 7% of patients with severe mitral stenosis.[23] Cardiac catheterization shows an elevated pulmonary artery wedge pressure, increased pulmonary vascular resistance, and an increased pressure gradient across the mitral valve. With severe stenosis, the mitral valve diastolic pressure gradient may exceed 25 mmHg, resulting in transudation of fluid into the alveolar walls.[29]

As pregnancy progresses, previously asymptomatic patients may become symptomatic. The following guidelines are essential for successful management.

1. During pregnancy physical activity should be restricted. With severe stenosis and pulmonary congestion, hospitalization and complete bed rest may be necessary.

2. If bed rest and medical management are unsuccessful, closed commissurotomy or, rarely, mitral valve replacement may be necessary.[30]

3. Rapid ventricular rates are not tolerated. Either sinus tachycardia or atrial fibrillation with a rapid ventricular response will decrease the time needed for diastolic flow across the stenotic valve orifice, resulting in significant decreases in cardiac output and increases in pulmonary vascular pressures.[26] Sinus tachycardia may be precipitated by pain, anxiety, hypercarbia, acidosis, light general anesthesia, or fever. Arrhythmia treatment includes elimination of the precipitating event, avoidance of drugs that produce tachycardia (atropine, scopolamine, ketamine,

pancuronium, and terbutaline), and administration of incremental doses of beta-adrenergic blocking agents.

When atrial fibrillation with a rapid ventricular response results in hemodynamic instability, direct-current electrical cardioversion starting with 25 watt-seconds of power is indicated as safe during pregnancy.[31] Digoxin therapy, 0.5 mg IV initially, followed by 0.25 mg every 2 hours to a full dose of 0.25 to 0.5 mg daily, can then be used to slow the ventricular response.[26] Beta-adrenergic blocking agents (propranolol and esmolol) can also be used to acutely decrease the rapid ventricular response should cardioversion be unavailable immediately.[26]

4. Large increases in central blood volume are not tolerated. Overhydration, overtransfusion, Trendelenburg position, and intermittent autotransfusions by uterine contractions may result in acute increases in pulmonary artery pressure and precipitate pulmonary edema, atrial fibrillation, or right heart failure.[26]

5. Rapid decreases in systemic vascular resistance are not tolerated. Since stroke volume is fixed, a decrease in systemic vascular resistance is compensated for by an increase in heart rate. As discussed previously, such tachycardias may result in decreased cardiac output, increased pulmonary artery pressure, pulmonary edema, and right heart failure. Beta-adrenergic agents such as ephedrine and epinephrine may increase heart rate and should be avoided.[26]

Alpha-agonists will restore systemic vascular resistance but may result in reduced uterine blood flow in therapeutic doses and should be avoided (Chapter 2). A metaraminol infusion (10 mg/250 ml of normal saline) will increase systemic vascular resistance and restore cardiac output at lower heart rates with less effect on uterine blood flow than phenylephrine or methoxamine.[32]

6. Pulmonary hypertension should be controlled. Hypercarbia, hypoxia, acidosis, hyperinflation of the lungs, and even attempted Valsalva's maneuvers associated with the urge to push can increase pulmonary vascular resistance and should be avoided. Pulmonary vasodilators and inotropic drugs like dobutamine may be required during the puerperium to relieve pulmonary hypertension and improve left ventricular performance.

7. Anticoagulation may be indicated if atrial fibrillation occurs.[33] Aspirin has been shown to be an effective anticoagulant with few side effects in pregnant patients with mitral valve grafts and atrial fibrillation.[33]

8. Rheumatic fever prophylaxis should be given during pregnancy, and subacute bacterial endocarditis prophylaxis is advised during delivery.[30]

For labor and delivery, segmental lumbar epidural anesthesia provides excellent pain relief and eliminates the urge to push during the second stage of labor. Overhydration and rapid hydration should be avoided. Hypotension should be treated by left uterine displacement, cautious intravenous fluid loading, and administration of small doses of metaraminol.

Cesarean section can be accomplished under either epidural blockade or general anesthesia. Spinal anesthesia should be avoided because of its acute reduction of systemic vascular resistance. With epidural anesthesia, epinephrine is usually omitted from the local anesthetic mixture, and a T_4 level can be established slowly by incremental top-up doses. Monitoring of arterial pressure, central venous pressure, and/or pulmonary artery pressure is often required to determine volume requirements and changes in systemic vascular resistance.

When general anesthesia is indicated, agents that produce maternal tachycardia must be avoided. With mild stenosis, a thiopental induction and 0.5% halothane or 1.0% enflurane maintenance are usually well tolerated. Succinylcholine, vecuronium, or atracurium can be utilized for muscle relaxation, but pancuronium, a vagolytic, should be avoided. When mitral stenosis is severe, anesthetic induction with inspired halothane or intravenous fentanyl induction may provide better maternal cardiovascular stability but offer increased risks of maternal aspiration during halothane insufflation or neonatal depression from maternal narcotics.[26] Epidural narcotics will provide excellent pain relief after operative delivery.

MITRAL REGURGITATION

Mitral regurgitation is the second most common form of heart disease during pregnancy.[28] Because patients usually remain asymptomatic for 30 to 40 years, most parturients with mitral regurgitation do well during pregnancy. The complication most frequently encountered is infective endocarditis (8.5%), followed by pulmonary congestion (5.5%), atrial tachycardia (4.3%), and pulmonary embolism (2.8%).[23]

Over time, the left atrium dilates because of regurgitant flow of blood across the incompetent valve from the left ventricle into the left atrium. Left atrial pressure increases late in the course of the disease and for a time protects the pulmonary vasculature from damaging back pressure.[26] Eventually pulmonary artery and wedge pressures also increase, resulting in pulmonary congestion and edema. Left ventricular dilation occurs secondary to its increased preload, and forward ejection of blood can be significantly reduced. With time, right ventricular hypertrophy also develops.

During pregnancy, the progressive increase in intravascular volume may exacerbate pulmonary hypertension and pulmonary congestion (Chapter 2). Pain, apprehension, and uterine contractions will increase systemic vascular resistance, promoting regurgitant backward flow across the incompetent valve at the expense of forward flow from the left ventricle. This may result in acute left heart failure and pulmonary edema.[26]

The regurgitant valve produces a pansystolic murmur that has been described as having a blowing quality. It is loudest at the cardiac apex but can radiate to the left axilla or infrascapular area. As left atrial pressure rises, pulmonary vascular congestion, pulmonary edema, and pulmonary hypertension eventually develop. Atrial fibrillation develops in about one-third of patients.[26] As pregnancy advances and intravascular volume increases, symptoms of dyspnea on exertion, orthopnea, and paroxysmal nocturnal dyspnea may appear.

Most patients will remain asymptomatic throughout pregnancy and delivery. Symptomatic patients will need invasive monitoring, including arterial and pulmonary artery monitoring during labor, delivery, and recovery. The following guidelines are important for the successful management of the parturient with mitral regurgitation:

1. Increases in systemic vascular resistance result in increased mitral regurgitation and decreased cardiac output. Low-dose sodium nitroprusside can be used to produce afterload reduction and decrease regurgitation. Sympathetic blockade from epidural anesthesia is also beneficial in reducing afterload and improving forward ejection.[26]

2. Atrial fibrillation can produce left ventricular failure and is treated with either electrical countershock or digoxin therapy. Anticoagulation with heparin therapy is recommended during pregnancy for parturients with atrial fibrillation.

3. Bradycardia is poorly tolerated. Since stroke volume is relatively fixed, cardiac output is determined primarily by heart rate.

4. Myocardial depressants are poorly tolerated. Even small doses of potent myocardial depressants, such as thiopental, may result in left ventricular decompensation.

5. Pulmonary artery monitoring is very useful in acute mitral insufficiency since the V wave size on the pulmonary occlusive pressure wave correlates well with increased regurgitation.[26]

6. Dopamine may be needed to provide left ventricular inotropic support and augment glomerular filtration and urinary output.

7. Rheumatic fever and subacute bacterial endocarditis prophylaxis should be administered to these patients.[30]

Lumbar epidural anesthesia is recommended for labor and vaginal delivery. The concomitant sympathetic blockade will reduce systemic vascular resistance and improve forward blood flow. Ephedrine is useful in treating hypotension in addition to cautiously increasing intravascular fluids during wedge pressure monitoring and providing left uterine displacement.

Should cesarean section be required, epidural anesthesia is preferred to general anesthesia. Spinal anesthesia should be avoided since the acute changes in afterload and the large amounts of intravenous fluids required to restore blood pressure may be poorly tolerated by the parturient. Ketamine should be avoided as an induction agent since the resulting tachycardia and vasoconstriction can decrease cardiac output. As indicated, thiopental may produce significant myocardial depression by its direct effects on contractility and peripheral vascular resistance and should be used cautiously. For general anesthesia, intravenous narcotics with oxygen and nitrous oxide may produce the least myocardial depression although they may result in neonatal depression.[26]

AORTIC INSUFFICIENCY

Aortic insufficiency is a valvular heart disease that usually remains asymptomatic for 7 to 10 years after the development of valvular regurgitation.[28] Since symptoms usually begin in the fourth and fifth decades of life, most women with the disease have uncomplicated pregnancies.

Left ventricular volume overload occurs progressively and is dependent on the pressure gradient between the left ventricle and the aorta, the duration of diastole, and the degree of valve incompetence.[33] Although the left ventricle dilates, end-diastolic pressure may remain normal for years. Once failure begins, cardiac output decreases, end-diastolic pressure increases, and pulmonary edema develops.[34] Physiologic changes in pregnancy lead to an increase in heart rate and a decrease in systemic vascular resistance, which is beneficial to these patients (Chapter 2). This benefit is balanced against the increase in intravascular volume, which can lead to decompensation. During labor, the increases in systemic vascular resistance produced by pain, apprehension, and uterine contractions can result in left ventricular dysfunction.

Most patients are asymptomatic. A widening pulse pressure with diastolic hypotension and bounding pulses accompanies moderate aortic insufficiency. A blowing diastolic murmur can be heard at the left sternal border along the second through fourth intercostal spaces. ECG changes include increased QRS amplitude, inverted T waves, and ST segment depression. Atrial fibrillation is rare unless mitral valve disease is also present.[26] Chest radiographs will reveal left ventricular dilation.

The same precautions for mitral insufficiency also apply for aortic insufficiency. Pulmonary artery hypertension is a late sign, but an acute increase in pulmonary wedge pressure indicates significant left ventricular failure.

The anesthetic management of aortic insufficiency is similar to that previously described for mitral insufficiency. Lumbar epidural anesthesia is recommended for labor and delivery because the afterload reduction provided reduces regurgitant flow and improves cardiac output.

AORTIC STENOSIS

Aortic stenosis is the most infrequent valvular lesion during pregnancy, affecting only 0.5% to 3% of parturients.[23, 35] Since most patients become symptomatic during their fifth or sixth decade of life, asymptomatic parturients are usually not at increased risk.[23] Symptomatic aortic stenosis during pregnancy, however, results in a significant increase in both maternal and fetal morbidity and mortality.[23, 28]

The stenotic valve restricts forward ejection from the left ventricle. When the valve orifice area narrows to less than 1 cm^2 from the normal orifice cross-sectional area of 2.6 to 3.5 cm^2, left ventricular end-diastolic pressure increases.[36] Symptoms of dyspnea and syncope usually appear when the orifice area is reduced to 0.75 cm^2.[36] In time, left ventricular hypertrophy and elevated left ventricular pressures produce ischemia. Tachycardia increases myocardial work and reduces the time needed for filling a stiff left ventricle and allowing it to eject blood across a pressure gradient.

Aortic stenosis produces a loud systolic murmur best heard in the second right intercostal space and frequently radiating into the neck. Dyspnea on exertion and angina occur as the stenosis progresses. Left ventricular hypertrophy and left bundle branch block may be seen on the ECG. Chest radiographs show left ventricular enlargement. Heart catheterization demonstrating a systolic pressure gradient of 50 mmHg or more between the aorta and left ventricle indicates severe aortic stenosis.[37]

During pregnancy, mild stenosis may become functionally severe and symptoms may develop. When this occurs, invasive monitoring, including radial artery and pulmonary artery catheterization, is indicated. The following precautions will serve as a general guide to the perinatal management of the parturient with aortic stenosis:

1. Sudden decreases in systemic vascular resistance are not tolerated. The normal compensation for a decrease in systemic vascular resistance is to increase stroke volume and heart rate. Since stroke volume is fixed in aortic stenosis, tachycardia will decrease diastolic filling and reduce cardiac output. As indicated in managing mitral stenosis, systemic vascular resistance should be maintained in parturients with aortic stenosis. Metaraminol provides the least reduction in uterine blood flow when vasopressor therapy is indicated.

2. Bradycardia will also reduce cardiac output. Since stroke volume is fixed, optimal cardiac output is dependent on normal heart rates.

3. Decreased preload is detrimental to left ventricular output. If the left ventricular end-diastolic volume is inadequate, stroke volume and

cardiac output will decrease. An adequate preload must be maintained by judicious fluid therapy directed by intracardiac filling pressures. Aortocaval compression by the uterus can markedly affect blood pressure, especially in the supine position (Chapter 2).[26]

Since sympathetic blockade may result in decreased systemic vascular resistance, increased heart rate, and decreased preload, regional anesthesia is usually not advised. If it is attempted, epidural local anesthetics should be administered gradually by small intermittent injections during continuous monitoring of pulmonary artery pressures and cardiac output. General anesthesia is indicated for cesarean section and is best accomplished with oxygen/nitrous oxide and narcotic-relaxant techniques. Halogenated agents may cause profound myocardial depression and should be avoided in parturients with severe left ventricular dysfunction (ejection fraction < 0.5).[26]

CONGENITAL HEART DISEASE

Most patients with congenital heart disease undergo corrective surgery before their reproductive years. Nevertheless, some patients with congenital heart disease escape detection and remain relatively asymptomatic until pregnancy. The classification of congenital heart disease includes septal defects, congenital valvular defects, and vascular lesions.

Ventricular Septal Defects. Most patients with large ventricular septal defects (VSDs) have surgical treatment before their reproductive years. However, small VSDs with minimal left-to-right shunt persist in 7% of parturients with congenital heart disease.[38] These women are usually asymptomatic. With labor and delivery, elevations in systemic vascular resistance during contractions and attempted Valsalva's maneuvers will result in increases in left-to-right shunting, pulmonary hypertension, and increased right ventricular workloads. Patients with large uncorrected VSDs during pregnancy may have mortality rates as high as 40%.[23, 28]

Increases in heart rate, intravascular volume, systemic vascular resistance, and cardiac output during pregnancy may exacerbate left-to-right shunting in parturients with VSDs. Pulmonary artery and wedge pressures increase and left ventricular dysfunction often develops. If systemic vascular resistance is decreased suddenly, a right-to-left shunt may occur, resulting in hypoxia and cyanosis.[26]

A VSD produces a pansystolic murmur that is loudest in the fourth or fifth intercostal space. With a large VSD, expiratory splitting of the second heart sound may be heard in the same areas.

Asymptomatic patients with small VSDs usually do not require invasive monitoring perinatally. The symptomatic patients should have arterial and pulmonary artery catheters inserted to monitor vascular pressures, resistances, and cardiac output. The following are important considerations for appropriate perinatal management of these patients:

1. Avoid increases in the heart rate. An increased heart rate may result in an increase in left-to-right intracardiac shunt.

2. Avoid increases in systemic vascular resistance that also increase shunting.

3. Avoid sudden decreases in systemic vascular resistance that may reverse existing shunts and cause hypoxia and peripheral cyanosis.

4. Avoid events that result in a sudden increase in pulmonary artery pressure that may also produce cyanotic shunts.

During labor and delivery, continuous lumbar epidural anesthesia removes pain and reduces elevations in systemic vascular resistance. To prevent an abrupt fall in systemic vascular resistance, small doses of local anesthetics should be incrementally administered. Should a cyanotic right-to-left shunt develop, systemic vascular resistance can be increased with metaraminol.

Induction of general anesthesia with small doses of thiopental sodium followed by inhalation agents and narcotics will minimize myocardial depression. Continuous monitoring of the pulmonary artery pressures, wedge pressures, cardiac output, and systemic vascular resistance is necessary to determine if afterload reduction, afterload elevation, or inotropic agents are needed to support cardiac output.

Atrial Septal Defects. Atrial septal defect (ASD) is the most common congenital defect. It occurs in 17.5% of adults.[23, 38, 39] Parturients with uncorrected ASDs usually remain asymptomatic throughout pregnancy, with maternal and fetal mortality rates of 1% to 12%.[23, 35, 38]

The left-to-right shunt of an ASD causes increased pulmonary blood flow. In addition, atrial enlargement may lead to supraventricular tachydysrhythmias. Normal increases in blood volume, heart rate, and cardiac output during pregnancy can increase left-to-right shunting.

A systolic ejection murmur with splitting of the second heart sound may be heard at the left upper sternal border. The ECG often shows right axis deviation and may show supraventricular tachycardia. Chest radiographs often show right heart enlargement and prominent pulmonary vascularity.

In addition to the considerations mentioned for patients with VSDs, parturients with ASDs do not tolerate supraventricular tachycardias (SVTs). An acute onset of SVT producing hypotension may require cardioversion followed by digitalization.

Tetralogy of Fallot. Tetralogy of Fallot (TOF) is the most common type of cyanotic congenital heart disease and accounts for approximately 15% of all congenital heart abnormalities.[24] It consists of an intraventricular septal defect, pulmonary stenosis, an overriding aorta, and right ventricular hypertrophy. In the past, few women with TOF lived to child-bearing age, but palliative and corrective surgery have increased long-term survival. Parturients with uncorrected TOF may have mortality rates as high as 12% and fetal death rates as high as 36%.[35] Although maternal mortality is not increased in patients with corrected TOF, fetal mortality rates remain as high as 25%.[40]

The pulmonary stenosis of TOF results in right-to-left shunting through the intraventricular septal defect. Right ventricular contractility and systemic vascular resistance maintain pulmonary blood flow and, when decreased, will increase right-to-left shunting with hypoxia and peripheral cyanosis. Right ventricular outflow obstruction can also be caused by infundibular hypertrophy common to TOF. Increased myocardial contractility may produce increased pulmonary infundibular obstruction and result in increased right-to-left shunting.

TOF causes cyanosis, decreased exercise tolerance, and dyspnea. Sudden decreases in systemic vascular resistance, increases in myocardial contractility, and concomitant increases in pulmonary outflow tract obstruction will precipitate acute episodes of hypoxia, cyanosis, and intense dyspnea, known as hypercyanotic or TET spells. Physical examination often demonstrates clubbing of the digits and a systolic thrill at the left sternal border in the second or third intercostal space. The ECG demonstrates right axis deviation, and the chest x-ray film shows cardiac enlargement with normal pulmonary markings. Cardiac catheterization will demonstrate the right-to-left shunt with decreased pulmonary artery pressure.

The parturient with uncorrected TOF will require invasive monitoring during labor and delivery, including arterial and central venous pressure catheters. The following considerations are important in the management of these patients:

1. Decreases in systemic vascular resistance will increase the right-to-left shunt, exacerbating hypoxia and cyanosis.

2. Decreases in venous return or circulating volume reduce right ventricular output and increase right-to-left shunt.

3. Myocardial depression and excessive myocardial contractility are poorly tolerated.

Regional anesthesia must be used with extreme caution since rapid decreases in systemic vascular resistance can result in profound maternal and fetal hypoxia. Labor and delivery may be managed with systemic narcotics, pudendal block, and local anesthetic infiltration. For cesarean section, general anesthesia is recommended over regional anesthesia. Invasive monitoring is necessary for constant blood pressure and central venous pressure determinations. Myocardial depression must be minimized, and normal venous return must be maintained. Inhalational anesthetics are usually tolerated as well as narcotics and nitrous oxide. If infundibular stenosis is present, tachycardia and increased myocardial contractility will not be well tolerated. Pulse oximetry will provide early warning of decreased peripheral oxygen saturation from increases in right-to-left shunt. Desaturation must be treated rapidly by increasing oxygen delivery and systemic vascular resistance. If infundibular hypertrophy is significant and hypercyanotic spells persist, heart rate and infundibular spasm can be controlled with beta-blockade.[26]

Eisenmenger's Syndrome. Eisenmenger's syndrome is a constellation of cardiac disorders affecting approximately 3% of all patients with congenital heart disease.[39] Features of the syndrome include pulmonary hypertension, right-to-left intracardiac shunting, and cyanosis. The shunt may be at atrial, ventricular, or aortopulmonary levels, depending on the location of the anatomic defect. Most patients with Eisenmenger's syndrome have a poor prognosis; maternal mortality is as high as 60% and fetal mortality is between 30% and 54% for parturients with VSDs.[41, 42] Termination of pregnancy is usually advised for parturients with VSDs and Eisenmenger's syndrome.

Right-to-left shunting is determined by the size of the circulatory communication, the relationship between pulmonary and systemic vascular resistances, and the contractile state of the heart.[26] Pregnancy is poorly tolerated since the progressive decrease in systemic vascular resistance will increase the right-to-left shunt. Increases in heart rate, stroke volume, and pulmonary artery pressure will also increase right-to-left shunting and decrease pulmonary blood flow.

Patients usually seek treatment for dyspnea and peripheral cyanosis. Intrauterine growth retardation secondary to chronic lack of oxygen is common. The type of murmur depends on the location of the shunt.[26] Electrocardiography usually shows right ventricular hypertrophy, and chest radiographs demonstrate right ventricular enlargement with prominent pulmonary vascular markings.

These patients are at increased risk and must be monitored throughout pregnancy for arterial oxygen desaturation. During labor and delivery invasive monitoring is required, and the following recommendations are helpful for management:

1. Decreases in systemic vascular resistance and venous return are poorly tolerated. Adequate crystalloid replacement and maintenance of hematocrit are necessary to prevent further O_2 desaturation.[26]

2. A maternal hematocrit greater than 60% and/or oxygen saturation below 80% are poor prognostic indicators.[30]

3. Acute elevations in pulmonary vascular resistance should be minimized.

The anesthetic management of parturients with Eisenmenger's syndrome is the same as that for TOF.

MISCELLANEOUS HEART DISEASE: PRIMARY PULMONARY HYPERTENSION

Primary pulmonary hypertension mainly afflicts young women of child-bearing age and has a maternal death rate of 50% or more, especially in association with Eisenmenger's syndrome.[41, 43] Pregnancy is contraindicated. Elective termination of unplanned pregnancy is recommended because of high mortality.[41, 43]

The main pathophysiologic abnormality is pulmonary hypertension with pressures exceeding 30/15 mmHg and mean pulmonary artery pressures often exceeding 25 mmHg.[44] Medial hypertrophy and intimal fibrosis of the pulmonary vasculature develop in response to chronic pulmonary hypertension and result in increased right ventricular pressure. The right ventricle hypertrophies and, in time, fails. Left ventricular dysfunction and decreased cardiac output follow.[44] Tricuspid insufficiency usually occurs and prominent A waves in the jugular veins can usually be observed. Cardiac changes during pregnancy and postpartum may lead to acute right ventricular failure with circulatory collapse and death.

Patients have dyspnea and fatigue with poor peripheral pulses. A systolic ejection murmur over the pulmonary valve is usually heard. Electrocardiography shows right ventricular hypertrophy and signs of right atrial enlargement. Chest radiographs usually show cardiac enlargement with a prominent pulmonary artery shadow. Heart catheterization is diagnostic, indicating pulmonary hypertension with a normal wedge pressure.

Cardiac catheterization is important and permits assessment of the severity of pulmonary hypertension, the reactivity of the pulmonary vasculature to vasodilators, and the presence of right ventricular failure. At the time of planned delivery, systemic arterial and pulmonary artery pressure monitoring is recommended. Additional recommendations include:

1. Strict limitations of exercise are necessary. If signs of right heart failure develop, hospitalization with strict bed rest is mandatory.

2. Anticoagulation should be considered.

3. Acute increases in pulmonary vascular resistance due to hypoxia, hypercarbia, lung hyperinflation, pharmacologic vasoconstrictors, acidosis, and stress should be minimized.

4. Decreases in both systemic vascular resistance and right ventricular preload are poorly tolerated.

5. Intravascular fluid overload is also poorly tolerated, and the increased venous return common in the postpartum period may lead to acute decompensation.[44]

Any anesthetic may be dangerous. Regional anesthesia with local anesthetics is especially dangerous because of acute decreases in systemic vascular resistance and should be avoided. Spinal and epidural opiates have been used for labor analgesia but are ineffective for surgical procedures. For labor, the use of spinal or epidural narcotics in combination with intravenous narcotics will provide pain relief but may result in neonatal respiratory depression.

General anesthesia is recommended for cesarean section. Induction with thiopental and succinylcholine may result in acute increases in pulmonary artery pressure and produce acute right heart failure. Inhalational induction in combination with intravenous narcotics may result in the greatest cardiovascular stability. Since the risk of aspiration is increased, continuous cricoid pressure after the loss of consciousness and pretreatment with oral antacids and H_2-receptor blocking drugs is recommended.

Elevations of central venous pressure and pulmonary artery pressures are initial signs of right ventricular decompensation. Specific causes of acute right-sided failure including light anesthesia, hypoxia, acidosis, and hypercarbia should be sought out and corrected. Inotropic agents such as dopamine or isoproterenol may improve cardiac output, and low-dose sodium nitroprusside or phentolamine may improve pulmonary blood flow.

Vascular Disease

EMBOLIC EVENTS

Embolic events are among the leading causes of maternal mortality.[45, 46] The clinical presentation, diagnosis, treatment, and prognosis depend on the type of material embolized, the size of the emboli, and the target organs affected. The three types of embolic events that can occur during pregnancy are thrombotic, amniotic, and air embolizations. Embolic events can occur during both cesarean section and vaginal delivery. Air may be the most frequently embolized material, followed by thrombus, with amniotic fluid being the rarest of all materials significantly embolized. Both amniotic and air emboli tend to be present in labor or in association with delivery, with thrombotic embolism usually confined to the puerperium. The lungs are the most common targets for emboli, although any organ may be in jeopardy if an intracardiac shunt exists.

Thromboembolism. Thromboembolic conditions have been well documented since the early nineteenth century.[47] Risk factors include increased maternal age and parity, obesity, cesarean section, prolonged bed rest during pregnancy, estrogen therapy for lactation suppression, blood type other than O, and antithrombin III (AT III) deficiency.[48, 49]

The etiology of thrombosis is best described in terms of Virchow's classic triad: vessel wall trauma, venous stasis, and alterations in the coagulation mechanism.[47] All of these factors may contribute to the increased risk of thromboembolism in the pregnant or postpartum patient (Chapter 2). Vessel wall injury appears to be unnecessary for the initiation of thrombosis since thrombosis can occur without a clear history of vessel trauma. However, trauma to the calf or pelvic veins in the parturient may contribute to the increased incidence of thrombosis, especially pelvic thrombophlebitis after cesarean section.[50]

The most common clinical presentation of a thrombolytic disorder in pregnancy is pulmonary thromboembolism. This produces complex alterations in pulmonary mechanics and circulatory function. These changes depend on the quantity and size of the pulmonary embolus, the sites of pulmonary artery obstruction, and the presence of preexisting cardiopulmonary diseases. A single small embolus may have no effect, whereas a large thrombus may straddle the pulmonary artery bifurcation or may break up and shower both lungs with multiple small emboli. With a unilateral pulmonary thromboembolus, the right lower lobe is the area affected most frequently. A large saddle embolus may cause fatal obstruction of the proximal pulmonary circulation. Pulmonary embolism does not always result in pulmonary infarction. The ratio of infarct to emboli is about 1 to 10. Recurrent pulmonary emboli often result in pulmonary hypertension.

Since the pulmonary arteries receive right ventricular output, an embolus in the main pulmonary artery or in its major branches can significantly lower left ventricular filling and output. In patients with limited cardiac reserve, the resulting reduction in coronary artery blood flow is poorly tolerated. The right ventricle is comparatively thin-walled and becomes an early target for increased right ventricular pressures. Right coronary blood flow does not seem to decrease during embolization; rather, it seems to increase secondary to local autoregulation. It may take a longer time to develop right ventricular failure, depending on the preexisting cardiovascular status. With a massive pulmonary embolism of any type, acute cardiovascular collapse, hypotension, and refractory shock may occur.

Respiratory changes of pulmonary thromboembolism include ventilation/perfusion inequalities with hypoxemia, bronchoconstriction, surfactant loss with atelectasis, and regional pulmonary edema. Venoarterial and intrapulmonary shunting contribute to the profound hypoxemia. Bronchoconstriction has been attributed to hypocarbia and to release of humoral factors, such as serotonin, histamine, and bradykinin. The hypoxemia of pulmonary thromboembolism is not fully corrected by oxygen administration, indicating severe intrapulmonary shunt.

Clinical manifestations of pulmonary embolism are nonspecific, and the diagnosis is frequently missed even in patients with segmental or larger vessel occlusion. Presenting signs include shortness of breath, chest pain often described as dull substernal tightness, altered sensorium, cough, hemoptysis, sweating, syncope, and tachycardia. A sudden gasp during mechanical ventilation may be the first indication of an intraoperative pulmonary embolus. Common physical findings include tachypnea at 30 to 40 shallow breaths per minute, decreased breath sounds, rales, tachycardia, and pyrexia. Pain, tenderness, swelling, and warmth of the phlebitic limb, including Homan's sign, are also highly significant findings. A chest x-ray film may offer evidence confirming the diagnosis and pinpoint the location of the embolus by showing ipsilateral atelectasis, diminished vascular markings, diaphragmatic elevation, and pleural effusion. The electrocardiogram may show changes consistent with right ventricular strain or failure and tachydysrhythmias. Both chest x-ray film and ECG may, however, be normal even in the presence of a large pulmonary embolus. Moser[51] states that the chief value of the chest x-ray film and ECG in assessing suspected pulmonary thromboembolism is to rule out other causes of chest pain, such as pneumothorax, rib fracture, tumor, pneumonia, or primary cardiac disease.

Treatment of pulmonary embolism is designed to support the circulation and prevent extension of thrombosis or recurrence of emboli by systemic anticoagulation.[52] Surgical thrombectomy may be indicated in very few selected cases. Oxygen therapy is essential, and tracheal intubation for mechanical ventilation is usually necessary. Maternal O_2 tension should be maintained at 70 to 100 mmHg to prevent fetal hypoxia. Intravenous morphine will relieve pain and anxiety. Fluid status should be monitored closely to prevent right ventricular overload, and pulmonary edema, congestive heart failure, and cardiogenic shock should be treated with diuretics and inotropic agents.

Anticoagulation is the cornerstone of therapy for pulmonary embolism.[53] After one thromboembolic event, there is a 12% risk of another embolus during the same pregnancy and a 5% to 10% risk of recurrent thromboembolism with subsequent pregnancies.[49, 54] Initial anticoagulation should be with intravenous heparin, since its effect is immediate. Heparin is a large mucopolysaccharide molecule with a molecular weight of nearly 20,000 daltons. It acts by binding antithrombin III, heparin cofactor, to inhibit the formation of thrombin. The lack of thrombin prevents the conversion of fibrinogen to fibrin. Heparin also increases the level of activated factor X inhibitor, which interferes with the production of thrombin from prothrombin. Heparin also inhibits the activation of factor IX, Christmas factor. Heparin prevents the formation of further thrombi but does not lyse clots already present. Heparin has a short half-life of 1.5 hours and is administered by continuous intravenous infusion for pulmonary thromboembolism. A simple heparin protocol recommended by Bolan[54] is as follows:

1. Draw a baseline complete blood count (CBC), prothrombin time (PT), partial thromboplastin time (PTT), and platelet count.
2. Give a loading dose of 5000 units of heparin by intravenous bolus.
3. a. Prepare heparin infusion with a concentration of 100 units/ml by adding 50,000 units of heparin to 500 ml of normal saline.
   b. Start continuous heparin infusion at a rate of approximately 1000 units/hour. Alternatively, the formula of 5 to 20 units/kg/hour may be used to calculate the initial infusion rate.
   c. Adjust infusion rate to achieve a PTT of two to three times the control. Check the PTT after any change in infusion rate and once or twice daily after the infusion is fixed.
   d. Control the flow rate of heparin infusion with the use of an electronic infusion pump.
4. Check the CBC and urinalysis every other day to monitor for occult hemorrhage.

The greatest risk of heparin therapy is occult hemorrhage, which may occur with an incidence ranging from 4% to 33%.[55] In addition, heparin may cause allergic skin reactions, alopecia, osteoporosis, and thrombocytopenia.

The oral agent most commonly used for systemic anticoagulation is sodium warfarin (Coumadin), a competitive inhibitor of vitamin K. Warfarin is a small molecule (molecular weight = 1000 daltons) that crosses the placenta readily and may anticoagulate a fetus with immature liver enzyme systems and cause birth defects if administered during the first trimester. Warfarin therapy in the late third trimester can cause fetal bleeding before or after delivery. Bonnar[56] reports an overall fetal mortality rate of between 15% and 30% in women taking oral anticoagulants during pregnancy. Most investigators no longer recommend the use of warfarin at any point during pregnancy because of these adverse effects.

For patients on heparin therapy at the time of labor and delivery, fetal hemorrhage is not a risk factor because maternal heparin does not anticoagulate the fetus. The half-life of heparin is short, and often there is no need to reverse the anticoagulant effects, especially if delivery is anticipated more than 4 to 6 hours after the last heparin injection. The usual recommendation is simply to stop administering heparin as soon as the patient goes into labor or to omit the heparin dose on the morning of induction or elective cesarean section. If an emergency delivery or cesarean section is indicated during heparin therapy, protamine, a heparin antagonist, may be administered. Each milligram of protamine neutralizes 100 units of heparin. The calculated dose of protamine should be administered slowly intravenously at a rate of 50 mg per 5-minute period.

The role of surgery in the treatment of thromboembolic disease during pregnancy is limited. Procedures that have been performed include femoral vein or vena cava interruption, thrombectomy, and pulmonary embolectomy. Embolectomy should be reserved for parturients with massive saddle emboli that are often fatal before heparin therapy can take effect. The mortality from embolectomy is high (about 80%), especially during pregnancy.[57]

Anesthetic management of parturients with pulmonary thromboembolism depends on the time of onset of the disease process. When thromboembolism occurs before delivery, the primary management goal is to provide anesthesia for an anticoagulated patient. When pulmonary embolism occurs during labor, the goal is to provide resuscitation including airway establishment, ventilation, oxygenation, inotropic support, heparin anticoagulation, and rapid delivery, if indicated. The goal of anticoagulation is to prolong the PTT 1.5 to 2.5 times normal control values. Many fear that such anticoagulation significantly increases the risks of regional anesthetics such as epidural and spinal blocks.[58] Epidural, subdural, and subarachnoid bleeding resulting in spinal cord compression and permanent neurologic dysfunction has been reported following regional blocks in anticoagulated patients.[58]

As with any anesthetic, the risks of regional blocks in anticoagulated parturients must be balanced by the benefits to the mother and fetus. Although neurologic sequelae of regional anesthetics are rare, spinal or epidural hematomas can produce catastrophic consequences. Vascular trauma often occurs during needle placement, especially during epidural blocks. Phillips and colleagues[59] reported a 3% incidence of bloody tap during epidural and spinal blocks and noted a 6% incidence when multiple needle passes were made. Inadvertent epidural vein cannulation occurs with an incidence of 1% to 10% during epidural blocks.[60] Even in patients receiving minidose heparin therapy, there are no case reports or prospective studies that provide assurances that spinal and epidural techniques are completely safe.[61]

Considerations for general anesthesia include careful manipulation of the lips and oral mucosa, atraumatic endotracheal intubation, avoidance of nasal instrumentation, avoidance of central venous lines unless necessary for inotropic therapy, and close observation for excessive intraoperative and postoperative bleeding.

Amniotic Fluid Embolism. Amniotic fluid embolism is a rare, unpredictable, and usually unpreventable obstetric catastrophe. It is initiated by entry of amniotic fluid into the maternal circulation and is characterized by the sudden onset of severe dyspnea, tachypnea, and cyanosis during labor, delivery, or the early puerperium.

Amniotic fluid embolism was first reported by Meyer[62] in 1926. It was reported again in an experiment on laboratory animals by Warden[63] in

1927. The importance of this condition and these early studies was not established until 1941, when Steiner and Lushbaugh[64] noted the clinical and pathologic findings in eight women who died suddenly during or just after labor. Schneider and coworkers[65] in 1968 showed that the lethal qualities of human amniotic fluid when infused intravenously into dogs were greatly enhanced by the addition of meconium.

The incidence of amniotic fluid embolism has been reported to be between 1 in 8,000 and 1 in 80,000 pregnancies.[64, 66, 67] The mortality rate is very high. Although it is a rare occurrence, amniotic fluid embolism still remains a leading cause of maternal and fetal death. In 1979, Morgan[68] reviewed 272 cases of amniotic fluid embolism reported in the United Kingdom for a combined mortality rate of 86%, with 25% of the deaths occurring within the first hour of the onset of symptoms. Even with optimal critical care management a high mortality rate persists.

Factors predisposing to amniotic fluid embolism include advanced maternal age, multiple pregnancy, macrosomic fetus, and short labor with tetanic contractions often stimulated by oxytocin.[69] Other potential causative factors suggested include fetal demise, meconium staining of amniotic fluid, amniotomy, preeclampsia, cesarean section delivery, abruptio placentae, placenta previa, ruptured uterus, amniocentesis, insertion of an intrauterine pressure catheter, and pregnancy at term with the presence of an intrauterine device. Morgan[68] has, however, only documented significant association between amniotic fluid embolism and advanced maternal age. In order for amniotic fluid embolism to occur, the amniotic fluid must enter the maternal circulation. Currently, there are three recognized conditions that permit this to occur: amniotomy, laceration of the endocervical or uterine vessels, and a pressure gradient sufficient to force amniotic fluid into the maternal circulation.

The two life-threatening consequences of amniotic fluid embolism, cardiopulmonary collapse and DIC, may occur in sequence or, more commonly, together. Amniotic fluid embolism causes acute pulmonary hypertension with a sudden reduction of blood flow to the left heart, decreased left ventricular output, and subsequent peripheral vascular collapse. The sudden development of pulmonary hypertension precipitates acute cor pulmonale and congestive heart failure with pulmonary edema. Ventilation/perfusion mismatching occurs, as in pulmonary thromboembolism, and produces hypoxemia and tissue hypoxia.

The toxicity of intravenously infused amniotic fluid appears to vary remarkably depending on its particulate matter, especially meconium.[70] Meconium includes shed fetal squamous cells or squames, fetal hairs, vernix caseosa, and mucin. If cor pulmonale and cardiogenic shock are not immediately fatal, massive hemorrhage from DIC soon becomes evident. The etiology of DIC is controversial. Evidence suggests that a thromboplastin-like activity of amniotic fluid causes widespread intravascular deposition of fibrin clots with activation of the fibrinolytic system. Such processes defibrinate the blood[71] producing afibrinogenemia, coagulopathy, and hemorrhage.[72] Trophoblasts also possess powerful thromboplastin-like effects. Systemic embolization of trophoblastic material may play an even greater role in the coagulopathy of amniotic fluid embolism than has been appreciated to date.

The most significant pathologic findings at autopsy are limited to the lungs. Grossly, the lungs show evidence of pulmonary edema in 70% of the cases.[73] Alveolar hemorrhage and pulmonary embolism of amniotic fluid materials are present. Embolic particles in the lungs, especially squames and trophoblasts, often confirm the diagnosis, but may be missed because of their small size.[72] Amorphous debris, epithelial squames, trophoblasts, and mucin often lodge in small arteries, arterioles, and capillaries of the lungs.[71] Since uterine trauma is a significant factor in pathogenesis because it provides direct venous access to the maternal circulation, signs of uterine laceration or rupture should be sought.[73] Acute right ventricular dilation is usually present. Amniotic fluid elements are sometimes found in uterine vessels, right atrium, and right ventricle. Histologic evaluation of other end organs confirms the magnitude of embolization, with particulate matter evident in the maternal brain, kidneys, liver, and spleen.

In a small percentage of patients, the onset of symptoms may begin before labor. The majority of patients, however, develop symptoms during the latter part of the first stage of labor or, to a lesser extent, during birth.[68] There have been two cases of amniotic fluid embolism in association with delivery of the placenta, and one case occurred 32 hours postpartum.[68] In one series, 45% of cases were associated with placental abruption of varying degrees. Many authorities believe abruptio placentae to be one of the primary catalysts in the development of amniotic fluid embolism.

In a review of amniotic embolism cases, potential predisposing conditions already present or developing during labor and delivery include, in order of frequency, severe amnionitis, moderate to severe pregnancy-induced hypertension, cephalopelvic disproportion, and traumatic midforceps delivery. Prodromal symptoms may include sudden chills, shivering, sweating, anxiety, and coughing followed by signs of respiratory distress, shock, cardiovascular collapse, and convulsions. All patients were conscious during the onset of symptomatology.[73] Respiratory distress as evidenced by cyanosis, tachypnea, and bronchospasm frequently culminates in fulminant pulmonary edema. Hypoxemia produces cyanosis and accounts for air hunger, restlessness, convulsions, and coma. Reflex tachypnea results from oxygen desaturation and cardiovascular collapse. Hypotension and tachyarrhythmias ensue and often progress to cardiac arrest. Convulsions may be an early manifestation of central nervous system ischemia and may be rapidly followed by coma and death. If the patient survives the initial episode, exsanguinating hemorrhage from DIC and uterine atony ensue. In all cases studied, bleeding was never documented as an initial indication of amniotic fluid embolism.[73]

The differential diagnosis of amniotic fluid embolism includes air embolism, aspiration pneumonitis, eclamptic convulsions and coma, local anesthetic toxicity, acute left heart failure, cerebrovascular accident, and hemorrhagic shock. A definitive diagnosis is usually made at postmortem examination by demonstration of amniotic fluid material in the maternal circulation and lungs. In living patients, definitive diagnosis can be made by identification of lanugo or fetal hairs, fetal squames, and trophoblasts in an aspirate of blood from the right heart or pulmonary circulation.[74] Fetal squames have even been recovered in the maternal sputum in some cases.[75] Additional diagnostic tools for confirmation of amniotic fluid embolism include (1) chest x-ray film, which may show right atrial and ventricular enlargement, a prominent proximal pulmonary artery, and pulmonary edema; (2) lung scan, which may demonstrate some areas of reduced radioactivity in the lung fields; (3) central venous pressure (CVP), with an initial rise due to pulmonary hypertension and eventually a profound drop due to severe hemorrhage; and (4) deranged measurements of coagulation activity. Procoagulant activity is increased normally in pregnancy (Chapter 2). However, with amniotic fluid embolism and DIC, blood fails to clot rather than clot readily, platelet counts decrease, afibrinogenemia occurs, PT and PTT lengthen, and fibrin degradation products appear in plasma.

The best management of amniotic fluid embolism is to prevent it. Trauma to the uterus should be avoided during any manipulation, especially insertion of an intrauterine pressure catheter or amniotomy. Incision of the placenta during cesarean delivery should also be avoided if possible.[68] Since one of the most frequent predisposing factors is considered to be tumultuous labor, excessively strong and frequent uterine contractions should be controlled by administration of intravenous beta-adrenergic tocolytics[68] or magnesium sulfate. In addition, oxytocic drugs may precipitate tetanic uterine contractions and should be used appropriately and judiciously.

In most cases, no therapy has proved effective. Whenever unexplained cyanosis and shock develop during labor, a diagnosis of amniotic fluid embolism should be considered.[76] Assuming accurate diagnosis is made before death, cardiopulmonary resuscitation, blood volume replacement, and early treatment of coagulopathy should be instituted quickly.

Resuscitation should begin with endotracheal intubation and mechanical ventilation with high inspired oxygen concentrations and positive end-expiratory pressure (PEEP) to increase functional residual capacity and improve oxygenation. Excessive PEEP may, however, produce a decrease in cardiac output and venous return. Some authorities feel that hyperbaric O_2 or cardiopulmonary bypass for extracorporeal oxygenation would be worthwhile in treating the severe tissue hypoxia accompanying amniotic fluid embolism.[75] To prevent and/or recognize further deterioration, careful monitoring is essential in managing parturients with amniotic fluid embolism. Arterial lines allow monitoring of arterial blood gases and chemistries; central venous or pulmonary artery catheters allow monitoring of cardiac status and circulatory volume.

At present, there is no clear regimen of drug therapy that reverses the symptoms and complications of amniotic fluid embolism. Drug therapy and other treatments have been supportive to date and aimed at improving ventilation/perfusion ratios, maintaining adequate blood pressure, and treating DIC.

Terbutaline therapy may offer both bronchodilation and tocolysis to undelivered parturients with live fetuses. Isoproterenol, also a tocolytic, relieves pulmonary vasoconstriction and improves cardiac function but causes peripheral vasodilation that can exacerbate hypotension. Dopamine may be preferable to isoproterenol because it improves cardiac function and increases mesenteric and renal perfusion unless infused in large doses. Aminophylline therapy for bronchodilation and cardiac stimulation and enhanced diaphragmatic contractility is controversial due to accompanying tachycardia. Hydrocortisone in doses up to 2 g/24 hours may reduce pulmonary vasospasm and pulmonary edema and augment hemodynamic responses to inotropic agents like dopamine, epinephrine, and norepinephrine. In the event of heart failure, digitalization with a rapidly acting agent is recommended.[77] Diuretics can be used if pulmonary wedge pressure is elevated. Indomethacin has been effective in treating severe pulmonary hypertension in laboratory animals and may be considered for use in a desperate situation with high mortality.

Hypotension should be treated first by left uterine displacement if the patient is undelivered. This can be accomplished easily by insertion of a wedge under the right hip (Chapter 2, Fig. 2–3). The vasopressor of choice is ephedrine because it does not decrease uterine perfusion (Chapter 2). However, if the fetus has expired or been delivered, isoproterenol or dobutamine can be used. The intravenous fluid of choice should be lactated Ringer's solution since its pH approximates that of blood. The volume of infusion will depend on filling pressures, as monitored by CVP or Swan-Ganz catheters. If acidosis is present, sodium bicarbonate should be administered and will also augment hemodynamic response to inotropic agents.

Treatment of the bleeding diathesis will require blood replacement with fresh whole blood if available or with blood components including fresh-frozen plasma, cryoprecipitate, and platelets. Heparin therapy for

DIC is controversial, with no clear studies supporting or contraindicating its use.

Uterine bleeding in a postpartum patient can often be controlled by massage and intravenous oxytocin. If uterine bleeding persists, one should consider careful exploration for retained placenta, retained fetal membranes, cervical tears, or uterine lacerations. Like oxytocin, methylergonovine is also a strong uterine stimulant that can be given very slowly by IV push. The use of prostaglandins (Hemabate) to control hemorrhage is controversial and may aggravate bronchospasm and pulmonary hypertension. The use of epsilon-aminocaproic acid (Amicar) and aprotinin (Trasylol) is not well documented in treatment of DIC associated with amniotic embolus, but these agents can be used when rapid reversal of the lytic state is indicated just before delivery. If the fetus is still viable, aprotinin (Trasylol) may prove to be the drug of choice since it does not cross the placenta. Aminocaproic acid readily crosses the placenta and is teratogenic as well.[77]

When amniotic fluid embolism occurs, the accompanying respiratory distress, cardiovascular collapse, and bleeding diathesis are contraindications to any regional anesthetics. With severe shock, general anesthetics must be administered with extreme caution. Since immediate delivery is necessary, emergency cesarean section is usually required. The choice of anesthetic agents will depend on the patient's condition, and aggressive cardiopulmonary resuscitation may be all that the anesthesiologist can provide. Anesthetic agents that produce the least myocardial depression should be administered and usually include narcotics, relaxants, and amnesics in preference to volatile inhalational agents.

Venous Air Embolism. The phenomenon of air embolism has been recognized since the Napoleonic Wars when Baron Larrey observed that cavalry officers suffering saber wounds of the head and neck frequently died not as a result of blood loss but because of air bubbles clogging the right heart and pulmonary circulation.[78] By 1885, Senn had described in great detail the pathophysiology of air entrainment from cranial veins. He not only noted the presence of air in the heart and pulmonary vessels, but also observed that it could be removed by aspiration through rubber catheters that had been inserted into the right heart via the neck veins.[79]

Until recently, it was considered highly unlikely that venous air embolism (VAE) could occur during a cesarean or vaginal delivery. This is due in part to the difficulty encountered in making the diagnosis. In fatal cases, the reports and autopsy evidence may not be sufficiently detailed to permit certain diagnosis. In nonfatal cases, no clinical signs and symptoms are specific for VAE. Previous attempts to determine the incidence of VAE at delivery were based on reports of maternal deaths. Data from England and Wales indicate seven deaths from VAE in approximately 750,000 live births,[46] for a maternal mortality of approximately 1 in 100,000 live births.[80] In most recent published statistics for maternal deaths in the United States,[45] 25 deaths (about 1%) were thought to be due to VAE, although the circumstances of these deaths were not disclosed in detail.

Recent studies by Malinow and coworkers[81] and Fong and colleagues[82] indicate that although maternal death from VAE may be a rare event, the occurrence of VAE during cesarean section may be more common than previously appreciated. Using a precordial Doppler signal change as evidence of an air embolic event, Malinow and coworkers[81] noted positive Doppler changes in 52% (46 of 89) of cesarean patients. Fong and colleagues[82] monitored patients with both precordial Doppler and precordial two-dimensional echocardiography and noted a 71% incidence of changes consistent with VAE during general anesthesia for cesarean section and a 39% incidence of such changes during epidural anesthesia for cesarean section.

Certain conditions must exist for VAE to occur. As noted by early experimentation, there must be a vascular access, usually venous, and a gradient between the surgical incision and the right heart to promote the movement of air from outside the body into the heart and lungs.[83] Gradients as small as 5 cm have been shown to result in the entrainment of large amounts of air (up to 200 ml).[84]

Certain features of pregnancy and parturition make VAE possible.[80] These include the following:

1. Uterine sinuses may entrain air during placental separation.
2. Uterine manipulation, manual extraction of the placenta, and incision of the uterus may all result in the opening of uterine venous sinuses, all potential conduits for air entry.
3. Negative intra-abdominal and uterine venous pressures created by the knee-chest and Trendelenburg positions can increase gravitational gradients draining the uterine venous sinuses.
4. Douching during pregnancy has been associated with VAE.

In a review of 45 fatal cases and two nonfatal cases, the following factors were noted.[85] The average age was 32 years, with seven of the patients (15%) delivered by cesarean section with either no labor or incomplete labor. Among the laboring patients with VAE, 12 patients presented during the first stage, 12 during the second stage, and 14 during the third stage. The most frequently associated finding was placenta previa, which occurred in 24% of patients. Manual extraction of the placenta was performed in eight patients.

VAE has also been reported during the puerperium.[85] In 10 patients VAE occurred 24 hours postpartum; of these 10 cases, five occurred with the patient in the knee-chest position, a therapy employed at that time (1960) for retroversion and subinvolution of the uterus. Other factors felt to be associated with postpartum VAE included vaginal douching and packing of the uterus.

When air enters the central venous circulation, it may embolize to the lungs directly or to the heart and brain through intracardiac shunts, like a patent foramen ovale, to cause significant maternal morbidity and mortality. The severity of VAE will depend on the patient's general condition, the rate of air entrainment, the type of entrained gas, and the total volume of gas introduced. The prolonged continuous entrainment of about 1 to 3 ml/kg/min for as long as 1 to 2 minutes could result in fatal VAE.[84] In the presence of N_2O during general anesthesia, a smaller volume of air could be rapidly doubled by the addition of N_2O to the air mixture to produce fatal VAE.

When massive VAE occurs, air collects in the right ventricle to create an air lock between the right ventricle and the pulmonary artery.[86] This air lock causes foaming of blood, valve dysfunction, and an acute decrease in right ventricular stroke volume. Central venous pressures increase and pulmonary artery pressures decrease. Since pulmonary blood flow has ceased, oxygenation is impaired and anoxia results. Left ventricular filling is severely diminished and cardiac output drops. Without immediate intervention, cardiac arrest is inevitable. Boyer and Curry[87] have shown that bronchospasm accompanies these circulatory changes.

In nonfatal cases, small emboli do not produce an air-trapping effect but instead enter the pulmonary circulation to produce pulmonary hypertension and ventilation/perfusion mismatching.[79] Paradoxical embolization of air across a patent foramen ovale has resulted in coronary and cerebral VAE in parturients.[88]

Signs of VAE include gasping ventilatory efforts, chest pain, increases in central venous pressure, ECG changes, hypotension, changes in heart sounds, cyanosis, and cardiac arrest.[89] Symptoms of chest pain and/or dyspnea will depend on the venous air volume embolized. Malinow and colleagues[81] found a significant relationship between unsolicited complaints of chest pain and/or dyspnea during cesarean section and the occurrence of positive Doppler changes. The chest pain was described as retrosternal, heavy, nonradiating, and lasting 5 to 10 minutes. In addition, 20% of parturients with Doppler changes complained of dyspnea, and 8% complained of both chest pain and dyspnea. Chest pain was not associated with the type of anesthetic or with surgical exteriorization of the uterus for hysterotomy repair.[81]

The concomitant hypoxemia, ventilation/perfusion mismatch, and increased dead space ventilation will be reflected in decreased oxygen saturation by pulse oximetry and decreased end-tidal CO_2 as measured by capnography. These changes can be verified by blood gas analysis. A precordial ultrasonic Doppler monitor is capable of detecting as little as

0.1 ml of intracardiac air.[90] It has been found that Doppler changes occur in about 50% of all patients undergoing elective cesarean delivery under regional anesthesia.[89] Precordial Doppler monitoring is uncomplicated. The role of precordial Doppler and two-dimensional echocardiography during routine cesarean section for early detection of venous air embolism is still undefined. It has been suggested that precordial Doppler monitoring should be considered for cases at risk for air embolism such as profound hypovolemia, abruptio placentae, or placenta previa.[80]

As in amniotic fluid embolism, the best management of VAE is prevention. Although no studies clearly document reliable techniques to prevent VAE, elimination of such etiologic factors as uterine irrigation, vaginal insufflation, knee-chest position, and extreme Trendelenburg positions during the peripartum period has been suggested.[85] It has been further suggested that obstetricians avoid placing traction on the uterus and exteriorizing the uterus for repair, since traction and exteriorization distend venous sinuses, increasing the risk of VAE.[85] Fong and associates[82] reported that VAE could occur at any time during cesarean section, regardless of anesthetic technique.

Downing and coworkers[91] challenge many of these recommendations and claim that modest head-up patient posture (5° to 10°) did not influence the occurrence of VAE. In addition, they were unable to substantiate the very high incidence of "definite" VAE reported in previous studies.[81, 82, 89] Their findings also differed from these reports with regard to the distribution of VAE in relation to operative events, with the highest incidence of VAE occurring at placenta delivery rather than during hysterotomy[81] or uterine closure.[82] In any event, large uterine sinuses will lie open and be vulnerable to the entry of air from an empty uterus after placental separation.

When VAE occurs, immediate treatment is necessary and may include the following[89]:

1. Prevent further air embolization by placing the patient in reverse Trendelenburg position with a 15° left-sided tilt. This position tends to prevent air from entering the right ventricle, therefore allowing easier aspiration from the superior vena caval–right atrial junction via a central catheter. Lowering the uterus eliminates gravity drainage and the negative pressure gradient between the uterine venous sinuses and the central venous circulation. The surgical field should also be flooded with normal saline to reduce and prevent further entrainment of air.

2. Discontinue N_2O and provide 100% oxygen.

3. Start immediate cardiopulmonary resuscitation if cardiovascular collapse occurs.

4. Advance a catheter to the superior vena caval–right atrial junction from a central vein or peripheral vein and aspirate as much air as possible.

5. If neurologic symptoms develop, precordial echocardiogram and brain computed tomography scan should be performed to search for possible paradoxical air embolism. If left atrial and cerebral air is present, hyperbaric oxygen therapy may reduce air bubble size, both in the heart and in the brain.

There are no studies providing conclusive evidence that any particular anesthetic technique should be either avoided or advocated in VAE. Epidural and spinal anesthesia without adequate volume preloading could predispose the patient to VAE by lowering central venous pressure and increasing the uterine to right atrial "negative" venous pressure gradient. Parturients appear to be at greater risk of clinically significant VAE under general anesthesia.[82] Any reduced risk with regional anesthesia may be attributed to generous volume loading prior to induction of epidural or spinal anesthesia. Patients in a recent study[82] also received 70% N_2O with solubility characteristics that could expand small, insignificant air emboli into larger, clinically significant emboli. Further investigation is needed to determine whether N_2O administration for general anesthesia increases the risk of VAE during cesarean section.

ARTERIAL VESSEL DISORDERS

Coronary Thrombosis and Myocardial Infarction. Coronary artery disease sufficient to cause a myocardial infarction (MI) is uncommon in women of reproductive age. In 68 reported cases of MI during pregnancy there was a 35% mortality rate.[92] Of these 68 patients, only 13% were documented to have coronary artery disease prior to pregnancy. In two-thirds of the women the MI occurred during the third trimester. Mortality for these women was 45%, as compared with 23% in those suffering MI during the first or second trimesters. Thus, the increased hemodynamic burden imposed on the parturients' cardiovascular system in pregnancy may unmask early coronary artery disease in some women and worsen the prognosis for those suffering infarction, especially during the third trimester. The fetus of a woman surviving MI during pregnancy is at increased risk of spontaneous abortion and unexplained stillbirth, possibly related to severe uteroplacental insufficiency.

Antepartum care of women with prior MI includes bed rest to minimize myocardial O_2 demands and nitrates for angina. Convalescence prior to delivery is recommended since delivery within 2 weeks of infarction is associated with increased mortality.[93] Induced delivery under controlled circumstances after a period of hemodynamic stabilization is also recommended. Labor in the lateral recumbent position, O_2 administration, epidural analgesia, and hemodynamic monitoring with pulmonary artery and arterial catheters, pulse oximetry, end-tidal CO_2 analysis, and maternal and fetal ECG monitoring are suggested.

Numerous reports of successful cardiovascular surgery during pregnancy are seen today, including successful correction of most types of congenital and acquired cardiac disease (Chapter 3).[93] Closed mitral valve commissurotomy has been replaced by open valvuloplasty with more favorable perinatal results.[94]

Early reports of cardiopulmonary bypass during pregnancy indicated a fetal wastage of up to 33%.[94] Initiation of cardiopulmonary bypass is followed generally by fetal bradycardia, correctable by high flow rates.[95, 96] With the use of continuous electronic fetal heart rate monitoring, the flow rate can be adjusted to avoid or correct fetal hypoperfusion and bradycardia, reducing fetal mortality to less than 10%.[96] Maternal mortality is highly dependent on the specific nature of the open heart procedure being performed and does not appear to be increased significantly by pregnancy. High-flow/high-pressure normothermic perfusion and continuous electronic fetal heart rate monitoring have produced optimal results for the fetus.[93]

The anesthetic plan for parturients with recent MI should be individualized according to the specific needs of the patient and continues to be somewhat controversial. Aglio and Johnson[97] prefer continuous epidural anesthesia. Hands and colleagues[98] advocate continuous epidural anesthesia for either vaginal or cesarean delivery and recommend a T_3 level using lidocaine, bupivacaine, or 2-chloroprocaine, in conjunction with an opioid, such as fentanyl. Hemodynamic stress evoked by each uterine contraction is effectively diminished with the use of a high-level, continuous epidural anesthesia. Another benefit from continuous epidural anesthesia noted by Hands and coworkers[98] was less blood loss in the event that a planned vaginal delivery failed and cesarean section became necessary. In addition, the epidural catheter can be used for excellent postoperative pain management. If continuous epidural anesthesia is not utilized, Hands and colleagues[98] recommend continuous spinal anesthesia titrated slowly to prevent sudden profound sympathetic blockade with hemodynamic instability.

Epinephrine should not be used to treat hypotensive episodes because of its tachycardic effect, which increases myocardial O_2 demand. Instead, phenylephrine administered incrementally offers less risk of tachycardia and hypertension. With careful titration of local anesthetics and volume preloading, maternal blood pressure and uteroplacental perfusion can be maintained during continuous epidural or spinal anesthesia.[99]

Should there be an absolute contraindication to regional anesthesia in parturients with recent MI, rapid induction of general anesthesia with high-dose opioids is recommended. Risks associated with general anesthesia include trauma from difficult tracheal intubation, neonatal narcosis, and need for postoperative mechanical ventilation of the parturient and/ or neonate. General anesthesia does not effectively control postdelivery pain, especially if the patient was delivered by cesarean section or after generous episioproctotomy for vaginal delivery. Other undesired effects associated with parenteral administration of analgesia and general anesthesia include a decrease in mobility, predisposing the patient to venous stasis and thrombus formation, hypoventilation, aspiration pneumonitis, atelectasis, and decreased intestinal motility with bowel distention and ileus.

After delivery the patient should remain as pain-free and comfortable as possible in an intensive care setting with all previously mentioned monitoring devices left in place (with the exception of the fetal monitor). This is best provided by continuous epidural analgesia using low concentrations of bupivacaine with fentanyl. Oxygen should be continued and mechanical ventilatory assistance provided, if required. High concentrations of oxytocin or ergot alkaloids should not be administered owing to risks of fluid overload from water retention and hypertension from peripheral vasoconstriction. Shivering should be prevented with warmed intravenous solutions and warming blankets. Intravenous low doses of opioids will also alleviate shivering should it develop despite preventive efforts.

Once the patient has recovered from the delivery, she should undergo thorough cardiac assessment including cardiac angiography, reassessment of left ventricular function by echocardiography, contrast or radionuclide ventriculography, and exercise stress testing. Data gained from these procedures will enable the physician to advise the patient regarding exercise, antianginal and anticoagulant therapy, coronary revascularization, and subsequent pregnancy.

While basic care is essentially the same as for any other patient with acute MI, certain considerations for the parturient with recent MI necessitate alterations in management. Teratogenic drugs, like warfarin, should be avoided. If anticoagulation is necessary, heparin is the drug of choice since it is rapidly metabolized and can be reversed by protamine. The fetus should be shielded during all radiographic procedures. After 24 weeks of gestation, the fetus may be delivered in the event of sudden maternal deterioration and inevitable demise. Invasive monitoring is helpful throughout labor, delivery, recovery, and the postpartum period. The least hemodynamically stressful approach for delivery should be chosen after detailed discussion with the patient and family. Limits as to the length of time labor will be permitted prior to operative intervention must be clearly defined should a vaginal delivery be contemplated. Ideally, if vaginal delivery is anticipated or induction of labor is planned, the patient should labor in a fully equipped operating room, set up for rapid cesarean section. A team approach to the patient's needs should be coordinated by the cardiologist, obstetrician, perinatologist, and anesthesiologist.

Marfan's Syndrome. Marfan's syndrome is an autosomal dominant disorder characterized by generalized weakness of connective tissue and cardiovascular anomalies, including cystic medial degeneration with aneurysmal dilation and dissection of the thoracic aorta. Coexisting ocular problems and skeletal abnormalities are common along with excessive length of the long bones (arachnodactyly) and cystic disease of the lungs.

Maternal mortality and morbidity are greatly increased in Marfan's syndrome.[100, 101] Rupture of splenic and aortic aneurysms occurs more often during pregnancy in patients with Marfan's syndrome due to medial necrosis in vessel walls and physiologic increases in cardiac output. In addition, mitral or aortic regurgitation occurs 60% more frequently during pregnancy in parturients with Marfan's syndrome.[102] Some authorities feel that pregnancy places Marfan patients at such peril that elective termination of the pregnancy is indicated.[103, 104] Prognosis remains best when individualized according to serial echocardiographic assessment of aortic root and postvalvular dilation, with pregnancy termination reserved for parturients with enlarging aortic aneurysms or severe aortic regurgitation. Radiographic assessment is not as effective as echocardiography in evaluating aortic root dilation[102] and, therefore, should not be used as the sole indicator of advancing disease. If the aortic root diameter is less than 40 mm, the mortality is less than 5%.[105] If this diameter is greater than 40 mm or if a regurgitant aortic valve is identified, the mortality rate approaches 50%.[105]

Perinatal management is directed toward maintaining normal intravascular pressures throughout pregnancy by prescribing strict bed rest and oral beta-blockers, like propranolol.[106] During labor, continuous epidural anesthesia and low forceps extraction shorten the second stage and minimize Valsalva's maneuvers, which acutely increase intravascular pressures.[101, 103, 104] Propranolol therapy is continued throughout labor, delivery, and the postpartum period. Endocarditis prophylaxis may be indicated due to mitral valve prolapse or aortic regurgitation.

If cesarean section is necessary, retention sutures are used to close the abdomen because of connective tissue weakness and laxity. Regional anesthesia is preferred for vaginal delivery or cesarean section in patients with normal intravascular pressures because it provides for normal to slightly reduced systolic blood pressure and eliminates reflex pushing and attempted Valsalva's maneuvers. Continuous fetal heart rate monitoring during the induction of regional anesthesia should be employed to determine the acceptable degree of systolic hypotension. If general anesthesia is selected for cesarean section, an inhalation technique with halothane is suggested, as hypertension and tachycardia will be less likely and the force of left ventricular ejection of blood against a dilated aorta may be decreased.

Aortic dissection or rupture with severe hemorrhage should always be anticipated. Two large-bore intravenous catheters should be inserted prior to elective delivery, and capabilities for massive whole blood transfusion and rapid resuscitation should be at hand. A cadiovascular surgical team should be consulted and remain on standby for delivery of patients with large aortic aneurysms.

HYPERTENSIVE DISORDERS

Chronic Hypertension. Hypertensive diseases of pregnancy affect approximately 10% of all pregnancies. Causes of hypertension may include renal disease, toxemia, chronic hypertension, or, more rarely, coarctation of the aorta and pheochromocytoma. For the most part, pregnancies complicated by hypertension progress well, with prognosis determined by the degree of vascular involvement and antihypertensive treatment.[107, 108]

Chronic hypertension implies a disease state antedating pregnancy. Chronic hypertension is often suspected if the diastolic pressure remains greater than 80 mmHg throughout the second trimester.[108]

Pregnancy can complicate preexisting hypertension or superimpose new forms of hypertension.[107, 108] Pregnancy will increase intravascular volume, place greater demands on the heart, increase systemic vascular resistance, and limit end-organ perfusion (Chapter 2).

A detailed history and physical examination should be obtained. If chronic hypertension is suspected, laboratory tests, ECG, and chest x-ray film will rule out chronic renal disease, pheochromocytoma, aortic coarctation, and end-organ damage, especially to the heart and kidneys. Abdominal ultrasound will confirm the estimated date of confinement and determine baseline fetal growth and development should any intra-uterine growth retardation occur in later pregnancy.[109] Biophysical profile and nonstress testing are also reliable means of assessing fetal status.

The most widely used antihypertensive drug for parturients with chronic hypertension is alpha-methyldopa, which centrally inhibits adrenergic transmissions from the medulla and hypothalamus. In addition, methyldopa reduces both central and peripheral norepinephrine levels at an average dose of 500 mg three times daily.

Hypertension affects nearly all organ systems and may greatly compromise pregnancy. It may have no effect on the fetus or cause multiple stillbirths. If preeclampsia is superimposed on chronic hypertension, fetal morbidity and mortality are five times greater than with either disease alone.[107, 108] Abruptio placentae is also more common in chronic hypertensive pregnancies.

Perinatal management of a parturient with chronic hypertension involves (1) maintaining an airway and adequate oxygenation, (2) controlling blood pressure by using left lateral tilt or right hip wedge to eliminate aortocaval compression (Chapter 2, Fig. 2–3), and (3) intravenous hydralazine, 2.5 to 5 mg, to maintain diastolic pressure of approximately 90 mmHg. Segmental epidural block is recommended with 1500 ml of Ringer's lactate solution for prehydration. Vasopressors should not be included in the epidural test and top-up doses and should be avoided altogether if possible. Invasive monitoring with arterial, central venous, and pulmonary artery catheters may be necessary for delivery of parturients with severe hypertension.

For cesarean section, either regional or general anesthesia is acceptable, with care taken to prevent acute drops in blood pressure. For general anesthesia, a halogenated agent may be added to blunt any hemodyanamic response to tracheal intubation. Sodium nitroprusside or phentolamine may be indicated to manage an acute hypertensive crisis.

Pregnancy-Induced Hypertension. Preeclampsia or, more commonly, pregnancy-induced hypertension (PIH) is a common complication of gestation. It is one of the most common causes of maternal death in obstetrics and is associated with a significant increase in perinatal morbidity and mortality.[45, 46] Before 1972, the term *toxemia* was used to describe all hypertensive disorders associated with pregnancy. In 1972, the American College of Obstetrics and Gynecology formulated the new definitions and classifications currently in use. PIH is divided into three categories: hypertension alone, preeclampsia, and eclampsia.

A diagnosis of hypertension alone is based on the onset of hypertension before 20 weeks' gestation without proteinuria or edema. A diagnosis of preeclampsia is based on the onset of hypertension with proteinuria and/ or edema after 20 weeks' gestation. Any earlier onset of these signs may suggest a molar pregnancy. Preeclampsia is almost exclusively a disease of the primigravida.[110] It most frequently affects women at the extremes of reproductive age, i.e., less than 20 years of age or greater than 35 years of age. The disease occasionally occurs in the multipara with uterine overdistention, vascular disease, or chronic renal disease.[111] Eclampsia is the combination of preeclampsia and neurologic disorders, such as seizure activity, increased intracranial pressure, or stroke.

Diagnostic criteria for PIH include either blood pressure 140/90 mmHg or greater constituting an increase of either 30 mmHg systolic or 15 mmHg diastolic over baseline values. Observation of these criteria on at least two occasions 6 or more hours apart establishes the diagnosis of mild PIH. The diagnosis of severe PIH is established either when the blood pressure exceeds 160/110 mmHg with proteinuria of 5 g/24 hours or more or when vascular end-organ damage occurs with headache, scotomata, oliguria, or renal failure.

The diagnosis of preeclampsia has traditionally required the identification of PIH plus proteinuria or generalized edema. Many authorities concur that edema, even of the hands and face, is such a common finding in pregnant women that its presence should not validate the existence of preeclampsia any more than its absence should exclude the diagnosis.[111] Proteinuria is an important sign of preeclampsia. Proteinuria is defined as the presence of 300 mg or more of protein in a 24-hour urine collection or a protein measurement of greater than 1 g/L in at least two random urine specimens collected 6 hours or more apart. It is important to note that the degree of proteinuria may fluctuate widely over any 24-hour period, even in severe cases. The addition of proteinuria to hypertension during pregnancy markedly increases the risk of perinatal mortality.

Preeclampsia develops throughout pregnancy and involves most end-organ systems, especially the fetoplacental unit. Decreased uterine blood flow may result in fetal growth retardation, chronic fetal hypoxia, and fetal death.[110]

In the placental bed, arteriolar vasospasm causes decreased fetal perfusion. Eventually, some placental vessels clot off from continuous vasospasm and thrombosis and produce calcified placental infarcts. Fetal outcome depends on early prenatal care.

When the diagnosis of preeclampsia is established, biweekly nonstress tests (NSTs) provide noninvasive monitoring of fetal well-being and permit early delivery of the fetus in jeopardy. With clinical deterioration as demonstrated by proteinuria or neurologic dysfunction, a contraction stress test (CST) or oxytocin challenge test (OCT) will permit more precise evaluation of fetal well-being. Late decelerations of fetal heart rate indicate the need for prompt delivery.

PIH is often associated with inadequate or no prenatal care, multiple gestation, diabetes mellitus, polyhydramnios, and hydatidiform mole. Eclampsia is an extension of preeclampsia, but in many cases preeclampsia never advances to eclampsia either because the disease is mild or because obstetric treatment forestalls progression to eclampsia. Grand mal seizure activity may first appear during labor or postpartum.[112] Seizure activity that occurs more than 48 hours postpartum is more likely associated with an underlying central nervous system lesion rather than with eclampsia.[113]

Preeclampsia–eclampsia has unknown etiology but requires the presence of chorionic villi. An immunologic rejection of fetal tissues by the mother may cause placental vasculitis with ischemia. Such a theory supports the common occurrence of PIH in nulliparas and in conditions associated with an abnormally large mass of trophoblastic tissue, such as molar pregnancy. Recent studies have documented an abnormal maternal immune responsiveness in preeclampsia.[114, 115]

Placental ischemia results in the release of placental renin, which triggers an increase in plasma angiotensin activity. Widespread arteriolar vasoconstriction results in hypertension, tissue hypoxia, and endothelial damage. Platelets adhere to sites of endothelial damage, promoting coagulopathies, such as thrombocytopenia and DIC. Angiotensin-directed aldosterone secretion promotes sodium and water retention. Placental ischemia causes tissue necrosis and release of thromboplastin with fibrin deposition in vasoconstricted glomeruli. Increased renal permeability to albumin and other plasma proteins results.

Placental prostaglandins and their role in the pathogenesis of PIH are being explored.[116] Decreased placental production of prostaglandin E (PGE_1), a potent vasodilator, fails to balance the hypertension and volume loading directed by an overstimulated renin-angiotensin system. Prostacyclin (PGI_2) produces vasodilation, increased uterine blood flow, decreased uterine activity, and platelet inhibition. Thromboxane opposes these effects. In a normal pregnancy, thromboxane production and prostacyclin production are equal. In a pregnancy associated with PIH, thromboxane is produced in much greater quantities than prostacyclin, creating unopposed vasoconstriction.[117]

In the cardiovascular system, intense generalized vasospasm produces hypertension, decreased end-organ perfusion, and tissue and cellular hypoxia. Fluid translocation from intravascular to interstitial compartments is promoted by the combination of high capillary hydrostatic pressures from generalized vasospasm and low colloid oncotic pressures from protein loss. In severe PIH, increased capillary permeability adds to tissue edema. Hypovolemia, hemoconcentration, and increased blood viscosity are end results that, like vasospasm, limit organ and tissue perfusion.

Vasospasm increases total peripheral resistance and cardiac afterload, increasing cardiac work and myocardial O_2 extraction. Swan-Ganz catheterization during early labor often demonstrates high cardiac output and increased left ventricular stroke work index, signs of a hyperdynamic myocardial state. The usual increases in cardiac output during labor and the early puerperium do not occur in preeclamptic patients. Increased sensitivity of the peripheral and possibly pulmonary vasculature to endogenous and exogenous vasopressors may exacerbate the hypertensive response to anxiety, pain, and noxious stimuli.

Mild preeclampsia produces minimal change in respiratory function. In severe cases, exaggerated mucosal edema occurs in the upper airway, larynx, trachea, and bronchi.[118] Increased tracheobronchial secretions and pulmonary congestion predispose the mother to pneumonitis. A mild to moderate alveolar/arterial oxygen gradient often develops, but significant hypoxemia is uncommon unless aspiration pneumonitis or heart failure occurs.

Renal blood flow and glomerular filtration rate decrease, sodium excretion diminishes, and ischemic glomeruli leak albumin into the urine.[111] Plasma colloid oncotic pressure falls,[119] occasionally to values as low as 10 mmHg, making pulmonary edema more likely. Damaged glomeruli with fibrinoid deposits often permit the passage of erythrocytes with hematuria. Renal tubular dysfunction is manifested by inability to concentrate sodium or secrete uric acid. Tubular epithelial degeneration (glomeruloendotheliosis) is often noted at postmortem and confirms clinical findings of tubular dysfunction. The degree of renal compromise in PIH can be monitored by determining daily creatinine clearances and serum uric acid levels. A creatinine clearance <75 ml/min with a serum uric acid level >7.5 mg/dl suggests severe renal compromise. Renal cortical necrosis characterized by oliguria, anuria, and azotemia occasionally occurs, especially when hemorrhagic shock complicates PIH.

Central nervous system manifestations of PIH include hyperreflexia, seizures, convulsions, stroke, and coma. Total cerebral blood flow remains normal, but an increase in cerebral vascular resistance occurs and resets cerebral autoregulation. When blood pressure exceeds autoregulatory limits, cerebral capillary integrity is lost and the brain swells from interstitial leakage of fluid and blood. Cerebral edema occurs primarily in eclamptic patients and ranks second to intracranial hemorrhage as a major cause of maternal death in PIH.[120]

Intervillous blood flow is reduced by vasoconstriction and/or occlusive lesions in decidual arteries. Histologic examination of the placenta often shows nodular ischemia with infarcts. Supporting tissue necrosis may lead to rupture of fetal cotyledons with fetomaternal hemorrhage or abruptio placentae.

Chesley[121] reported that mean plasma volume in women with mild preeclampsia was 9% below normal, and, in those with severe disease, plasma volume was as much as 30% to 40% below normal. The inverse relationship between intravascular volume and severity of hypertension is confirmed with CVP measurements. Patients with diastolic blood pressures greater than 110 mmHg often have CVP measurements of 0 to −4 cm H_2O and may require a volume infusion to raise the CVP to normal. A significant reduction in maternal plasma volume as manifested by subnormal CVP may actually precede the development of preeclampsia in previously normotensive parturients.

Preeclampsia is a "hyperviscosity syndrome" because it is associated with elevated plasma viscosity and hemoconcentration. Hyperviscosity decreases peripheral blood flow to tissues and cells. Placental blood flow through the villous capillary network is reduced, producing chronic fetal hypoxia, malnutrition, and growth retardation.

Earlier output studies with pulmonary artery catheters suggested that patients with severe preeclampsia were hyperdynamic.[118] These investigations were, however, conducted during labor or in the postpartum period after treatment had already been instituted. In a study[122] of 10 hypertensive and four healthy pregnant ewes near term and not in labor, initial hemodynamic measurements included low pulmonary capillary wedge pressures, low cardiac outputs, increased systemic vascular resistances, and elevated heart rates consistent with low-output states in untreated hypertensives. Volume expansion in the hypertensive ewes resulted in a significant rise in pulmonary capillary wedge pressures and cardiac index, while systemic vascular resistances and maternal heart rates decreased. Volume expansion also significantly reduced mean arterial pressure, mainly by decreasing systolic pressure, a beneficial effect of volume expansion on elevated blood pressure noted by many.[122] Subsequent treatment with hydralazine did not alter pulmonary capillary wedge pressure but further increased cardiac index and decreased systemic vascular resistance.[122] Such data indicate that volume expansion in severe preeclampsia will improve maternal tissue perfusion. In addition, Joyce and Loon[123] have shown a dramatic increase in urine output following volume replacement with 25% albumin in severe preeclamptics.

Medical treatment of mild PIH includes bed rest in lateral decubitus position, sedation when necessary, and observation of blood pressure, fluid balance, weight gain, and central nervous system irritability. Diuretic therapy is discouraged since it decreases an already contracted intravascular volume, causes fetal hypovolemia and glucose intolerance, and reduces placental perfusion. Severe salt restriction, a previously popular treatment, facilitates hypovolemia and further increases the production of renin, angiotensin, and aldosterone. Frequent evaluation of fetal well-being is performed using ultrasound, NSTs, CSTs, or OCTs.

In severe PIH, the purpose of therapy is to (1) prevent convulsions; (2) prevent intracranial hemorrhage; (3) prevent abruptio placentae; (4) correct hematologic, cardiovascular, and respiratory aberrations; and (5) terminate the pregnancy when most feasible. Definitive therapy is delivery of the placenta. In severe cases, aggressive management should continue for at least 24 to 48 hours after delivery to prevent postpartum eclampsia.

Convulsions are prevented with magnesium sulfate to decrease irritability in peripheral and central nervous systems. The drug's peripheral site of action is at the neuromuscular junction where it limits the release of acetylcholine by the presynaptic nerve terminal, decreases the sensitivity of the motor end-plate to acetylcholine, and depresses the excitability of muscle membranes. The resulting neuromuscular blockade alleviates hyperreflexia and increases maternal sensitivity to neuromuscular blocking agents. These effects can be reversed with either calcium gluconate or calcium chloride in 1-g intravenous doses. Therapeutic serum magnesium levels range between 4 and 6 mEq/L. Magnesium overdose causes loss of deep tendon reflexes, myocardial depression, respiratory paralysis, and cardiac arrest. Magnesium therapy produces mild to moderate peripheral vasodilation with some blood pressure reduction, direct smooth muscle relaxation with tocolysis, and increased uterine blood flow.

Magnesium ions cross the placenta readily and may lead to fetal and neonatal hypermagnesemia. There is a poor correlation between magnesium concentrations in umbilical cord blood and the incidence of low Apgar scores and neonatal respiratory depression. No deleterious effects of maternal magnesium sulfate therapy have been seen in nonasphyxiated full-term neonates.[112] Neonatal respiratory depression previously attributed to magnesium therapy in earlier studies was probably due to asphyxia and/or prematurity.[112]

When magnesium determinations are not readily available, assessment of deep tendon reflexes and urine output (>30 ml/hour) will monitor and direct therapy. If seizure prophylaxis with magnesium fails, seizures can be stopped with intravenous thiopental, 50 to 75 mg, or diazepam, 5 to 10 mg. This dose of thiopental may cause less fetal-neonatal depression than diazepam and produces minimal cardiovascular effects in the mother. Use of diazepam should be avoided if delivery is imminent because of its depressant effects on the neonate.

Antihypertensive therapy in preeclampsia lessens the risk of maternal cerebrovascular accidents and improves placental perfusion. Plasma volume expansion also helps to fulfill these goals of antihypertensive therapy. Hydralazine given intravenously produces an effect within 10 to 15 minutes and has a relatively short half-life. Hydralazine causes reflex tachycardia; elevates cardiac output; and increases renal, hepatic, coronary, and cerebral blood flow. In PIH, hydralazine's effect on uterine blood flow depends on the degree of uterine vasodilation achieved by blood pressure control. At present, little is known regarding the response of uterine vasculature to hydralazine or other vasodilators. Therefore, to prevent excessive blood pressure reduction and to maintain uterine blood flow, hydralazine is given in 2.5- to 5-mg doses spaced at least 10 minutes apart until diastolic pressure reaches 90 to 100 mmHg or the mean arterial pressure is reduced by 15% to 20%. In severely hypertensive parturients with diastolic pressures of 110 mmHg or greater, continuous pressure monitoring by arterial and Swan-Ganz catheters simplifies and directs antihypertensive therapy. Maternal O_2 inhalation, lateral decubitus position, and continuous electronic fetal heart rate (FHR) monitoring are also important during vasodilator therapy. Trimethaphan, a ganglionic blocker, is particularly useful in hypertensive emergencies complicated by cerebral edema and increased intracranial pressure, as trimethaphan does not cause cerebral vasodilation. Succinylcholine-induced neuromuscular blockade may, however, be prolonged by trimethaphan's inhibition of plasma pseudocholinesterase.

Epidural anesthesia for labor and delivery is recommended for parturients with PIH, providing there is no clotting abnormality or plasma volume deficit. In normovolemic patients, epidural anesthesia causes an acceptable reduction in blood pressure and a significant improvement in placental perfusion. James and Davies[124] showed that in preeclamptic patients, epidural anesthesia reduced mean arterial pressure without altering cardiac index, pulmonary vascular resistance, central venous pressure, or pulmonary capillary wedge pressure. There was a slight but statistically insignificant reduction in systemic vascular resistance.[124] With the use of radioactive xenon,[125] it was shown that following induction of epidural analgesia the intervillous blood flow rose, sometimes by as much as 75%. By relieving labor pains and decreasing maternal catecholamine levels, epidural anesthesia prevents wide swings in maternal blood pressure and obviates the need for narcotics that could promote maternal cardiorespiratory depression and neonatal neurologic depression.

Unlike epidural anesthesia for preeclamptic patients, spinal anesthesia should be used with great caution, if at all, because of sudden and severe sympathetic blockade. However, recently the use of minute doses of intrathecal and epidural narcotics has provided good analgesia with few side effects in parturients with PIH.[126]

For cesarean section, the level of regional anesthesia should extend to T_3–T_4, making adequate fluid replacement and left uterine displacement even more vital. Should hypotension occur, its correction will require a reduced dose of ephedrine, 2.5 to 5.0 mg IV, in view of the increased sensitivity to vasopressors among preeclamptics. General anesthesia in preeclamptics has its own particular hazards. Rapid-sequence induction and tracheal intubation to prevent aspiration may be difficult due to edema of the tongue, epiglottis, or pharynx. In parturients with impaired coagulation, laryngoscopy may cause profuse oral bleeding, which obscures the larynx. Marked systemic and pulmonary hypertension precipitated by tracheal intubation or extubation may increase the risk of cerebral hemorrhage and pulmonary edema. Such detrimental changes are best minimized with antihypertensives, such as trimethaphan or nitroprusside. Ketamine should be avoided due to its vagolytic and hypertensive effects. As noted, magnesium sulfate may prolong the neuromuscular blocking effects of all muscle relaxants. Therefore, relaxants should be administered in small titrated doses and their blocking effects should be monitored with a nerve stimulator to avoid overdosage. General anesthesia is indicated in acute emergencies such as fetal distress or abruptio placentae and in patients who do not meet the criteria for epidural anesthesia.

PIH is a disease of unknown etiology that carries a substantial risk of morbidity and mortality for the mother and her fetus. It affects practically every maternal organ system and is associated with hemodynamic alterations that lead to placental and tissue hypoperfusion. Treatment at present is largely symptomatic. In severe cases, invasive monitoring should be utilized to monitor maternal hemodynamic status and guide drug therapy. The anesthesiologist significantly contributes to patient management by providing maternal pain relief, resuscitating depressed neonates, and providing critical care therapy.

HELLP Syndrome. Pritchard and associates in 1954[127] were the first to describe a syndrome of hemolysis, elevated liver enzymes, and low platelet counts in three eclamptic patients. Since then, others have reported similar cases associated with PIH. In 1982, Weinstein[128] coined the term HELLP to describe this syndrome. Although Weinstein considers the HELLP syndrome a unique variant of PIH, others question its existence. Greer and colleagues[129] suggested that more sensitive laboratory tests would identify an associated coagulopathy and that the HELLP syndrome is in fact PIH with mild DIC. Hematologic and hepatic changes unique to the HELLP syndrome and not discussed under PIH are presented here.

HELLP syndrome is associated with poor maternal and fetal outcomes, with maternal mortality ranging from 3.5% to 24%. In addition, such patients are at greater risk of liver rupture, DIC, abruptio placentae, and acute renal failure.[130] Perinatal mortality is equally high, ranging from 100 to 367 perinatal deaths/1000 live births, with such excessive mortality due primarily to placental infarcts, abruptio placentae, intrauterine growth retardation, intrauterine asphyxia, and prematurity. Thrombocytopenia and leukopenia occur in 25% to 30% of neonates of mothers with HELLP syndrome. As in PIH, a humoral mechanism may be involved in the etiology of the HELLP syndrome.[131]

Inadequate uterine perfusion appears to play an important role in the etiology of PIH and HELLP syndrome. A possible mechanism initiating the process may be a developmental defect of the spiral arteries of the uterus. Typically in the HELLP syndrome, the muscular walls of these vessels are invaded by trophoblasts and rendered unable to contract. In PIH, this invasion is incomplete, and the spiral arteries retain their ability to contract. The end-result is an ischemic process that produces placental necrosis and the release of tissue thromboplastin and renin into the maternal circulation in both PIH and HELLP.[132]

In HELLP, an alteration of the renin-angiotensin system occurs, which causes vasospasm with generalized tissue hypoxia and vascular endothelial damage. Aldosterone secretion also increases and causes sodium and water retention. Maternal coagulation system activation and enhanced platelet aggregation at sites of endothelial damage result in the deposition of fibrin in the basement membranes of the smaller vessels. Overall, a generalized capillary leak shifts fluids and electrolytes into the extracellular space. Albumin loss into the tissues produces a decrease in colloid oncotic pressure, hypovolemia, hemocentration, and increased blood viscosity.

In the liver, fibrin is deposited in the hepatic sinusoids, obstructing hepatic blood flow. The liver swells, stretching Glisson's capsule and producing epigastric and right upper quadrant pain. Hemorrhagic periportal necrosis, subcapsular hemorrhages, and spontaneous liver rupture in extreme cases may occur. Serum levels of liver enzymes rise with serum glutamic-oxaloacetic transaminase (SGOT) values of 700 units/ml or higher. Infrequently, acute hepatic failure and jaundice will appear. Maternal hypoglycemia is a particularly grave prognostic finding of unknown etiology.

Hemolysis in HELLP is consistent with microangiopathic hemolytic anemia with red blood cell fragmentation in response to vascular endothelial damage and fibrin deposition. The peripheral blood smear contains burr cells, crenated and distorted red cells with spiny border projections, and schistocytes, irregularly shaped red cell fragments.[133] Peripheral destruction of platelets produces thrombocytopenia, and an increase in bone marrow megakaryocyte activity suggests rapid platelet turnover.[133] In addition, recent studies suggest associated platelet activation as well as platelet dysfunction in HELLP.[134]

Definitive therapy for parturients with HELLP is delivery. Prior to delivery, control of the disease is the goal. Pregnancy is usually allowed to continue as long as there is no apparent evidence of fetal and/or maternal compromise. Medical management is directed toward cardiovascular stabilization, maintenance of intravascular volume, prevention of intracranial hemorrhage, and control of central nervous system irritability.

A significant portion of HELLP patients will require an operative delivery for fetal distress. In Weinstein's series of 57 patients with HELLP,[135] 29% of multiparous patients and 79% of primigravida patients were delivered by cesarean section.[135]

Invasive monitoring in parturients with HELLP is based on the following assumptions: (1) the nature of the illness is critical; (2) the severity of illness is often not apparent initially; and (3) most parturients with HELLP will deliver operatively and need precise hemodynamic control. Continuous lumbar epidural analgesia is the anesthetic technique of choice in patients with PIH.[136] However, epidural analgesia in patients with HELLP syndrome may be limited by the presence of a significant coagulopathy. The advantages of epidural anesthesia include excellent analgesia for labor and delivery and a decrease in circulating catecholamines. Epidural analgesia also avoids the depressant effects associated with systemic medication in both the mother and the fetus. Concomitant sympathetic blockade produces vasodilation and a decrease in systemic vascular resistance. In addition, cardiac output and uteroplacental blood flow are increased. Without prehydration, however, epidural analgesia may produce profound hypotension in a hypertensive and hypovolemic preeclamptic patient.

When delivery is anticipated, intravenous magnesium sulfate therapy is begun for its anticonvulsant effects, its mild vasodilatory, sedative, and tocolytic effects, and its combined actions that increase uterine blood flow. Side effects associated with magnesium sulfate therapy in HELLP include increased maternal and fetal sensitivity to muscle relaxants, with fetomaternal respiratory depression, neonatal hypotonia, and apnea. As noted, these effects can be reversed by administration of calcium.

If antihypertensive therapy is indicated, hydralazine, a smooth muscle relaxant, is the drug of choice because it increases uteroplacental perfusion and renal blood flow to a greater extent than other antihypertensives.[122] Hydralazine does not, however, offer fine control of blood pressure as do other agents, especially trimethaphan, nitroprusside, and nitroglycerin. These agents do not increase uteroplacental perfusion to the same extent as hydralazine, and other problems may be associated with their use, such as cyanide toxicity with nitroprusside and methemoglobinemia with nitroglycerin. Such agents may be used to blunt the pressor response to laryngoscopy and to control postpartum blood pressure.[137] The goal of antihypertensive therapy in HELLP is to maintain a maternal diastolic blood pressure between 90 and 110 mmHg, since diastolic pressures below 90 mmHg are often associated with inadequate uteroplacental perfusion. The best indicator of adequate uteroplacental perfusion during antihypertensive therapy is a continuous recording of a normal FHR pattern. Inadequate perfusion will be reflected by significant changes in the FHR pattern.

When delivery is planned, invasive monitoring should be instituted prior to the administration of any anesthetic. The patient is put in a supine position with left lateral uterine displacement (approximately 15° to 20°), continuous FHR monitoring is continued, and supplemental oxygen by nasal cannula is administered. Small amounts of fentanyl, 50 to 100 μg, may be administered intravenously prior to central venous cannulation. If epidural analgesia is used, the catheter is placed with the patient on her side. The preferred form of anesthesia for delivery is continuous lumbar epidural. Hemodynamic profiles are obtained prior to the induction of anesthesia and at set intervals following the administration of local anesthesia. If needed, 25% albumin is administered to maintain wedge pressures between 6 and 10 mmHg. Epidural dosing proceeds slowly with a 2- to 3-ml test dose of 1% plain lidocaine. Top-up doses follow with 0.25% plain bupivacaine and 50 μg of fentanyl to each 10 ml of local anesthetic solution. If a long labor is anticipated, a continuous epidural infusion of 0.125% bupivacaine with fentanyl, 2 μg/

ml, can be used. For short labors, intermittent dosing is continued with 0.25% bupivacaine without fentanyl.

If regional anesthesia is contraindicated, labor pain is managed with systemic medication. Additional pain relief at delivery can be accomplished with pudendal/local infiltration combined with mask analgesia (30% to 40% N_2O). Low dose ketamine (0.25 mg/kg body weight) may be used cautiously to supplement N_2O analgesia if blood pressure is adequately controlled. Several authors have recommended low-dose halogenated agents for additional analgesic effects.[138, 139] If the patient loses consciousness, endotracheal intubation and general anesthesia should be instituted.

Spinal anesthesia for cesarean section is contraindicated in patients with HELLP syndrome because of the hazards associated with sudden hypotension from rapid and extensive sympathetic block. Induction of general anesthesia in patients with PIH may be associated with the release of endogenous catecholamines at laryngoscopy for tracheal intubation producing severe exacerbations of blood pressure. There may also be increases in systemic vascular resistance, pulmonary artery pressure, and PCWP and a decrease in cardiac output and uterine perfusion. Pretreatment with curare is usually not required if the patient is receiving magnesium sulfate. Mask O_2 is administered prior to induction of anesthesia. Oral endotracheal intubation is accomplished with a rapid-sequence induction with sodium thiopental (3 to 4 mg/kg; 300 mg maximum) and succinylcholine (1 to 1.5 mg/kg) during cricoid pressure. After delivery, anesthesia may be deepened with additional thiopental sodium, narcotics, or low-dose halogenated agents.

If time, adequate fluid replacement, and normal coagulation status permit, continuous lumbar epidural anesthesia is also preferred for cesarean delivery. At our institution, 2% plain lidocaine and fentanyl, 100 μg in 20 ml of local anesthetic, are used. The patient is placed supine with left lateral uterine tilt and continuous fetal heart rate monitoring. An epidural test dose of 2 to 3 ml is administered and additional 2- to 3-ml top-up doses are administered at 3- to 5-minute intervals during continuous monitoring of systemic pressure, pulmonary artery pressure, and PCWP. If systemic blood pressure decreases, 25% albumin is administered as needed to maintain PCWP at 6 to 10 mmHg. Additionally, small amounts of intravenous ephedrine, 2.5 to 5 mg, may be used to raise blood pressure. Adequate anesthesia levels are achieved in 20 to 30 minutes.

Parturients with HELLP syndrome are often critically ill, and their infants are often born prematurely and asphyxiated. The best perinatal management includes thorough preanesthetic evaluation, knowledge of the pathophysiologic processes involved, and precise medical, obstetric, and anesthetic therapy.

CEREBROVASCULAR ACCIDENTS

Parturients with preexisting hypertension, diabetes, vasculitis, and atherosclerosis are predisposed to more frequent occurrences of cerebro-vascular accidents (CVAs). Predisposing pathophysiologic conditions include fragile cerebral feeding vessels, as in aneurysms and arteriovenous malformations (AVMs), hyperviscosity states producing cerebrovascular thrombosis, as in preeclampsia and sickle cell disease, or altered cere-brovascular permeability, as in the HELLP syndrome and DIC. Long-term morbidity is less frequently associated with cerebral venous occlusion, although arterial occlusions have a better initial prognosis.

Subarachnoid hemorrhages (SAHs) from a ruptured AVM or aneurysm account for nearly 10% of maternal deaths. If the SAH is due to aneurysm, its occurrence is most common during the third trimester. Labor will generally follow SAH from aneurysmal rupture.[140–142] Symptoms include sudden onset of severe headache, nausea, vomiting, nuchal rigidity, and often coma. Patients with normal neurologic examinations still have a 15% chance of death from rebleeding. The more disoriented and stuporous the patient, the greater the incidence of mortality.

The diagnosis of SAH or CVA is made by computed tomographic head scan showing an intracranial infarct or hemorrhage and by cerebral angiogram, lumbar puncture, and electroencephalogram. CVA from an arterial occlusion is not common in pregnancy but occurs more frequently than venous occlusion, especially during the latter half of pregnancy and in the puerperium. The onset of neurologic symptoms is abrupt and frequently not associated with headache. Usual symptoms include speech and gait difficulties, motor loss, and sensory deficits. Seizure and loss of consciousness rarely occur.

Recovery from CVA is slow and often complicated by residual deficit. If seizure or coma develop, the prognosis is guarded. Vaginal delivery without stress or bearing down is preferable to more hazardous cesarean section for abdominal delivery.

Perinatal management of parturients with CVA includes seizure control, blood pressure regulation, and intracranial pressure reduction. With SAH, sedation should be administered to alleviate anxiety and enable the patient to tolerate strict bed rest in a quiet environment.

Intact intracranial aneurysm diagnosed during pregnancy is managed neurosurgically by craniotomy and clipping under general anesthesia with deliberate hypotension using nitroprusside or trimethaphan.[142, 143] During and after the procedure, the parturient should have a wedge placed under the right hip, and the FHR should be monitored continuously. Tocolytic therapy may be necessary postoperatively. Should vaginal delivery become imminent, regional analgesia and outlet forceps are utilized to prevent second-stage expulsive efforts. For cesarean delivery, regional anesthesia is advisable to monitor neurologic and mental status and to prevent extreme fluctuations in blood pressure.

Respiratory Conditions and Complications

ACUTE ASTHMA EXACERBATIONS
DURING PREGNANCY

A patient with acute asthma often has wheezing, shortness of breath, and chest tightness frequently precipitated by an upper respiratory infection with changing sputum characteristics, fever, and chills. Initial history-taking seeks causative factors and prior or current corticosteroid use. In addition, upper respiratory infections, allergens, aspirin therapy, dyes, noxious inhalants, and even strenuous exercise or cold air exposure can trigger asthmatic attacks.[144]

Physical examination includes assessment of pulse, blood pressure, respiratory rate, and pulmonary function. A pulse rate over 120/minute, respiratory rate over 30/minute, forced expiratory volume over 1 second (FEV_1) less than 1 L, pulsus paradoxus over 18 mmHg, moderate to severe dyspnea, accessory muscle use, and severe wheezing are all signs of life-threatening disease and need for hospitalization.[145] Combinations of inspiratory and expiratory wheezes indicate more lower airway obstruction than expiratory wheezes alone. Asthma in its most severe forms causes few wheezes because little air moves through markedly constricted airways.

Arterial blood gas analysis rapidly identifies hypoxemia and directs O_2 therapy to prevent fetal hypoxia. Blood gas analysis also identifies acute respiratory alkalosis, which can also impair O_2 delivery to the fetus. With mild asthma, arterial CO_2 tension is normal or slightly reduced. With more severe asthma, hypercarbia and marked hypoxemia are common.[146] Both hypoxemia and respiratory alkalosis will be improved by O_2 therapy. Chest x-ray films will rule out signs of accompanying pneumonia or pneumothorax.[147] Peak expiratory flow rates and FEV_1/ FVC (forced vital capacity) ratios are useful, especially when compared with previous values and followed serially throughout an attack and its treatment.

In the pregnant patient, nebulizer treatment is begun with a bronchodilator, such as isoetharine, 0.5 ml of 1% solution in 1.5 ml of saline, and can be repeated every 1 to 2 hours as needed. Intravenous aminophylline infusion should also be started. If the patient is currently taking a theophylline preparation,, no loading dose is necessary. If not, aminophylline, 5.6 mg/kg, is administered intravenously over 30 minutes with no more than 400 mg as a loading dose. If the admission theophylline level is subtherapeutic, a partial aminophylline loading dose may be given. Once the loading dose is completed, a continuous aminophylline infusion is begun at 0.5 mg/kg/hour. A theophylline blood level, obtained after 10 to 12 hours of therapy, will confirm therapeutic ranges of 10 to 14 µg/ml. Additional management includes intravenous hydration with 0.45 normal saline at a rate of 100 to 125 ml/hour and O_2 at a rate of 2 to 3 L/minute. O_2 should be titrated carefully if the patient has CO_2 retention (Paco$_2$ >45 mmHg) with a Venturi mask that can deliver accurate, low-dose O_2. An arterial Po$_2$ of 70 to 100 mmHg should be maintained during O_2 therapy.

Corticosteroid therapy is indicated if clinical examination and spirometry (FEV$_1$ remaining less than 1 L) show no improvement after 2 to 4 hours, if the patient gives a history of current or recent corticosteroid use, or if the attack has been going on for several days before medical attention. Methylprednisolone, 25 mg IV, is administered every 4 hours for an acute attack. If corticosteroids are used, this regimen is continued until the attack is resolved. Oral corticosteroids are administered concomitantly at an initial dose of prednisone, 60 mg daily. If the patient remains free of wheezing, this dose is reduced by 20 mg at 4-day intervals until a daily dose of 20 mg is achieved. From this point, corticosteroid dose is tapered weekly by 5 mg until it is discontinued or until the lowest dose that prevents wheezing is attained. An alternate-day regimen is preferable to a daily regimen if oral corticosteroids cannot be tapered completely. Inhaled corticosteroids will sometimes facilitate tapering of oral corticosteroids. However, they should not be added until wheezing is controlled, since they do not penetrate bronchoconstricted airways effectively. Corticosteroids should be continued indefinitely without hesitation because adequate control of asthma is essential for optimal fetal and maternal outcome.

Antibiotics are indicated for pneumonia or bacterial superinfections, which often precipitate acute attacks. For infectious bronchitis, oral ampicillin or cephalosporin is used unless the sputum culture directs a more specific antibiotic. A 10-day course of therapy is recommended.

An outpatient bronchodilator program is also initiated as the acute attack begins to resolve and oral corticosteroids have been started. Oral theophylline also replaces intravenous aminophylline therapy. In making this transition, the 24-hour intravenous aminophylline dose is recorded. Since 85% of aminophylline is theophylline, a 24-hour theophylline dose can be calculated. This 24-hour dose can be divided into two or three daily oral doses of a long-acting theophylline preparation, with the first oral dose administered as the intravenous aminophylline infusion is being slowly discontinued. An oral beta-mimetic, such as terbutaline, 2.5 to 5.0 mg tid, may be added to the theophylline if needed to provide tocolysis and synergistic bronchodilation. An inhaled bronchodilator, such as metaproterenol, 2 puffs qid, may be a helpful adjunct to oral bronchodilator therapy. When beta-mimetic agents are combined, high-output congestive heart failure and postpartum uterine atony may occur and complicate the puerperium.

Although the treatment program presented will manage most asthmatic attacks, a subgroup of asthmatics will remain refractory to such therapy. The parturient with refractory asthma will be identified by hypercarbia rather than the expected hypocarbia during an asthma attack.[146] If the treatment plan above does not rapidly reverse airway obstruction, CO_2 retention, respiratory acidosis, and obtundation will result. Endotracheal intubation and mechanical ventilation will often be required. Mechanical ventilation in the severely asthmatic parturient is associated with significant morbidity and, in one study, a 38% mortality.[148] The severe asthmatic who requires high mean airway pressures to provide effective alveolar ventilation is at significant risk of pulmonary barotrauma.

To reduce complications of mechanical ventilation, Scoggin and colleagues[148] suggest that management should compromise (1) use of the largest endotracheal tube possible, at least 8.0 mm in outside diameter, to reduce expiratory air flow resistance; (2) delivery of constant tidal volumes with a volume ventilator; (3) humidifying the air delivered; (4) allowing adequate expiratory time by using the lowest rate that permits adequate CO_2 elimination; and (5) suppressing agitation and spontaneous ventilatory drive with sedatives and paralysis. Histamine-releasing drugs such as morphine and meperidine should probably be avoided as sedatives, and it should be noted that the benzodiazepines are teratogenic during organogenesis (see Chapter 1). If delivery occurs during pharmacologic paralysis, the neonate should be observed carefully for flaccidity and respiratory depression and may need short-term mechanical ventilation during reversal and resolution of placentally transferred maternal muscle relaxants.

Mediastinal emphysema can develop from the elevated airway pressures during spontaneous or mechanical ventilation from alveolar rupture with air dissection along vascular sheaths to the hilum and mediastinum.[149] Besides asthma, mediastinal emphysema can also occur during expulsive efforts of the second stage of labor, with hyperemesis gravidarum of early pregnancy, or after a bout of coughing.[149] The patient complains of sharp retrosternal pain often radiating to the shoulders and arms. On physical examination, subcutaneous emphysema is present, and a crunching noise (Hamman's sign) can be heard with each heart beat at the left sternal edge. Left pneumothorax is commonly associated with spontaneous pneumomediastinum. Treatment is with analgesia and O_2 therapy, air drainage of an associated pneumothorax by chest tube, and observation in an intensive care area. If tension builds in the mediastinum and causes cardiovascular compromise, air-releasing incisions over the sites of greatest subcutaneous air accumulation may be indicated.[149]

Labor and delivery of the parturient in asthmatic crisis will require several special considerations, including discontinuance of beta-mimetics, switching from oral to intravenous bronchodilators, and regulation of corticosteroid therapy to include an additional stress dose of glucocorticoid to avoid addisonian crisis. Hydrocortisone, 100 mg IM, should be administered at the onset of labor and repeated every 8 hours for 24 hours, when the patient may return to her prior oral steroid regimen.[150] Should general anesthesia become necessary for delivery, halogenated gases are preferable to intravenous agents because of their bronchodilatory properties.

PULMONARY EDEMA SECONDARY TO BETA-ADRENERGIC TOCOLYSIS

Although the precise mechanism of pulmonary edema associated with beta-adrenergic tocolytic therapy is not presently known, most patients display signs and symptoms of acute high-output left ventricular failure. Thus, by directly exaggerating the high-output cardiac state of pregnancy or by impairing compensatory mechanisms, it is possible that these agents could produce pulmonary edema (Chapters 2 and 7).

In addition to their anticipated tocolytic effects on myometrial contractility, the beta-mimetics will also stimulate $beta_2$-receptors in blood vessels and the bronchial tree and $beta_1$-receptors in the myocardium, liver, and adipose tissue. In fact, even the most selective $beta_2$-tocolytic will have some degree of $beta_1$-activity that can trigger a series of metabolic and cardiovascular changes culminating in heart failure and pulmonary edema.

Plasma volume expansion will occur shortly after initiation of intravenous beta-adrenergic tocolysis and result in significant contraction of red cell volume with a 6% mean reduction in hematocrit within 24 hours.[151] Such rapid expansion of intravascular volume is a prime factor in the ability of the beta-mimetics to create a hyperdynamic cardiac state. A simultaneous, marked decrease in urinary output is apparent within 2 hours of beta-mimetic tocolysis. Retention of water and electrolytes and oliguria are directed by excessive secretion of antidiuretic hormone (ADH) at the initiation of therapy. Interestingly, however, ADH plasma concentration returns to normal 6 hours after initiation of beta-adrenergic treatment, while oliguria persists for the duration of intravenous tocolysis. Plasma renin activity also increases markedly at the onset of therapy, but aldosterone concentration decreases to nonpregnant levels. This suggests that the retention of water and electrolytes characteristic of tocolytic therapy is not dependent on aldosterone. Most exogenously administered sodium will be retained by parturients undergoing tocolysis because of the sodium-retaining effects of beta-agonists. After discontinuation of intravenous therapy, diuresis begins within 1 hour in most patients.

Beta-adrenergic agents cause a marked drop in arterial vascular resistance that is often manifested by a decrease in diastolic blood pressure noted within 30 minutes of initiating therapy. Pulse pressure widens as the diastolic pressure decreases and the systolic blood pressure increases.[152] Peripheral vascular resistance falls as hemodilution from fluid retention decreases blood viscosity. Such a reduction in vascular resistance is another important factor in the ability of the beta-mimetics to create a hyperdynamic cardiac state.

Positive inotropic and chronotropic effects on the heart are produced by beta-mimetics.[152] There is a 50% to 60% increase in cardiac output from a combination of direct myocardial effects, decreased peripheral vascular resistance, and increased intravascular volume.[153, 154] This iatrogenic increase in cardiac output is superimposed on the physiologic 40% increase of normal pregnancy, and cardiac outputs over 10 L/minute have occurred in parturients undergoing tocolysis with beta-mimetics.[153]

The large and sudden increase in intravascular volume caused by intravenous therapy will also dilute plasma albumin and reduce colloid osmotic pressure.[155] Generous fluid therapy with dextrose-containing crystalloids will further reduce oncotic pressure in patients with low plasma albumin stores common to pregnancy itself (see Chapter 2).[156] Thus, a superimposition of drug actions expands blood volume, dilutes already low stores of plasma proteins, and reduces colloid osmotic pressure.

In addition, there is suggestive evidence that beta-mimetics have direct cardiotoxic effects similar to the catecholamines and can cause ischemic cardiomyopathy indistinguishable from that observed in patients with pheochromocytoma.[157] Anginal chest pains, pulmonary edema, and ischemic electrocardiographic changes have been reported during tocolytic therapy with beta-mimetics.[157]

Myocardial function may be impaired indirectly by beta-adrenergic agents as a result of reduction in intracellular potassium concentration. A significant decrease in plasma potassium concentration is seen within the first 30 minutes of intravenous beta-adrenergic treatment and will persist for the duration of treatment if not corrected. However, after beta-agonists are discontinued, the potassium level will quickly return to a normal range. Parturients who develop pulmonary edema during tocolytic treatment often have marked hypokalemia, suggesting increased sensitivity of the renin-aldosterone system to beta-agonists in these patients.[155]

Serum glucose increases markedly 30 minutes after starting intravenous tocolysis with beta-mimetics and is another factor promoting mobilization of fluids into the intravascular compartment. Metabolism of this glucose generates lactic acid, which further reduces total peripheral resistance.[158]

Early signs and symptoms of pulmonary edema are subtle and may be missed. Parturients receiving tocolytics should be observed for tachycardia and tachypnea without dyspnea, and auscultated frequently for scattered rales and rhonchi as the earliest signs of pulmonary edema. Agitation or restlessness often signifies hypoxia. Pulmonary edema is well established once shortness of breath is noticeable to both the physician and the patient. An early chest radiograph may show patchy infiltrates or may appear normal. As the disease progresses, total opacification of the lung fields may occur unless increased airway pressures are provided by mechanical ventilation.

Parturients should be sitting or in the left lateral decubitus position for blood gas sampling because PaO_2 is frequently reduced by 10 to 15 mmHg in the supine position. With pulmonary injury, the parturient's lung will preferentially eliminate the more soluble CO_2 rather than take up less soluble O_2, explaining the hypoxemia and normocarbia common to early pulmonary edema. In parturients with respiratory distress, a $PaCO_2$ greater than 45 mmHg is markedly abnormal and signifies that many alveoli are not being ventilated or perfused.

Another early change in the development of pulmonary edema during tocolysis is the appearance of interstitial pulmonary edema, which is often detected by a decrease in functional lung volume.[159] Serial measurements of vital capacity may offer a simple and sensitive method for assessing functional lung volume, for detecting the early development of pulmonary edema, and for directing early therapy.[159]

While the patient is receiving intravenous beta-adrenergic therapy, maternal weight, fluid intake and output, serum electrolytes, glucose, hematocrit, vital signs, fetal well-being, and signs and symptoms of pulmonary congestion should be evaluated frequently, preferably at least every 12 hours. Most cases of pulmonary edema during tocolysis appear to be secondary to iatrogenic hypervolemia.[159] Increasing maternal weight or decreasing hematocrit should be regarded as early signs of hypovolemia. Initial treatment is instituted with fluid restriction, reduction of tocolytic doses, and small doses of loop diuretics if fluid restriction and tocolytic regulation fail to rapidly restore normovolemia.

Intravenous tocolysis should be limited to 24 to 48 hours because the risk of cardiorespiratory complications increases with the duration of treatment. The large majority of patients with beta-adrenergic–associated pulmonary edema have developed this complication while in the intravenous phase of treatment. When contractions are not producing cervical dilatation, oral tocolytic therapy can replace intravenous tocolysis with fewer complications.

Tocolytic therapy should be discontinued if the patient develops chest pain, dyspnea, or rales. A maternal pulse rate of 100 to 120 beats/min is indicative of therapeutic blood levels of tocolytic agents and is associated with a low probability for the development of cardiorespiratory problems. A maternal pulse rate persistently above 120 beats/min indicates early cardiovascular toxicity and directs a rapid decrease in tocolytic dose to a safer level.

Parturients with multiple gestation often have preterm labor and are at greater risk of pulmonary edema during tocolysis.[160] Parturients receiving glucocorticoids to accelerate fetal pulmonary maturity may also be at greater risk of pulmonary edema during tocolysis, especially if a potent mineralocorticoid such as hydrocortisone is used. In addition, glucocorticoids may increase beta-adrenergic responsiveness by increasing beta-receptor concentrations in several tissues, including the lungs.[161] Preexisting anemia and hypokalemia during therapy should be corrected as both conditions predispose to arrhythmias during tocolysis.

Therapy for pulmonary edema during tocolysis includes discontinuing the tocolytic agent, ensuring adequate ventilation and oxygenation, correcting fluid imbalance and hypotension, and maintaining adequate cardiac output. Continuous fetal assessment should accompany maternal treatment and may direct early delivery. Alternative tocolytics like magnesium sulfate can be used or the parturient may be delivered prematurely without further tocolysis. In general, alternative tocolytics such as magnesium sulfate and calcium channel blockers may not be effective or may produce side effects that worsen pulmonary edema.

In most instances of pulmonary edema complicating tocolytic therapy, the expanded circulating volume can be contracted quickly by diuretics like furosemide, 20 mg IV stat and at 4-hour intervals until the intravascular volume is adequately reduced. In addition to its diuretic effect, furosemide will cause an immediate fall in effective circulating blood volume by increasing venous capacitance through vascular smooth muscle relaxation. This reduction in blood volume should ideally be followed with central venous and pulmonary artery pressure monitoring so that overshoot resulting in hypovolemia does not ensue. Serial determinations of the hematocrit, hourly fluid input, and urinary output are helpful. Expanded intravascular volume can be safely reduced to a point at which the hematocrit approximates that obtained before initiation of beta-adrenergic therapy.

Hypoxemic patients tolerate hypotension poorly. The treatment of hypotension in patients with pulmonary edema requires a knowledge of the circulating blood volume and ventricular filling pressures derived by central venous and/or pulmonary artery pressure monitoring. If the blood volume is high or normal, drugs that will raise blood pressure by increasing the force of myocardial contractions, such as dopamine or dobutamine, are effective.[162] If the blood volume is low, the best treatment is rapid intravascular expansion, preferably with fresh whole blood to increase both the oxygen-carrying capacity of the parturient's blood and colloid osmotic pressure.

Pulmonary artery catheterization is indicated in (1) situations in which there is reasonable evidence of underlying heart disease precipitating or aggravating pulmonary edema; (2) patients who do not respond to conventional therapy within 1 to 2 hours; (3) patients who require administration of intravenous fluids at doses substantially greater than those recommended (1500 to 1800 ml/24 hours); (4) cases complicated by hypoxia and hypotension or requiring mechanical ventilation; and (5) cases in which the degree of intravascular volume expansion is unclear. In patients who do not fulfill these conditions, maternal monitoring may be limited to observations of the vital signs, determination of blood gases, measurement of fluid intake and urine output, serial hematocrit determinations, and daily chest radiographs. With improvement, the tachypnea and tachycardia will decrease, blood gases will reflect better oxygenation and decreased CO_2 retention, hematocrit will rise, and chest infiltrates will resolve.

Termination of pregnancy will not significantly improve the respiratory status of a patient who develops pulmonary edema during tocolytic therapy. Vaginal delivery may increase O_2 requirements because of increased cardiac and uterine work.[163] Cesarean section adds all the risks of anesthesia and surgery to a critical situation. It is better to stabilize the patient first and deliver her later after transfer to an institution with facilities for both intensive maternal and fetal care.

The fetus of a hypoxic gravida is well adapted to short-term existence in such hostile environments. If the maternal hemoglobin concentration is 10 g/dl or more and the maternal PaO_2 is 65 mmHg or greater, fetal oxygenation will probably be adequate. The fetus eliminates hydrogen ions by producing CO_2 that is transferred to the mother through the placenta. When maternal $PaCO_2$ reaches a level close to that of the fetus (about 50 mmHg), the diffusion gradient for CO_2 from fetus to mother is impaired and fetal acidosis and death may ensue. Only effective maternal alveolar ventilation will maintain the necessary CO_2 gradient for fetal CO_2 elimination.

If maternal hypoxemia and acidosis are present when fetal distress is detected and the maternal problems are correctable, the fetus will benefit more from elimination of treatable maternal conditions than from a preterm delivery that may be unnecessary. If the maternal prognosis is poor, delivery should not be delayed because the fetus may have a better chance for survival in an outside environment rather than in an intrauterine setting of worsening hypoxia and respiratory acidosis.

Drug Abuse

Substance abuse during pregnancy is occurring at alarming rates and presents a wide range of problems for the abuser and her fetus. Perinatal drug abuse affects the well-being of the entire pregnancy, from prenatal care and fetal development to intrapartum management and postnatal neurobehavioral development. Perinatal drug abuse also influences anesthetic management for labor and delivery.

Drug abuse may include occasional recreational use, physical or psychological addiction, and inadvertent or suicidal overdose. Mothers abuse non-narcotic drugs more than narcotics, with hallucinogens and ethanol probably being the most frequently abused non-narcotics. There are additional dangers associated with parenteral administration of addictive substances including transmission of infectious diseases like hepatitis and acquired immunodeficiency syndrome, frequent overdose, and allergic reactions to adulterants. The drug abuser's unstable emotional state and insecure environment often prevent adequate nutrition and prenatal care. Fetal abuse by chemical assault has been alleged in litigation against repeat offenders.[164] Programs designed to handle a broad spectrum of needs in addition to perinatal care seem to provide more successful results when intervention for maternal drug abuse is made.[165]

Specific effects of illicit drugs on maternal physiology include altered fertility, placental integrity and function, and uterine blood flow. Placental drug metabolism resembles hepatic drug metabolism with restrictions in substrate specificity and enzyme quantity. Illicit drugs may induce fetal liver enzymes to biotransform naturally occurring substances, such as steroids, into teratogenic metabolites (see Chapter 1). Fetal effects occur primarily from the drug or its metabolic byproducts or secondarily from drug-induced functional changes.[166] Limited neonatal metabolizing capabilities prolong drug effects and increase the likelihood of infant intoxication and later withdrawal. Necessary treatment of maternal withdrawal with a specific drug agonist may additionally prolong neontal drug exposure.[167]

ALCOHOL

Due to the teratogenic effects of ethanol on the fetus, it is no longer used for its tocolytic effects. Acute alcohol intoxication inhibits hepatic cytochrome p450-dependent drug oxidation and increases levels of drugs predominantly excreted by hepatic oxidation, such as propranolol and lidocaine.[168] On the other hand, chronic alcohol abuse induces hepatic oxidizing enzyme systems.

Delirium tremens is life-threatening and necessitates immediate pharmacologic treatment despite the danger of drug exposure to the fetus. Treatment with phenobarbital and clonidine is preferred since benzodiazepines are teratogenic, paraldehyde will induce acidosis and potentiate central nervous system depression, and phenothiazines are teratogenic and cause tardive dyskinesias (see Chapter 1).

Alcohol has no effect on umbilical artery impedance, but alcohol ingestion does impair placental transfer of nutrients to the fetus. Placental metabolism of alcohol is similar to hepatic metabolism.[168] Daily or regular consumption of large amounts of alcohol produces intrauterine growth retardation, with developmental and functional defects occurring in a dose-dependent fashion. First-trimester alcohol overexposure causes functional deficits and developmental defects, and third-trimester abuse is associated with fetal growth retardation.[169] There is also an increased rate of spontaneous abortion in proportion to the amount of alcohol consumed.[169]

Acute or chronic fetal alcohol intoxication can depress the newborn. Neonatal ethanol withdrawal produces agitation, excessive crying, irritability, excessive perspiration, and seizures within 24 hours. Treatment consists of supportive care supplemented as necessary with phenobarbital, diazepam, or chlorpromazine.

Antenatal alcohol exposure can produce a syndrome now known as fetal alcohol syndrome, consisting of retarded growth with mental and motor performance deficits, craniofacial anomalies, and fetal or neonatal demise. Prominent facial dysmorphism includes a characteristically drawn appearance with hypoplastic midface, long and smooth philtrum, thin upper lip, and hypoplastic mandible. Variability of occurrence results in full expression in 1 or 2/1000 live births and partial expression in 3 to 5/1000 live births. It is estimated that 10% to 20% of mild and moderate mental retardation may be the result of maternal alcohol consumption during pregnancy.[169]

The alcoholic patient needs anesthetics tailored to suit her present state of pathophysiology. Narcotic analgesia may exacerbate hypoxia by cardiorespiratory depression. Narcotic and local anesthetic metabolism may be affected if liver function is impaired. Evaluation of neurologic deficit following regional anesthesia may be confused with myopathy or neuropathy. The risk of epidural hematoma may be increased due to alcohol-related coagulopathy. If the prothrombin time remains within normal limits, metabolism of amide-type local anesthetics is normal. However, decreased liver production of cholinesterase will prolong 2-chloroprocaine and procaine metabolism. Such factors should be considered before initiation of spinal or epidural anesthesia for cesarean section, since the mother and fetus will generally benefit by remaining conscious during the procedure.

MARIJUANA

Marijuana abuse produces sleepiness, ataxia, and decreased motor and cognitive ability by its effects on two prominent central nervous system neurotransmitters, acetylcholine and gamma-aminobutyric acid (GABA).[170] Chronic marijuana smokers may experience infertility from abnormal secretion of luteinizing hormone, follicle-stimulating hormone, and prolactin. Marijuana increases heart rate, myocardial workload, and plasma volume through its beta-mimetic effects, which are blocked by propranolol. Tetrahydrocannabinol (THC), the active ingredient in marijuana, is metabolized by the liver and stored in body fat with a serum half-life extending for days. Tolerance develops to some behavioral effects and, as with opiates, a larger dose is required to attain highs. Cross-tolerance usually does not develop with hallucinogens, but some may exist with ethanol.

As noted, marijuana abuse produces temporal disintegration, relaxation, and sleepiness.[170] Higher doses trigger paranoid feelings, delusions, and hallucinations. Mild sympathomimetic effects accompanying intoxication respond best to conservative management. Diazepam is preferable if sedation is needed, since chlorpromazine potentiates postural hypotension and barbiturates potentiate hallucinations. Both diazepam and chlorpromazine are teratogenic during organogenesis (see Chapter 1). No recognized withdrawal syndrome occurs; however, irritability, restlessness, insomnia, and nervousness may accompany discontinuation.

Marijuana smokers have chronic bronchitis and associated bronchoconstriction (usually worse than in cigarette smokers) and require the same anesthetic care as cigarette smokers. If cesarean section is required, regional rather than general anesthesia is recommended.

Sympathomimetic effects commonly produce tachycardia up to 140 beats/min. Some patients may have sufficient analgesia for vaginal delivery when they are severely intoxicated. If hypotension develops after epidural block, use of mephentermine rather than ephedrine may prevent further tachycardia. If general anesthesia is required, minimum alveolar concentration (MAC) will be reduced for all inhaled agents and there will be greater sensitivity to the cardiodepressant effects of sodium pentothal and halothane. Marijuana-induced microsomal dechlorinase will increase halothane metabolism.[171] Etomidate is the preferred induction agent because it does not aggravate bronchospasm and does not increase fetal depression. Dry mouth and tachycardia contraindicate the use of anticholinergics.

COCAINE

In addition to producing prolonged local anesthesia, cocaine accelerates and desynchronizes the electroencephalogram and increases blood pressure, respiration, and uterine tone. Chronic intranasal or parenteral use produces serious consequences including seizures, depression, and paranoia.[172] Cocaine-induced coronary artery spasm produces focal endothelial injury with platelet aggregation, platelet thrombosis, chronic intimal proliferation, and myocardial infarction.[173] Pseudomembranous enterocolitis and cerebrovascular accidents can occur at a young age.[174]

Many patients with acute cocaine intoxication or overdose appear to have suffered a myocardial infarction but actually die from seizures and respiratory failure. Beta-adrenergic blocking agents will control tachycardia. Unopposed alpha-adrenergic stimulation can produce hypertension and require treatment with nitroprusside.[175] Psychosis responds to neuroleptics or lithium, although the former does not reduce euphoria.[176] The so-called rewarding effects of cocaine result from acute activation of dopamine pathways, and cocaine's addicting effects result from dopamine depletion. Thus, administration of dopamine agonist drugs prevents cocaine craving.[177, 178]

Cocaine increases norepinephrine levels, decreases uterine blood flow and increases uterine contractility and tone. Abruptio placentae and tumultuous labor can occur immediately following administration of intranasal or intravenous cocaine.[179]

Cocaine abuse increases the frequency of spontaneous abortions during pregnancy, with incidences of 36% to 46%.[179] Intravenous cocaine abuse is associated with fetal and neonatal cerebral infarction.[180] In a study of pregnancy outcome, Chasnoff and coworkers[179] noted sudden infant death syndrome (SIDS) in one infant and prune belly syndrome in another whose mother abused cocaine at 5 weeks' gestation. Additionally, Brazelton neurobehavioral assessments of infants born to cocaine-addicted mothers reveal significant depression of interactive behavior and poor organizational response to environmental stimuli (see Chapter 9).[173]

Cocaine-abusing parturients require thorough evaluation for evidence of coronary artery disease, including ECG, cardiac enzyme analysis, and echocardiography. In addition to the usual cardiac screens, ECG leads II and V_5, ST segment trends, and transesophageal echocardiography can also detect early cardiac ischemia. The abuser's catecholamine depletion and sluggish response to ephedrine favor gradual epidural block over spinal block to avoid hypotension. Cocaine abusers have increased sensitivity to central nervous system depressants and decreased MAC for all inhaled agents. During induction of general anesthesia, etomidate produces less hypotension than thiopental. As for cardiac anesthetics, nitroglycerin and beta-adrenergic or calcium channel blockers may be indicated to control heart rate and prevent coronary vasospasm. Ketamine and N_2O should be avoided due to their sympathomimetic effects.

Since cocaine increases uterine contractility, preterm labor is a frequent occurrence in intoxicated addicts. The parturient may require little anesthesia, since cocaine produces systemic analgesia and rapid labor to delivery time. Epidural analgesia during labor will reverse systemic vasoconstriction and improve uterine blood flow. Additional local anesthetics may, however, potentiate cocaine toxicity by occupying cocaine-metabolizing hepatic enzyme systems. Since plasma cholinesterase does not significantly metabolize cocaine, 2-chloroprocaine is a better choice for epidural anesthesia than amide local anesthetics. The risk of local anesthetic toxicity is minimized with spinal anesthesia. However, depletion of intravascular volume and uncertain response to sympathomimetics like ephedrine, due to catecholamine depletion, increase the risk of uncorrectable hypotension with spinal anesthesia. In addition to the monitoring recommended for chronic cocaine abuse, central venous or pulmonary artery pressure monitoring facilitates correction of intravascular volume deficits in acute cocaine overdose.

General anesthesia is usually indicated in most cases of abruptio placentae. Acute cocaine intoxication during general anesthesia can precipitate myocardial infarction or be relatively benign.[181-183] With severe cocaine toxicity, especially "crack" cocaine overdose, maternal blood volume and pressure control with fluids, beta-blockers, and vasodilators must precede anesthetics. Thiopental induction will limit catecholamine release in response to tracheal intubation, but etomidate induction may prove safer with hypovolemia. Like cocaine, ketamine also blocks the re-uptake of norepinephrine and can potentiate the hemodynamic side effects of acute cocaine toxicity. N_2O also has sympathomimetic effects and can complicate maintenance of anesthesia during cocaine toxicity.[184] Additionally, patients with impaired coronary arterial flow should not receive N_2O. If ECG signs of myocardial ischemia appear, coronary vasodilators are indicated. Droperidol and thorazine may be used post delivery since they possess both sedative and alpha-adrenergic blocking effects and do not influence uterine contractility.

METHAMPHETAMINE

Like cocaine, amphetamines stimulate release and inhibit re-uptake of catecholamines peripherally and centrally, increasing blood pressure, respirations, and uterine tone, and suppressing appetite. Methamphetamine produces more central nervous system effects and fewer cardiovascular effects than does amphetamine. Tolerance to amphetamine develops only to central and not to cardiovascular effects; therefore, abuse results from cravings for mood elevation and fatigue reduction. Weight loss, bruxism, face picking, suspiciousness, stereotyped repetitious or disorganized behavior, and paranoid schizophrenia characterize chronic abuse. Psychotic symptoms appear more slowly than with cocaine. Users take increasing doses until aberrant behavior prevents them from obtaining additional drug. Within a few hours of cessation, they sleep for 12 to 18 hours, awakening hungry and depressed. Depression causes a new "run." Narcotics delay the "crash."

Overdose produces severe chest pain, toxic paranoid syndrome, seizures, unconsciousness, cardiovascular collapse, and death from respiratory failure. Toxic symptoms resemble those of cocaine toxicity and call for similar treatment. Ammonium chloride urine acidification accelerates excretion of amphetamines and their metabolites.

Amphetamines are teratogenic in animals and cause small-for-gestational-age infants in humans. In 25% of cases, amphetamine abusers deliver prematurely, and their neonates have a perinatal mortality rate of 7.5%.[185] Neonatal withdrawal causes excessive drowsiness and occasional seizures.

Known users require close surveillance with ultrasound for fetal growth disturbances and placental dysfunction. Nonstress and biophysical profile monitoring during gestation provides additional noninvasive assessment of fetal well-being for known amphetamine abusers.

The hazards of hypotension during conduction anesthesia are increased in amphetamine abusers because of a poor response to indirect-acting sympathomimetic agents. The dose requirements (ED_{50}) for intravenous and inhalation agents decrease.[184] For induction of general anesthesia, etomidate may cause less cardiovascular depression than thiopental sodium. Tracheal intubation for airway protection and mechanical ventilation is indicated in comatose patients. Preoperatively, antipsychotics and barbiturates help stabilize paranoid patients. Although coronary artery disease is less frequent with amphetamine abuse than with cocaine abuse, parturients still need monitoring for myocardial ischemia. The hypovolemic patient benefits from CVP monitoring. By comparison, cocaine levels invariably decrease with time, but continued gastric and intestinal absorption of oral amphetamine may actually increase its toxicity during labor. Epidural analgesia maintains or improves uterine blood flow. Since vasoconstriction and volume depletion characterize amphetamine toxicity, epidural anesthesia may be preferable to spinal block. Like inhaled anesthetics, amphetamines sensitize the myocardium to catecholamines. Thiopental induction may attenuate the hypertensive response to tracheal intubation, but etomidate is safer during hypovolemia. Some workers[182] report difficulty maintaining anesthesia with nitrous oxide and fentanyl in amphetamine abusers.

Neurologic Emergencies

AUTONOMIC HYPERREFLEXIA

Autonomic hyperreflexia is a disorder that develops in patients who have sustained spinal cord transection above T_5–T_6 levels. The syndrome is caused by a sudden release of catecholamines producing episodes of paroxysmal hypertension, throbbing headaches, cardiac arrhythmias, facial flushing, and perspiration.[186, 187] By monitoring these episodes, some laboring paraplegics are able to determine when a uterine contraction is occurring. In paraplegic patients, the splanchnic sympathetic bed is uninhibited by higher centers and therefore is bombarded by sympathetic stimuli from uterine contractions, a full bladder, pelvic examinations, and even rectal examinations or fecal impaction. In addition, the same stimuli can increase somatic hyperreflexia with flexor and extensor spasms and sustained clonus that make vaginal delivery difficult.

Beta-adrenergic blocking agents such as propranolol given intravenously (in 1-mg doses and repeated every 5 minutes until 8 to 10 mg has been given) are effective in treating cardic arrhythmias associated with autonomic hyperreflexia. Continuous lumbar epidural or spinal anesthesia maintained to a level of T_7–T_{10} is indicated for patients with this disorder. Either of these two forms of regional anesthesia effectively prevents both somatic and autonomic hyperreflexia associated with high thoracic spinal cord transection.

MYASTHENIC CRISIS

Myasthenia gravis, an autoimmune disease of the motor end-plates of striated muscles, is clinically manifested by fluctuating fatigability of skeletal muscles. Autoantibodies against postsynaptic acetylcholine receptors interfere with neuromuscular transmission, accelerate turnover of receptors, and lead eventually to irreversible deformation of postsynaptic membranes. Thymectomy and corticosteroid therapy will alter the immunogenesis of the disease process and promote rare spontaneous remissions. Treatment with cholinesterase inhibitors such as neostigmine and pyridostigmine stimulates both muscarinic and nicotinic acetylcholine receptors. Young women with generalized myasthenia gravis are advised to have a thymectomy and wait until the disease stabilizes before attempting to become pregnant.

Myasthenic women usually have uncomplicated childbirth since myometrial muscles are unaffected. In fact, myasthenia may improve during pregnancy because the alpha-fetoprotein antigen blocks the interaction of the antiacetylcholine receptor antibody with the receptor antigen. Ventilatory exhaustion is a problem encountered by some myasthenic parturients and should be anticipated during the later stages of pregnancy and labor. During pregnancy, serial determinations of vital capacity will detect the early onset of respiratory fatigue. Magnesium sulfate therapy is contraindicated because it will precipitate a myasthenic crisis by blocking presynaptic acetylcholine release.

If vaginal delivery is anticipated, regional anesthesia with lidocaine is recommended.[188] Procaine, 2-chloroprocaine, and other ester-type local anesthetics may become toxic when their hydrolysis by plasma cholinesterase is blocked by anticholinesterase therapy. Amide-type drugs, such as lidocaine, are inactivated in the liver and may prove safer for regional anesthesia. Inhalational agents are recommended for general anesthesia and usually obviate the need for muscle relaxants with effects that may be unpredictable and for relaxant reversal with anticholinesterases that can precipitate cholinergic crisis.

Cholinesterase inhibitors such as neostigmine are given intravenously to ensure absorption after labor has been established. The intravenous dosage of neostigmine and pyridostigmine administered to the laboring patient is one-thirtieth of the oral dose. Atropine (0.4 to 1.0 mg or more as required) should be given before intravenous administration of any cholinesterase inhibitors to prevent muscarinic side effects, especially bronchorrhea.

Myasthenic patients may develop rapidly progressive weakness and respiratory failure caused either by worsening of their myasthenia or by cholinergic crisis from anticholinesterase overdose. Prolonged labor or infection can also produce myasthenic crisis.

Other drugs that can block neuromuscular transmission are curare, aminoglycoside antibiotics, quinine, and quinidine.[188] Narcotic analgesia is not advisable since respiratory drive may become depressed. Hyperthyroidism and potassium depletion may contribute to muscle weakness.

Like a myasthenic crisis, a cholinergic crisis also causes weakness through a different mechanism of prolonged depolarization and later fatigue of neuromuscular end-plates. In cholinergic crisis, overstimulation of both muscarinic and nicotinic receptors occurs. Overstimulation of muscarinic acetylcholine receptors produces diarrhea, belching, vomiting, sweating, hypersalivation, bronchorrhea, fasciculations, and pallor. In normal lighting, pupils measuring less than 2 mm in diameter are often the forerunner of bradycardia and hypotension. Atropine sulfate (2 mg IV) is the treatment of choice and may be repeated hourly as needed. As noted, nicotinic receptor overstimulation produces weakness and respiratory muscle paralysis.

The differentiation between myasthenic and cholinergic crises is important but can be difficult. In either case, the trachea should be intubated and mechanical ventilation provided. During crisis, an edrophonium test may complicate initial management. Even though the effects of edrophonium are short, the additional cholinergic effects during crisis may be significant enough to produce cardiorespiratory collapse in cholinergic crisis. Patients with myasthenic crisis will usually strengthen after intravenous edrophonium; however, ventilation may be further compromised by excessive pulmonary secretions. Furthermore, a patient slipping into myasthenic crisis may have ingested additional acetylcholinesterases in the hope of increasing her strength.

When a crisis occurs, all medication should be discontinued for 24 hours. If the patient's vital capacity is below 1.2 L, or if she tires when ventilation is unassisted, controlled mechanical ventilation should be continued. If the patient is no stronger the following day, plasmapheresis will reduce circulating autoantibodies, improve respiratory muscle strength, and permit re-institution of anticholinesterase therapy. Most nonpregnant patients respond after three to five 2-L plasma volume exchanges.

MATERNAL HEMORRHAGIC EMERGENCIES

Although maternal mortality has been reduced dramatically by improved prenatal care, hospitalization for delivery, and the availability of blood and its components for transfusion, death from obstetric hemorrhage remains prominent in the majority of mortality reports. There are many causes of maternal hemorrhage but the most prominent include placenta previa, abruptio placentae, placenta accreta, and uterine rupture.

Placenta Previa

Placenta previa is defined as a placenta implanted in the lower uterine segment with varying degrees of encroachment on the internal cervical os. Depending on the degree of encroachment, the following types of placenta previa are described:

1. Central, total, or complete previa with the placenta completely covering the internal cervical os.
2. Partial or incomplete previa with the placenta covering only a portion of the internal cervical os.
3. Low-lying or marginal previa with the placental edge reaching but not extending beyond the margin of the internal cervical os. Since the type of placenta previa is influenced by the degree of cervical effacement and dilatation, this classification should be based on the findings at the initial examination.

The incidence of placenta previa varies from 0.1% to 1%[189, 190] and is highest in the multipara and older gravida. Placenta previa is three times more common in women over 35 years of age regardless of parity. When age is held constant, there is no association with parity. Once placenta previa occurs, the risk of its recurrence in a subsequent pregnancy is about 12 times greater than the general incidence. Accompanying placenta previa is an increase in fetal malpresentation. The frequencies of the different types of placenta previa are total, 20% to 31%; partial, 20% to 33%; and marginal, 37% to 60%.[189, 191, 192]

The precise cause of placenta previa is unknown. Predisposing factors may include previous uterine incisions, especially those in the lower uterine segments, leiomyomata distorting the contour of the uterus, endometritis, multiple gestation, and repeated therapeutic abortions.

The primary presenting symptom of placenta previa is painless vaginal bleeding. The bleeding most commonly occurs during the third trimester, although a small amount of bleeding can occur in the first and second trimesters. The initial bleeding is usually self-limiting and rarely fatal. Almost all initial bleeding episodes stop spontaneously. Subsequent bleeding episodes may recur at unpredictable times and may or may not be quite as severe. Uterine bleeding is rarely associated with death of the fetus. Uterine or abdominal pain is absent and the uterus, as a rule, is not tender but will become irritable with bleeding.

About 90% of patients with placenta previa have had at least one significant antepartum hemorrhage; 10% to 25% develop hypovolemic shock.[191, 192] Parturients with total previa develop shock more often and tend to bleed earlier and more profusely.[191, 192]

After an initial bleeding episode, ultrasound examination will pinpoint placental location. Repeated examinations are often required because the location of the placenta changes as the uterus enlarges.

If bleeding persists or increases, jeopardizing the pregnancy, emergency cesarean section is performed despite fetal gestational age. Regional anesthesia has no place in the management of the severely or persistently bleeding parturient. General anesthesia is the anesthetic of choice for the parturient in shock. Preparation for general anesthesia should include the administration of a nonparticulate antacid, insertion of two large-bore intravenous lines, and often CVP line insertion to monitor actual blood volume. Prior to induction, volume replacement with whole blood or its components is often required. The patient should be denitrogenated with 100% O_2 for 3 to 5 minutes prior to induction. If time does not permit 3 to 5 minutes of denitrogenation, then four deep breaths of 100% O_2 by the parturient prior to rapid-sequence induction of general anesthesia is indicated. Because of its sympathomimetic properties, ketamine is an excellent induction agent for a patient who is hypovolemic from previa hemorrhage.

Abruptio Placentae

Abruptio placentae is defined as a separation of the normally implanted placenta after the 20th week of gestation and before the birth of the fetus. Severe bleeding between the placenta and the decidua basalis results, and bleeding either escapes vaginally or is retained occultly between the uterus and the placenta. The etiology is unknown, but abruptio placentae is frequently associated with hypertension, multiparity, uterine abnormalities, abdominal trauma, sudden decompression of the uterus, short umbilical cord, tetanic uterine contractions, inferior vena caval occlusion, or maternal vascular disease.[193–196]

The incidence of abruptio placentae varies from 0.2% to 2.4%,[194,]

[197-199] with a significant increase associated with multiparous women but not with age. Over one-half of abruptions occur before the 36th week of gestation, and the incidence of recurrence in subsequent pregnancies is 11%.[194, 196, 200] When the abruption is accompanied by fetal death, there is a 30% chance that in a subsequent pregnancy the fetus will die with recurrent abruptio placentae.[196]

The clinical manifestations of abruptio placentae depend primarily on the degree of separation and the amount of hemorrhage. The condition is classically defined as mild, moderate, or severe. Mild forms of abruption are accompanied by vaginal bleeding, which may be confused with bloody show, and minimal uterine tenderness. The uterus may be slightly irritable, and there is usually no indication of fetal distress or maternal shock. The diagnosis is confirmed prenatally by ultrasound[201] or postpartum by placental examination showing an adherent retroplacental clot.

With moderate abruption, there is usually sudden onset of persistent abdominal pain accompanied by vaginal bleeding and hypertension. Fetal distress may or may not be evident, depending on the extent of the placental separation and the amount of maternal blood loss. The uterus is tender to palpation and contracts when manipulated, making fetal heart tones difficult to auscultate. If the membranes have been ruptured, the application of a scalp electrode will identify the fetal heart rate and allow precise fetal ECG monitoring.

In severe abruptio placentae, there is a sudden onset of intense persistent abdominal pain, often described as knife-like or tearing. The uterus is rigid and extremely tender. The fetus is usually dead and the mother is often in shock, the severity of which may be out of proportion to the visible vaginal bleeding because of concealed retroplacental bleeding. If prompt and effective management is not instituted, the patient will develop coagulopathy, renal failure, and refractory shock.

The most common complications associated with abruptio placentae are DIC, renal failure, and pituitary necrosis (Sheehan's syndrome). Specific blood coagulation defects commonly associated with an abruption include afibrinogenemia, thrombocytopenia, decreases in factors V and VIII, and increases in fibrin split products.

The obstetric management of abruptio placentae depends on the extent of the abruption, the maternal hemodynamic state, and the gestational age and status of the fetus. Regional anesthesia may be used for vaginal delivery in parturients with mild to moderate abruptio placentae but only in very specific situations involving (1) no hypovolemia, (2) no clotting abnormalities, and (3) no fetal distress. For imminent vaginal delivery, however, pudendal block supplemented with inhalation analgesia might be more satisfactory, quicker, and easier to accomplish than regional anesthesia.

For cesarean section, general anesthesia is indicated and requires two large-bore intravenous lines and a preoperative coagulation profile. Thiopental is a myocardial depressant, and ketamine is a uterine stimulant; each causes effects that may make either agent unsuitable as the sole induction agent. Heparin is not indicated for the associated coagulopathy (see DIC). Fresh-frozen plasma and platelet replacement are often necessary. Packed red cells or whole blood may be transfused as indicated by serial hematocrits.

Adherent Placenta

Adherence of the placenta to the uterine wall is much more likely to occur in association with placenta previa than with a normally implanted placenta. Such an abnormality might be expected with placenta previa[202] because of poorly developed decidua in the lower uterine segment. As a result, one or more cotyledons are firmly bound to the decidua or may even invade the myometrium. The abnormal adherence may involve the entire placenta (total placenta accreta), a few cotyledons (partial accreta), or a single cotyledon (focal placenta accreta). A precise classification of adherent placenta is as follows:

1. Placenta accreta—placental villi attach to the myometrium.
2. Placenta increta—placental villi invade the myometrium.
3. Placenta percreta—placental villi penetrate the entire thickness of the myometrium.

The frequency of adherent placenta is unknown. Significant morbidity and even mortality occur from severe hemorrhage, uterine perforation, and postpartum infection.[202] Successful treatment depends on immediate blood replacement therapy for severe hemorrhage and prompt hysterectomy. The diagnosis may be made antenatally using ultrasound techniques. In 1983, Pasto and associates[203] confirmed that the absence of a subplacental sonolucent or "hypoechoic retroplacental" zone is consistent with adherent placenta.

Uterine Rupture

Uterine rupture is a condition that may occur spontaneously in a uterus with no previous scars. It may be a traumatic rupture from blunt abdominal trauma or a chronic rupture through a previous cesarean section scar. It is customary to classify uterine rupture as complete or incomplete, depending on whether the laceration communicates directly with the peritoneal cavity or is separated from the cavity by the visceral peritoneum over the uterus. Rupture indicates that the uterine muscle has torn apart, while separation indicates a weakening of a uterine scar with progressive separation of myometrial muscle fibers.[204]

The probability of rupture of a classical cesarean scar is several times greater than that of a low transverse uterine scar. If a classical cesarean scar does rupture, it usually occurs before labor in about one-third of the cases. Classical scar rupture may occur several weeks before term, long before a repeat cesarean section would ordinarily be scheduled. Thus, scheduled abdominal delivery may not prevent classical scar rupture. Lower segment scars are confined to the noncontractile portion of the uterus and rarely, if ever, rupture before labor; only infrequently does rupture occur during labor.[204]

One factor that may lead to rupture is excessive oxytocin stimulation, particularly in multiparous women and in parturients with previous uterine scars. Other predisposing factors include rapid and tumultuous labor, multiparity with a weakness of the uterine wall, and uterine overdistention associated with twins, fetal macrosomia, or polyhydramnios.

The incidence of uterine rupture varies from 1 in 100 to 1 in 11,000 cases, with a maternal mortality at present of approximately 5% and a neonatal mortality of 50%.[204]

Signs and symptoms of the rupture may be initially silent but will progress to severe abdominal pain. The pain may suddenly decrease after an acute onset. The patient often exhibits a shock-like state out of proportion to visible blood loss. Hypotension and fetal distress will soon ensue.

If the parturient has an epidural anesthetic block at the time of the rupture, shock or severe bleeding may dictate conversion to general anesthesia by rapid-sequence technique for immediate cesarean section. If the patient is hemodynamically stable, thiopental sodium may be a satisfactory induction agent. Ketamine remains the drug of choice for anesthesia induction in parturients in shock. Two large-bore intravenous lines and possibly a central venous or pulmonary artery catheter will be needed for intravascular volume replacement and assessment during cesarean hysterectomy or cesarean delivery with uterine reconstruction.

Disseminated Intravascular Coagulopathy

DIC or defibrination consumption coagulopathy is a secondary fibrinolytic process that occurs most often as a complicating factor of a triggering disease, particularly placental and embolic complications of pregnancy.[205] Triggering disease processes may include abruptio placentae, placenta previa, amniotic fluid embolism, prolonged retention of a dead fetus, retained placenta, septic abortion, unsterile delivery, and eclampsia.[206, 207]

Pregnancy normally causes increases in the concentrations of many procoagulants, especially fibrinogen and factors VII, VIII, IX, and X (see

Chapter 2). Other plasma factors and platelets do not change remarkably. Plasminogen levels are increased considerably, but antepartum activity is normally decreased compared with the nonpregnant state. Various stresses initiate the conversion of plasminogen to plasmin, especially activation of the coagulation cascade.

Intravascular activation of the clotting cascade may be due to thromboplastin activation of the extrinsic pathway, collagen activation of the intrinsic pathway, protease activation of factor X, as in some neoplasias, and initiation of preprocoagulant activity by white blood cells.[208] Coagulation activates the lytic process with plasminogen converted to plasmin, which in turn lyses fibrinogen into its fibrin monomers, the fibrin split products. These split or degradation products may also contribute to coagulopathy by delaying fibrin polymerization, prolonging prothrombin time, or causing impaired clot stability and retraction. Fibrin split products are deposited in the microcirculation, cause ischemic damage to vital organs, and promote hemorrhage.

Hematologic sequelae of DIC include depletion of coagulation factors, thrombocytopenia, and activation of the fibrinolytic process. A marked decrease in fibrinogen and procoagulants is due to their consumption during intravascular coagulation and their rapid removal by the reticuloendothelial system. Thrombocytopenia is caused by the consumption of platelets at a rate greater than the bone marrow is able to compensate for. Active fibrinolysis occurs, fibrin split products abound, and plasminogen levels fall.[209] Normal hematologic changes of pregnancy, including hyperfibrinogenemia, increased platelet activity, and decreased fibrinolytic activity, may set the stage for DIC with fibrin deposition in the microcirculation during pregnancy (see Chapter 2).[210]

The parturient with DIC usually presents with unexplained bleeding, hemorrhagic shock, thrombosis, and conditions predisposing to DIC. Excessive bleeding from minor trauma sites, like venipunctures and perineal shave nicks, and spontaneous bleeding from the gums or nose often herald coagulopathy. Reduced plasma fibrinogen levels and thrombocytopenia help to confirm the diagnosis. In addition, prothrombin time, thrombin time, and partial thromboplastin time are significantly prolonged. Fibrin split products are increased and indicate the onset of secondary fibrinolysis. In mild DIC, ample procoagulant and platelet reserves may compensate for their slow consumption.

Hypofibrinogenemia is a serious condition that one may test at the bedside by drawing a blood sample and observing time to clotting as well as the size and consistency of the clot that forms. In DIC, a soft clot may form initially but may soften and dissolve over several minutes. If there is no apparent clot formation, afibrinogenemia is present and indicates advanced DIC.

Treatment of the underlying cause of DIC is the cornerstone of patient management. For patients in hypovolemic shock, intravascular volume and organ perfusion are restored by transfusion therapy and inotropic support. Activated coagulation factors and circulating fibrin and fibrin split products will be removed more promptly by the reticuloendothelial system when adequate organ perfusion is restored.

Once the uterus is completely emptied, DIC will begin to subside; for this reason, heparin use in obstetric DIC is quite controversial. Occasionally, DIC progresses even after uterine evacuation and requires low-dose heparin therapy at 500 units/hour.[205] Epsilon-aminocaproic acid (EACA, Amicar) therapy should be reserved for use in primary fibrinolysis and is contraindicated in DIC.

Vaginal delivery is preferable to cesarean section or hysterotomy in parturients with DIC because less blood loss can be anticipated. Ideally, operative intervention should be avoided if possible. Conduction anesthesia appears to be contraindicated in a parturient with severe hemostatic instability from DIC owing to the risk of epidural or subdural bleeding with significant neurologic sequelae. General anesthesia with rapid-sequence induction is indicated for the patient with DIC.

Vigorous support of the intravascular volume to adequately perfuse the vital organs is essential and may obviate the need for drugs and other fibrinolytic agents. The fluid of choice is lactated Ringer's solution. Blood components, such as fresh-frozen plasma and packed red cells as well as platelets and cryoprecipitate, will frequently be needed if severe hemorrhage has occurred.

UMBILICAL CORD ACCIDENTS

Faulty umbilical cord insertion and cord accidents have been responsible for many obstetric emergencies and fetal wastage. With the development of obstetric ultrasound, improved prenatal care, and fetal monitoring, some cord problems have been diagnosed antenatally and have permitted safer abdominal delivery. Common cord problems that may result in serious consequences for the fetus and neonate include short umbilical cord, prolapsed umbilical cord, and vasa previa.

The umbilical cord normally contains three vessels (two arteries and a vein) and is usually inserted centrally on the fetal surface of the placenta. The location of cord insertion is determined at the time of uterine implantation of the conceptus. Although variations occur, the umbilical cord averages about 55 cm in length. The cord must be sufficiently long to reach from its attachment to the vulva to allow for normal vaginal delivery.

Short Umbilical Cord

It is uncommon for the cord to be so short that it causes dystocia,[211] but in rare instances short cord has been the attributing cause of abruptio placentae, rupture of the cord, umbilical hernia, and even uterine inversion. Unfortunately, the diagnosis may not be confirmed until considerable damage has occurred; however, with the high reliability of ultrasound technology, short cord is being diagnosed antenatally and its complications can be prevented by elective cesarean section.

Prolapsed Umbilical Cord

Cord prolapse occurs when there is imperfect adaptation between the fetal presenting part and the pelvic inlet. Cord prolapse most frequently occurs with breech presentations, compound presentations, preterm or small fetus, and premature rupture of the membranes. When cord prolapse occurs, the presenting part can compress the cord against the pelvic inlet or cervical os, asphyxiating the fetus. Manual elevation of the presenting part off the prolapsed cord will relieve cord occlusion and permit safer abdominal delivery by emergency cesarean section during general anesthesia.

Vasa Previa

In vasa previa, velamentous insertion of the umbilical cord permits the umbilical vessels to cross the internal cervical os. Vasa previa presents considerable potential danger to the fetus since rupture of the membranes could lacerate one or more umbilical vessels, exsanguinating the fetus.[212] Vasa previa is often diagnosed by ultrasound or pelvic examination prior to labor and spontaneous rupture of membranes. Early diagnosis will permit delivery by elective cesarean section.

EMERGENCIES SECONDARY TO ANESTHETIC ADMINISTRATION

Hypotension

The most common complication of spinal or epidural anesthesia in the pregnant patient is hypotension from sympathetic blockage. Mild to moderate drops in maternal blood pressure that do not adversely affect the mother may have profound effects on uteroplacental perfusion and fetal well-being.

Despite the 40% increase in blood volume that occurs with normal pregnancy, the term parturient is particularly susceptible to hypotension during major conduction anesthesia (see Chapter 2).[213, 214] Compression of the inferior vena cava and aorta caused by the gravid uterus is present in most parturients lying in the supine position (see Chapter 2, Fig. 2–3).[215, 216] Vena caval compression not only impedes venous return to the heart, producing hypotension, but also increases uterine venous pressure and vascular resistance, which further decrease uterine blood flow. An increase in resting sympathetic tone partially compensates for the effects of aortocaval compression on maternal blood pressure. When sympathetic tone is suddenly removed by spinal or epidural blocks, marked falls in blood pressure may occur. In addition, diminished intravascular volume occurs with preeclampsia, antepartum bleeding, or fasting dehydration and may aggravate hypotension following regional anesthesia.

Most parturients will tolerate prolonged systolic blood pressures of 80 to 90 mmHg and maintain adequate, autoregulated end-organ blood flow. The fetus, however, is exquisitely sensitive to decreases in maternal arterial blood pressure because there is no uteroplacental autoregulation. Hypotension from spinal or epidural anesthesia will cause uterine blood flow to fall linearly with blood pressure.[217, 218] Fetal response to reduced uterine blood flow is dependent on the degree and duration of the reduction and the preexisting status of the uteroplacental circulation. If uterine blood flow is already inadequate, fetal asphyxia may develop.[219, 220] The exact degree and duration of hypotension necessary to cause fetal distress is variable. Several investigators have noted that a drop in maternal blood pressure greater than 20% from normal produced sustained episodes of fetal bradycardia and abnormal FHR patterns.[219] However, in all of these studies, the FHR returned to normal with correction of maternal hypotension.[219] In all cases of fetal bradycardia caused by hypotension related to sympathetic block from regional anesthesia, every effort should be made to correct the hypotension prior to delivery. Prophylactic measures to decrease or prevent hypotension from combinations of aortocaval compression and regional anesthesia at term are presented in Chapter 2.

Local Anesthetic Toxicity

Lidocaine, bupivacaine, and 2-chloroprocaine are the agents most commonly used for regional blocks in obstetrics. Each agent has advantages and potential disadvantages. Potential disadvantages may include (1) bupivacaine cardiotoxicity, (2) chloroprocaine neurotoxicity, (3) the neurobehavioral effects of lidocaine, and (4) the tocolytic effects of local anesthetic solutions containing epinephrine.

BUPIVACAINE CARDIOTOXICITY

Bupivacaine, a long-acting amide, is allegedly more cardiotoxic than shorter-acting amides like lidocaine.[221] Bupivacaine-induced seizures, often resulting from intravascular overdose, have been associated with cardiac arrest, profound metabolic acidosis, and death.[221] Whether or not bupivacaine is inherently more cardiotoxic than other local anesthetics remains a controversial topic still under investigation. Additional aspects of the controversy include the parturient's susceptiblity to the adverse effects of bupivacaine, prophylactic measures to reduce or eliminate bupivacaine toxicity, and the best management techniques for parturients with bupivacaine toxicity. Rosen's group[222] studied conscious adult sheep that were rapidly injected intravenously with pharmacologically equivalent doses of lidocaine or bupivacaine. Both local anesthetics produced similar central nervous system toxicity at equivalent doses. More cardiac arrhythmias, however, occurred after bupivacaine overdose. In subsequent studies, bupivacaine cardiotoxicity was enhanced significantly by prior establishment of hypercarbia, acidosis, and hypoxia in the experimental animals.[222]

Thus, in certain settings, bupivacaine appears to be potentially more cardiotoxic than lidocaine, probably due to its effects on cardiac sodium channels.[222] Both lidocaine and bupivacaine block sodium channels in nerves and in the heart. These channels open briefly during the upstroke of the action potential and are responsible for fast conduction in nerves and Purkinje fibers. Competitive blockade of sodium channels will slow or stop conduction of an action potential. This is the primary mechanism of action of local anesthetics at nerve membranes. Lidocaine blockade of cardiac sodium channels appears well tolerated by the heart and permits lidocaine's common use as an antiarrhythmic. In contrast, the action of bupivacaine on the heart is not as well tolerated.[223] When electrophysiologic differences between lidocaine and bupivacaine were compared, lidocaine was found to enter the cardiac sodium channel quickly and to leave it quickly.[223] In contrast, bupivacaine was found to be a fast-in and slow-out agent.[223] As a result, bupivacaine is a more long-lived cardiac sodium channel blocker than lidocaine, has greater cardiodepressant potential, and is not a safe antiarrhythmic.[223] A number of cardiac arrests associated with accidental intravascular injection of 0.75% bupivacaine in obstetric patients caused the U.S. Food and Drug Administration (FDA) to withdraw 0.75% bupivacaine for obstetric anesthesia.[224]

Despite its potential for cardiotoxicity, 0.125% to 0.5% bupivacaine still remains a very useful agent for epidural blocks in obstetric anesthesia. Bupivacaine produces high sensory block with minimal motor block, has a relatively long duration of action, and is effective for labor analgesia in concentrations as low as 0.125%. Bupivacaine 0.5% has been found effective for cesarean section.[224] Although bupivacaine 0.75% produced a more rapid onset of a denser block, the added hazard of the higher concentration now contraindicates its use in obstetrics.

To lessen the risk of local anesthetic toxicity, a number of prophylactic measures are recommended, including use of the minimum effective dose, cautiously aspirating for blood or cerebrospinal fluid through the epidural needle and catheter, using small test doses, and slowly administering the local anesthetic in fractional amounts.

Aspiration that does not yield cerebrospinal fluid or blood does not always eliminate the possibility of subarachnoid or intravascular injection. A small test dose of local anesthetics with monitoring of end-results, such as absence of spinal block and tachycardia, will confirm a truly negative aspiration test.[225] When using continuous epidural techniques, test doses given prior to loading and top-up doses will eliminate subarachnoid or intravascular injections caused by catheter-tip migration. A test dose containing 15 to 20 μg of epinephrine, if injected into a blood vessel, will cause tachycardia within 45 seconds. A sedated patient may exhibit only a transient increase in pulse rate of 20 or more additional beats/min for approximately 15 to 30 seconds. Parturients receiving beta-blockers may not respond to this amount of epinephrine with increased heart rate but instead may manifest only a transient increase in blood pressure. Finally, the local anesthetic solution should be administered slowly and in fractionated doses, rather than by rapid bolus injection.

Bupivacaine-induced seizure activity is managed with combinations of airway protection, effective ventilation, and anticonvulsants such as benzodiazepines for hypotensive parturients or barbiturates for normotensive parturients. For parturients near term, the uterus should be displaced to the left manually and the feet should be elevated to relieve aortocaval compression and facilitate venous return.

CHLOROPROCAINE NEUROTOXICITY

Chloroprocaine is an ester-type local anesthetic with a rapid onset and a brief duration of action. Very little chloroprocaine crosses the placenta because of its rapid hydrolysis by maternal plasma cholinesterases.[226–228] Although chloroprocaine has achieved great popularity in obstetric anesthesia, several case reports have described persistent nonspecific neurologic damage, prolonged sensory deficits, and prolonged motor deficits after inadvertent subarachnoid administration of large volumes of chloroprocaine.[229–231]

Chloroprocaine neurotoxicity appears to be dependent on the pH of the local anesthetic solution and its concentration of a preservative antioxidant, sodium metabisulfite.[231] Chloroprocaine solutions containing 0.2% sodium bisulfite with a pH near 3.0 produced irreversible nerve blocks in experimental animals.[232] Chloroprocaine solutions not containing sodium bisulfite with a pH near 3.0 produced a safe, transient nerve block. Gissen and associates[232] concluded that 2-chloroprocaine itself is not neurotoxic but that its preservative, bisulfite, in solution at low pH may produce severe neuropathy. The authors attributed the observed neurotoxicity to the effects of sulfur dioxide (SO_2) liberated from bisulfite dissolution in tissue at low pH.[232] The SO_2 diffuses across the nerve membrane and into the axon, where it is hydrated into sulfurous acid, which liquefies tissue by acidification. In addition, the subarachnoid injection of large volumes of local anesthetic solutions intended for epidural space injection may cause extrinsic spinal cord and spinal nerve root compression, limiting perfusion in a closed space and resulting in ischemic injury.[232]

At present, 2% and 3% bisulfite-free and methylparaben-free chloroprocaine solutions are recommended for caudal and epidural administration in all cases. For cesarean section, the initial total volume of preservative-free chloroprocaine injected should be limited to 15 to 25 ml. Local anesthetic agents other than chloroprocaine, preferably 1% lidocaine plain, should be used for skin and needle-track infiltration prior to epidural anesthesia with chloroprocaine. Chloroprocaine should not be used as an epidural test dose solution.

EPINEPHRINE AS AN ADJUVANT TO LOCAL ANESTHETICS IN OBSTETRICS

Epinephrine, a potent vasoconstrictor, is often added to local anesthetic solutions to limit systemic absorption and prolong duration of local anesthesia.[233-235] In addition, epinephrine is added to epidural test-dose solutions to produce transient maternal tachycardia should inadvertent intravascular catheterization occur.[225] Large doses or continuous infusions of epinephrine in laboring parturients will limit uterine perfusion by systemic vasoconstriction and uterine contractility by beta-mimetic tocolysis.[236-242] Even small doses of intravenous epinephrine, 10 to 20 µg, will produce transient decreases in uterine blood flow without limiting uterine contractions.[243] Despite its ability to produce a brief decrease in uterine blood flow, epinephrine-containing test doses do not limit the expulsive forces of labor and will accurately signal an unwanted intravascular injection by causing brief tachycardia. In addition to its use in epidural test-dose solutions, epinephrine in a dose of 2.5 to 5.0 µg/ml (1:400,000 to 1:200,000) may be added to local anesthetic solutions used to provide epidural anesthesia for cesarean section. Such doses of epinephrine will limit systemic absorption of the local anesthetic, protect the parturient and fetus from local anesthetic toxicity produced by rapid intravascular absorption, prolong the duration of a more profound motor block, and not interfere with a labor mechanism about to be ended by abdominal delivery.[238-242] The continuous injection or infusion of epinephrine-containing local anesthetic solutions during epidural analgesia for labor may result in a cumulative epinephrine dose that decreases uterine contractility and prolongs labor not augmented by oxytocin.[243]

Airway Complications

Endotracheal intubation may be difficult in obese parturients, and such difficulties are better anticipated beforehand rather than discovered after induction of anesthesia and loss of airway-protective reflexes. Careful positioning may facilitate endotracheal intubation in an obese parturient. The shoulders can be elevated to allow pendulous breasts to fall away from the neck and chin. Folded towels or foam doughnuts are used to support the occiput and place the slightly extended head in a sniffing position, which permits better access to the upper airway. The short-handled laryngoscope[244] or the adjustable-angle blade[245] may simplify laryngoscopy for direct tracheal intubation in obese parturients. In addition to limited airway access, laryngeal edema often complicates excessive weight gain in pregnancy[246] and preeclampsia (see Chapter 2).[247] Small-diameter (6.0- to 7.0-mm outside diameter) endotracheal tubes should be used for endotracheal anesthesia in such patients to avoid further airway swelling. Besides a variety of laryngoscopes and endotracheal tubes, additional specialized equipment should be available for unanticipated difficult airway management in parturients. Such specialized devices may include flexible fiberoptic laryngoscopes for fiberoptically directed tracheal intubation and cricothyrotomy kits for temporary transtracheal ventilation using high-pressure O_2 sources.[248]

Maternal and, subsequently, fetal hypoxia and acidosis will develop with alarming rapidity following maternal upper airway obstruction or failed tracheal intubation in unconscious parturients. A decreased functional residual capacity stores less O_2, and O_2 consumption is increased and CO_2 production is accelerated in all parturients, especially in those who are obese. A pulse oximeter often provides early warning of maternal O_2 desaturation during alveolar hypoventilation. Awake tracheal intubation may be indicated in elective situations or after failure of conventional intubation.[249]

Malignant Hyperthermia

When anesthetizing patients who are susceptible to malignant hyperthermia, pretreatment with oral dantrolene before induction of labor or cesarean section is recommended. Treatment regimens include oral dantrolene, 100 mg twice daily for 3 days, before elective induction of labor or 150 mg of oral dantrolene on admission in labor, followed by an additional 100 mg orally 6 hours later. Dantrolene crosses the placenta and has a fetal-maternal ratio of approximately 0.4 with no apparent adverse effects in neonates.[250] Other studies in which the drug was administered intravenously to awake pregnant ewes demonstrated the drug's maternal and fetal safety.[250] Maternal blood pressure and cardiac output increased slightly, but no significant changes were observed in maternal heart rate, central venous pressure, or uterine blood flow. FHR decreased 25% after 3 minutes but returned to normal within 10 minutes, and no clinically significant changes in maternal or fetal acid–base status were noted.[250]

Pseudocholinesterase Deficiency

Despite reduced serum cholinesterase activity during pregnancy, prolonged neuromuscular paralysis is rare following appropriate doses of succinylcholine (see Chapter 2).[251, 252] However, slightly prolonged paralysis rarely lasting more than 20 minutes has been reported in numerous parturients with genotypically normal but very low levels of serum pseudocholinesterase.[251–253] Dehydration, acidosis, diabetes mellitus, electrolyte abnormalities, magnesium, trimethaphan, and cholinesterase inhibitors may all depress serum cholinesterase activity and slightly prolong depolarizing neuromuscular block with succinylcholine.[252, 254] Monitoring muscle twitch and post-tetanic fasciculations with a nerve stimulator when succinylcholine is administered to parturients will prevent overdosing and risk of dual block.[255]

Like succinylcholine hydrolysis, chloroprocaine hydrolysis also depends on serum pseudocholinesterases. Chloroprocaine is rapidly hydrolyzed in parturients, even in those with significantly depressed cholinesterase activity, to its metabolic byproducts, especially para-aminobenzoic acid (PABA), the end-product of ester cleavage. PABA crosses the placenta freely but does not appear to cause appreciable fetal depression.[256] Chloroprocaine has a faster rate of plasma hydrolysis than the other commonly used local anesthetic esters, procaine and tetracaine.[256] Its in vitro plasma half-life is 21 seconds for maternal blood and 43 seconds for umbilical cord blood. Thus, chloroprocaine is unlikely to reach the fetus in appreciable amounts and, if any reaches the fetus, it is rapidly hydrolyzed by fetal serum cholinesterases.[256]

Aspiration Pneumonitis

Aspiration of acidic gastric contents during general anesthesia remains a major cause of maternal morbidity and mortality. Administration of an antacid prior to induction of anesthesia significantly raises gastric pH[257] but may give the parturient an alkaline, particulate meal to regurgitate and aspirate (see Chapter 2). Prophylactic measures to reduce the risk of regurgitation and aspiration of acidic gastric contents are presented in Chapter 2.

CONCLUSIONS

A variety of maternal and fetal emergencies from preexisting, congenital, or acquired causes may complicate pregnancy and require immediate critical care and, often, preterm delivery. An understanding of the pathophysiologic consequences of such emergencies will enable the perinatal management team to develop treatment plans that provide effective monitoring of the parturient and the fetus, indicate proper timing and method of delivery, and ensure better outcomes for both the mother and her newborn.

References

1. Bryant JW, Wheeler AS: The traumatized obstetric patient. In: James FM, Wheeler AS, Dewan DM (eds): Obstetric Anesthesia: The Complicated Patient, 2nd ed. Philadelphia: F. A. Davis, 1988, p 489
2. Montgomery TA, Lewis A, Hammersly M: Maternal deaths in California, 1957–1962. West J Med 100:412, 1964
3. Griswold RA, Collier HS: Blunt abdominal trauma. Int Abst Surg 112:309, 1961
4. Elliott M: Vehicular accidents and pregnancy. Aust NZ J Obstet Gynaecol 6:279, 1966
5. Crosby WM, Costiloe JP: Safety of lap belt restraint for pregnant victims of automobile collisions. N Engl J Med 284:632, 1971
6. Patterson RM: Trauma in pregnancy. Clin Obstet Gynecol 27:32, 1984
7. Eastman NJ: Medical and surgical management of threatened abortion. Chicago Med 64:9, 1961
8. Fort AJ, Harlin RS: Pregnancy outcome after non-catastrophic maternal trauma during pregnancy. Obstet Gynecol 35:912, 1970
9. Dyer I, Barclay DL: Accidental trauma complicating pregnancy and delivery. Am J Obstet Gynecol 83:907, 1962
10. Crosby WM: Traumatic injuries during pregnancy. Clin Obstet Gynecol 26:902, 1983
11. Breheny F, McCarthy J: Maternal mortality. Anaesthesia 37:561, 1982
12. Feller I, Tholen D, Cornell RG: Improvements in burn care, 1965–1979. JAMA 244:2074, 1980
13. Deitch EA, Clothier J: Burns in the elderly: An early surgical approach. J Trauma 23:891, 1983
14. Shepard T: Catalog of Teratogenic Agents, 2nd ed. Baltimore: Johns Hopkins University Press, 1980, p 164
15. Dilts P, Brinkman C, Kirschbaum T, et al.: Uterine and systemic hemodynamic interrelationships and their response to hypoxia. Am J Obstet Gynecol 103:138, 1969
16. Baxter CR, Shires GT: Physiological response to crystalloid resuscitation of severe burns. Ann NY Acad Sci 150:874, 1968
17. Barden TP: Premature labor. In: Bolognese RT, Schwarz RH, Schneider J (eds): Perinatal Medicine: Management of High Risk Fetus and Neonate, 2nd ed. Baltimore: Williams & Wilkins, 1982, pp 240–303
18. Pietsch J, Meaklins JL: Complications of povidone-iodine absorption in topically treated burn patients. Lancet 1:280, 1976
19. Szyfelbein SK: Anesthetic considerations for major burn surgery. In: Hershey SG (ed): ASA Refresher Courses in Anesthesiology, vol 8. Philadelphia: J. B. Lippincott, 1980
20. Gronert GA, Theye RA: Pathophysiology of hyperkalemia induced by succinylcholine. Anesthesiology 43:89, 1975
21. Loirat P, Rohan J, Baillet A, et al.: Increased glomerular filtration rate in patients with major burns and its effect on the pharmacokinetics of tobramycin. N Engl J Med 299:915, 1978
22. Sugrue D, Blake S, MacDonald D: Pregnancy complicated by maternal heart disease at the National Maternity Hospital, Dublin, Ireland, 1969 to 1978. Am J Obstet Gynecol 139:1, 1981
23. Szekely P, Snaith L: Heart Disease and Pregnancy. London: Churchill Livingstone, 1974, p 265
24. Szekely P, Snaith L: Atrial fibrillation and pregnancy. Br Med J 1:1407, 1961
25. Skaredoff MN, Ostheimer GW: Physiologic changes during pregnancy: Effects of major regional anesthesia. Reg Anesth 6:28, 1981

26. Mangano DT: Anesthesia for the pregnant cardiac patient. In: Shnider SM, Levinson G (eds): Anesthesia for Obstetrics. Baltimore: Williams & Wilkins, 1987, pp 345–381
27. Rapaport E: Natural history of aortic and mitral valve disease. Am J Cardiol 35:221, 1975
28. Burwell CS, Metcalfe J: Heart disease and pregnancy. Boston: Little, Brown, 1958, p 210
29. Ueland K, Akamatsu TJ, End M, et al.: Maternal cardiovascular dynamics. VI. Cesarean section under epidural anesthesia without epinephrine. Am J Obstet Gynecol 114:775, 1972
30. Otterson WN, Dunnihoo DR: Cardiac disease. In: Pauerstein CJ (ed): Clinical Obstetrics. New York, John Wiley & Sons, 1987, p 627
31. Schroeder JS, Harrison DC: Repeated cardioversion during pregnancy: Treatment of refractory paroxysmal atrial tachycardia during three successive pregnancies. Am J Cardiol 27:445, 1971
32. Ralston DH, Shnider SM, deLorimier AA: Effects of equipotent ephedrine, metaraminol, mephentermine, and methoxamine on uterine blood flow in the pregnant ewe. Anesthesiology 40:354, 1974
33. Brawley RK, Morrow AG: Direct determination of aortic blood flow in patients with aortic regurgitation. Circulation 35:32, 1967
34. Schlant RC, Nutter DO: Heart failure in valvular heart disease. Medicine 50:421, 1971
35. Mendelson CL: Cardiac Disease in Pregnancy. Philadelphia: F. A. Davis, 1960, p 177
36. Frank S, Ross J: The natural history of severe acquired valvular aortic stenosis. Am J Cardiol 19:128, 1967
37. Hurst JW: The Heart. New York: McGraw-Hill, 1978, p 152
38. Cannell DE, Vernon CP: Congenital heart disease and pregnancy. Am J Obstet Gynecol 85:744, 1961
39. Campbell M: The incidence and later distribution of malformations of the heart. In: Watson H (ed): Paediatric Cardiology. London: Lloyd-Luke, 1968, p 71
40. Meyer EC, Tulsky AS, Sigman P, et al.: Pregnancy in the presence of tetralogy of Fallot. Am J Cardiol 14:874, 1964
41. Jones AM, Howitt G: Eisenmenger syndrome in pregnancy. Br Med J 1:1627, 1965
42. Copeland WE, Wooley CF: Pregnancy and congenital heart disease. Am J Obstet Gynecol 86:107, 1963
43. Coleman PN, Edmunds AWB, Tregillus J: Primary pulmonary hypertension in three sibs. Br Heart J 21:81, 1959
44. Joyce TH, Palacios QT: Cardiac disease. In: James FM, Wheeler AS, Dewan DM (eds.): Obstetric Anesthesia: The Complicated Patient. Philadelphia: F. A. Davis, 1988, p 159
45. Kaunitz AM, Hughes JM, Grimes DA, et al.: Causes of maternal mortality in the United States. Obstet Gynecol 65:605, 1985
46. Turnbull AC: Report on Confidential Enquiries into Maternal Deaths in England and Wales 1979–1981. London: HMSO, 1986, p 30
47. Sabiston DC: Pathophysiology, diagnosis and management of pulmonary embolism. Am J Surg 138:343, 1979
48. Bergqvist A, Bergqvist D, Hallbrook T: Deep vein thrombosis during pregnancy: A prospective study. Acta Obstet Gynecol Scand 62:443, 1983
49. de Swiet M: Thromboembolism. Clin Haematol 14:643, 1985
50. Tawes RL, Kennedy PA, Harris EJ, et al.: Management of deep vein thrombosis and pulmonary embolism during pregnancy. Am J Surg 144:141, 1982
51. Moser KM: Diagnosis and management of pulmonary embolism. Hosp Pract 15:57, 1980
52. Kakkar V: The diagnosis of deep vein thrombosis using the I fibrinogen test. Arch Surg 104:152, 1972
53. Kalimada P, Rashad MN, Murthy BN, et al.: Pulmonary embolism: Hemodynamics, diagnosis, prophylaxis and management. Anesthesiol Rev 12:29, 1985
54. Bolan JC: Thromboembolic complications of pregnancy. Clin Obstet Gynecol 26:913, 1983
55. Salzman JG, Deykin K, Shapiro RM, et al.: Management of heparin therapy—a controlled prospective trial. N Engl J Med 292:1046, 1975

56. Bonnar J: Venous thromboembolism and pregnancy. Clin Obstet Gynecol 8:456, 1981
57. Bounameaux H, Vermylen J, Collen D: Thrombolytic treatment with recombinant tissue-type plasminogen activator in a patient with massive pulmonary embolism. Ann Intern Med 103:64, 1985
58. Barnes AB, Kanarek DJ, Greenfield AJ, et al.: Vena cava filter placement during pregnancy. Am J Obstet Gynecol 140:707, 1981
59. Phillips OC, Ebner H, Nelson AT, et al.: Neurologic complications following spinal anesthesia with lidocaine. Anesthesiology 30:284, 1969
60. Bromage PR: Epidural Anesthesia. Philadelphia: W. B. Saunders, 1978, p 229
61. Rao TL, El-Etr AA: Anticoagulation following placement of epidural and subarachnoid catheters: An evaluation of neurologic sequelae. Anesthesiology 55:618, 1981
62. Meyer JR: Embolis pulmonar-caseosa. Braz Med 2:301, 1926
63. Warden MR: Amniotic fluid as possible factor in etiology of eclampsia. Am J Obstet Gynecol 14:292, 1927
64. Steiner PE, Lushbaugh CC: Maternal pulmonary embolism by fluid as a cause of obstetric shock and expected deaths in obstetrics. JAMA 117:1245, 1941
65. Schneider CC, Henry MM, Chaplick MJ: Meconium embolism in vivo. Am J Obstet Gynecol 101:909, 1968
66. Liban E, Raz S: A clinocopathologic study of fourteen cases of amniotic fluid embolism. Am J Clin Pathol 51:477, 1969
67. Abouleish E: Amniotic fluid embolism: Report of a fatal case. Curr Res Anesth Analg 53:549, 1974
68. Morgan M: Amniotic fluid embolism. Anaesthesia 34:20, 1979
69. Courtney LD: Amniotic fluid embolism. Obstet Gynecol Surv 29:169, 1974
70. Frost AC: Death following intrauterine injection of hypertonic saline solution with hydatidiform mole. Am J Obstet Gynecol 101:342, 1967
71. Russell W, Nicholson J: Amniotic fluid embolism. A review of the syndrome with a report of 4 cases. Obstet Gynecol 26:476, 1965
72. Kitzmiller JL, Lucas WE: Studies on a model of amniotic fluid embolism. Obstet Gynecol 39:626, 1972
73. Peterson EP, Taylor HB: Amniotic fluid embolism: an analysis of 40 cases. Obstet Gynecol 35:787, 1970
74. Lumley J, Owen R, Morgan M: Amniotic fluid embolism. A report of 3 cases. Anaesthesia 34:33, 1979
75. Schaerf RH, DeCampo T, Civetta J: Hemodynamic alterations and rapid diagnosis in a case of amniotic fluid embolus. Anesthesiology 46:155, 1977
76. Phillips OC, Weigel JE, McCarthy JJ: Amniotic fluid embolus. Fundamental considerations and a report of cases. Obstet Gynecol 24:431, 1964
77. Mulder JI: Amniotic fluid embolism. An overview and case report. Am J Obstet Gynecol 152:430, 1985
78. Lesky E: Notes on the history of air embolism. German Med Monthly 6:159, 1961
79. Senn N: An experimental study of air-embolism. Ann Surg 2:197, 1885
80. Davies DE, Digwood KI, Hilton JH: Air embolism during cesarean section. Med J Aust 1:644, 1980
81. Malinow AM, Naulty JS, Hunt CO, et al.: Precordial ultrasonic monitoring during cesarean delivery. Anesthesiology 66:816, 1987
82. Fong J, Gadalla F, Pierri MK, et al.: Incidence of venous air embolism during cesarean section. Anesthesiology 69:A655, 1988
83. Maroon JC, Goodman JM, Horner TG: Detection of minute venous air emboli with ultrasound. Surg Gynecol Obstet 127:1236, 1968
84. Albin MS, Carroll RG, Maroon JC: Clinical considerations concerning detection of venous air embolism. Neurosurgery 3:380, 1978
85. Nelson PK: Pulmonary gas embolism in pregnancy and the puerperium. Obstet Gynecol Surv 15:449, 1960
86. Durant TM, Long J, Oppenheimer MJ: Pulmonary (venous) air embolism. Am Heart J 33:269, 1947
87. Boyer NH, Curry JJ: Bronchospasm associated with pulmonary embolism. Arch Intern Med 73:403, 1944
88. Wong RT: Air emboli in the retinal arteries. Arch Ophthalmol 25:149, 1941
89. Robinson DA, Albin MS: Parturition and venous air embolism. Obstet Anesth Dig 7:38, 1987

90. Michenfelder JD, Miller RH, Gronert GA: Evaluation of an ultrasonic device (Doppler) for diagnosis of venous air embolism. Anesthesiology 36:164, 1972
91. Downing JW, Karuparthy VR, Husain FJ, et al.: Posture and the incidence of venous air embolism during cesarean section. Anesthesiology 71:A910, 1989
92. Hankins GDV, Wendel GD, Leveno KJ, et al.: Myocardial infarction during pregnancy: A review. Obstet Gynecol 65:139, 1985
93. Bernal JM, Miralles PJ: Cardiac surgery with cardiopulmonary bypass during pregnancy. Obstet Gynecol Surv 41:1, 1986
94. Ueland K: Cardiovascular surgery and the OB patient. Contemp OB/GYN, Oct 1984, p 117
95. Koh KS, Friesen RM, Livingstone RA, et al.: Fetal monitoring during maternal cardiac surgery with cardiopulmonary bypass. Can Med Assoc J 112:1102, 1975
96. Werch A, Lambert HM, Cooley D, et al.: Fetal monitoring and maternal open heart surgery. South Med J 70:1024, 1977
97. Aglio LS, Johnson MD: Anaesthetic management of myocardial infarction in a parturient. Br J Anaesth 65:258, 1990
98. Hands ME, Johnson MD, Saltzman DH, et al.: The cardiac, obstetric and anesthetic management of pregnancy complicated by acute myocardial infarction. J Clin Anesth 2:258, 1990
99. Ramanathan S, Grant GJ: Vasopressor therapy for hypotension due to epidural anesthesia for cesarean section. Acta Anesthesiol Scand 32:559, 1988
100. McAnulty JH, Metcalfe J, Ueland K: Heart disease and pregnancy. In: Hurst JW (ed): The Heart, 5th ed. New York: McGraw-Hill, 1983, p 1527
101. Ueland K: Cardiovascular diseases complicating pregnancy. Clin Obstet Gynecol 21:429, 1978
102. Pyeritz RE, McKusick VA: The Marfan syndrome: Diagnosis and management. N Engl J Med 300:772, 1979
103. McAnulty JH, Metcalfe J, Ueland K: General guidelines in the management of cardiac disease. Clin Obstet Gynecol 24:773, 1981
104. Murdoch JL, Walker BA, Halpern BL, et al.: Life expectancy and causes of death in the Marfan syndrome. N Engl J Med 286:804, 1972
105. Pyeritz RE: Maternal and fetal complications of pregnancy in the Marfan syndrome. Am J Med 71:784, 1984
106. Slater EE, DeSanctis RW: Dissection of the aorta. Med Clin North Am 63:141, 1979
107. Szekely P, Snaith L: Heart Disease and Pregnancy. London: Churchill Livingstone, 1974, p 286
108. Sullivan JM: Blood pressure elevation in pregnancy. Prog Cardiovasc Dis 16:375, 1974
109. Spargo B, McCartney CP, Winemiller G: Glomerular capillary endotheliosis in toxemia of pregnancy. Arch Pathol 68:593, 1959
110. Speroff L: An autoregulatory role for prostaglandins in placental hemodynamics: Their possible influence on blood pressure in pregnancy. J Reprod Med 15:181, 1975
111. Chesley LC: Hypertensive Disorders in Pregnancy. New York: Appleton-Century-Crofts, 1978, p 445
112. Aldrete JA: Clinical implications of magnesium therapy. In: Shnider SM, Moya F (eds): The Anesthesiologist, Mother and Newborn. Baltimore: Williams & Wilkins, 1974, p 128
113. Borges LF, Gucer G: Effect of magnesium on epileptic foci. Epilepsia 19:81, 1978
114. Pritchard JA, Bretten AL: Clinical and laboratory studies in severe abruptio placentae. Am J Obstet Gynecol 97:681, 1967
115. Beecham JB, Watson WJ, Clapp JF: Eclampsia, preeclampsia, and disseminated intravascular coagulation. Obstet Gynecol 43:576, 1974
116. Demers LM, Gabbe SG: Placental prostaglandin levels in preeclampsia. Am J Obstet Gynecol 126:137, 1976
117. Walsh SW: Preeclampsia: An imbalance in placental prostacyclin and thromboxane production. Am J Obstet Gynecol 152:335, 1985
118. Bonica JJ, Figge DC: Toxemia. In: Bonica JJ (ed): Principles and Practice of Obstetric Analgesia and Anesthesia. Philadelphia: F. A. Davis, 1969, p 1127
119. Benedetti TJ, Carlson RW: Studies of colloidal osmotic pressure in pregnancy induced hypertension. Am J Obstet Gynecol 135:308, 1979
120. Hibbard LT: Maternal mortality due to acute toxemia. Obstet Gynecol 42:263, 1973

121. Chesley LC: Plasma and red cell volumes during pregnancy. Am J Obstet Gynecol 112:440, 1972
122. Ring G, Krames E, Shnider SM, et al.: Comparison of nitroprusside and hydralazine in hypertensive pregnant ewes. Obstet Gynecol 50:598, 1977
123. Joyce TH III, Loon M: Preeclampsia: Effect of albumin 25% infusion. Anesthesiology 55:A313, 1981
124. James FM III, Davies P: Maternal and fetal effects of lumbar epidural analgesia for labor and delivery in patients with gestational hypertension. Am J Obstet Gynecol 126:195, 1976
125. Joupilla R, Joupilla P, Hollmen A, et al.: Epidural analgesia and placental blood flow during labor in pregnancies complicated by hypertension. Br J Obstet Gynaecol 86:969, 1979
126. Abboud T, Dailey PA, Schnider SM, et al.: Sympathoadrenal activity, maternal, fetal, and neonatal responses after epidural anesthesia in the preeclamptic patient. Am J Obstet Gynecol 144:915, 1982
127. Pritchard JA, Weisman R Jr, Ratnoff OD, et al.: Intravascular hemolysis, thrombocytopenia, and other hematologic abnormalities associated with severe toxemia of pregnancy. N Engl J Med 280:89, 1954
128. Weinstein L: Syndrome of hemolysis, elevated liver enzymes and low platelet count: A severe consequence of hypertension in pregnancy. Am J Obstet Gynecol 142:159, 1982
129. Greer IA, Gameror AD, Aalker JJ: HELLP syndrome: Pathologic entity or technical inadequacy. Am J Obstet Gynecol 152:113, 1985
130. Killam AP, Dillard SH Jr, Patton RC, et al.: Pregnancy induced hypertension complicated by acute liver disease and disseminated intravascular coagulation. Am J Obstet Gynecol 123:823, 1975
131. Sigai BM, Taslimi MM, El-Nazar A, et al.: Maternal-perinatal outcome associated with the syndrome of hemolysis, elevated liver enzymes and low platelets in severe preeclampsia-eclampsia. Am J Obstet Gynecol 155:501, 1986
132. Goodlin RC, Cotton DB, Hasslein HC: Severe edema-proteinuria-hypertension gestosis. Am J Obstet Gynecol 132:595, 1978
133. Lopez-Llera M, Espinosa M, DeLeon MO, et al.: Abnormal coagulation and fibrinolysis in eclampsia. A clinical and laboratory correlation study. Am J Obstet Gynecol 124:681, 1976
134. Clark SL, Phelan JR, Allen SH, et al.: Antepartum reversal of hematologic abnormalities associated with the HELLP syndrome. A report of three cases. J Reprod Med 31:70, 1986
135. Weinstein L: Preeclampsia/eclampsia with hemolysis, elevated liver enzymes and thrombocytopenia. Obstet Gynecol 66:657, 1985
136. Newsome LR, Bramwell RS, Curling P: Severe preeclampsia, hemodynamic effects of lumbar epidural anesthesia. Anesth Analg 65:31, 1986
137. Craft JB, Co EG, Yonekura ML, et al.: Nitroglycerin therapy for phenylephrine-induced hypertension in pregnant ewes. Anesth Analg 59:494, 1980
138. Gutsche BB, Cheek TG: Anesthetic considerations in preeclampsia/eclampsia. In: Shnider SM, Levinson G (eds): Anesthesia for Obstetrics, 2nd ed. Baltimore: Williams & Wilkins, 1984, p 225
139. Hodgkinson R, Husain FJ, Hayaski RH: Systemic and pulmonary blood pressure during caesarean section in parturients with gestational hypertension. Can Anaesth Soc J 27:389, 1980
140. Hunt HB, Schifrin BS, Suzuki K: Ruptured berry aneurysms and pregnancy. Obstet Gynecol 43:827, 1974
141. Robinson JL, Hall CS, Sedzimir CB: Subarachnoid hemorrhage in pregnancy. J Neurosurg 36:27, 1972
142. Robinson JL, Hall CS, Sedzimir CB: Arteriovenous malformations, aneurysms, and pregnancy. J Neurosurg 41:63, 1974
143. Minielly R, Yuzpe AA, Drake CG: Subarachnoid hemorrhage secondary to ruptured cerebral aneurysm in pregnancy. Obstet Gynecol 53:64, 1979
144. Scherter CB, Polnitsky CA, Matthay RA: Chronic obstructive pulmonary diseases (asthma, bronchitis, emphysema, bronchiectasis and cystic fibrosis). In: George R, Light R, Matthay R, (eds): Chest Medicine. New York: Churchill Livingstone, 1982, p 229
145. Fischl MA, Pitchenik A, Gardner LB: An index predicting relapse and need for

184   *Perinatal Management of Maternal and Fetal Emergencies*

hospitalization in patients with acute bronchial asthma. N Engl J Med 305:789, 1981
146. Franklin W: Treatment of severe asthma. N Engl J Med 290:1469, 1974
147. Findley LJ, Sahn SA: The value of chest roentgenograms in acute asthma in adults. Chest 80:535, 1981
148. Scoggin CH, Sahn SA, Petty TL: Status asthmaticus: A nine-year experience. JAMA 238:1158, 1977
149. Hague WM: Mediastinal and subcutaneous emphysema in a pregnant patient with asthma. Br J Obstet Gynaecol 87:440, 1980
150. Turner ES, Greenberger PA, Patterson R: Management of the pregnant asthmatic patient. Ann Intern Med 93:905, 1980
151. Kirkpatrick C, Quenon M, Desir D: Blood anions and electrolytes during ritodrine infusion in preterm labor. Am J Obstet Gynecol 138:523, 1980
152. Bieniarz J: Cardiovascular effects of beta adrenergic agonists. In: Anderson A, Beard R, Brudenell JM, et al. (eds): Pre-term Labor. London: Royal College of Obstetricians and Gynaecologists, 1977, p 188
153. Bieniarz J, Ivankovich A, Scommegma A: Cardiac output during ritodrine treatment in premature labor. Am J Obstet Gynecol 118:910, 1974
154. Wagner JM, Morton MJ, Johnson KA, et al.: Terbutaline and maternal cardiac function. JAMA 246:2697, 1981
155. Cotton DB, Strassner HZ, Lipson CG, et al.: The effects of terbutaline on acid-base, serum electrolytes, and glucose homeostasis during the management of preterm labor. Am J Obstet Gynecol 141:617, 1981
156. Robertson EG, Cheyne GA: Plasma biochemistry in relation to oedema of pregnancy. J Obstet Gynaecol Br Commonw 79:769, 1972
157. James TN: On the cause of sudden death in pheochromocytoma, with special reference to the pulmonary arteries, the cardiac conduction system and the aggregation of platelets. Circulation 54:348, 1976
158. Haddy FJ, Scott JB: Metabolic factors in peripheral circulatory regulation. Fed Proc 34:2006, 1975
159. Benedetti T, Johansen T, Luthey D: Prediction of respiratory insufficiency during premature labor inhibition with betasympathomimetics (Abstract.) Proc Soc Perinat Obstet (San Antonio), 1962, p 69
160. Katz M, Robertson PA, Creasy RK: Cardiovascular complications associated with terbutaline treatment for preterm labor. Am J Obstet Gynecol 139:605, 1981
161. Cheng JB, Goldfein A, Ballard PL, et al.: Glucocorticoids increase pulmonary beta adrenergic receptors in the fetal rabbits. Endocrinology 107:1646, 1982
162. Herbert P, Tinker J: Inotropic drugs in circulatory failure. Intensive Care Med 6:101, 1980
163. Metcalfe J, Ueland K: Maternal cardiovascular adjustments to pregnancy. Prog Cardiovasc Dis 16:363, 1974
164. Condon JT: The spectrum of fetal abuse in pregnant women. J Nerv Ment Dis 174:509, 1986
165. Marsh JC, Miller NA: Female clients in substance abuse treatment. Int J Addict 20:995, 1985
166. Lucier GW, Lui EM, Lamartiniere CA: Metabolic activation/deactivation reactions during perinatal development. Environ Health Perspect 29:7, 1979
167. Committee on Drugs of the American Academy of Pediatrics: Neonatal drug withdrawal. Pediatrics 72:895, 1983
168. Rice PA, Nesbitt RE Jr, Cuenca VG, et al.: The effect of ethanol on the production of lactate, triglycerides, phospholipids, and free fatty acids in the perfused human placenta. Am J Obstet Gynecol 155:207, 1986
169. Smith IE, Coles CD, Lancaster J, et al.: The effect of volume and duration of prenatal ethanol exposure on neonatal physical and behavioral development. Neurobehav Toxicol Teratol 8:375, 1986
170. Husain S, Khan I: An update on cannabis research. Bull Narc 37:3, 1985
171. Berman ML, Bochantin JF: Effect of delta-9 tetrahydrocannabinol (marihuana) on liver microsomal dechlorinase activity: A preliminary report. Anesth Analg 51:929, 1972
172. Washton AM, Tatarsky A: Adverse effects of cocaine abuse. Natl Inst Drug Abuse Res Monogr Ser 49:247, 1984

173. Howard RE, Hueter DC, Davis GJ: Acute myocardial infarction following cocaine abuse in a young woman with normal coronary arteries. JAMA 254:95, 1985
174. Fishel R, Hammamoto G, Barbul A, et al.: Cocaine colitis: Is this a new syndrome? Dis Colon Rectum 28:264, 1985
175. Ramoska E, Sacchetti AD: Propranolol-induced hypertension in treatment of cocaine intoxication. Ann Emerg Med 14:1112, 1985
176. Scott ME, Mullaly RW: Lithium therapy for cocaine-induced psychosis: A clinical perspective. South Med J 74:1475, 1981
177. Dackis CA, Estroff TW, Sweeney DR, et al.: Bromocriptine treatment for cocaine abuse: The dopamaine depletion hypothesis. Int J Psychiatry Med 15:125, 1985
178. Dackis CA, Gold MS: Pharmacological approaches to cocaine addiction. J Subst Abuse Treat 2:139, 1985
179. Chasnoff IJ, Burns WJ, Schnoll SH, et al.: Cocaine use in pregnancy. N Engl J Med 313:666, 1985
180. Chasnoff IJ, Bussey ME, Savich R, et al.: Perinatal cerebral infarction and maternal cocaine use. J Pediatr 108:456, 1986
181. Barash PG, Kopriva CJ, Langou R, et al.: Is cocaine a sympathetic stimulant during general anesthesia? JAMA 243:1437, 1980
182. Chiu YC, Bricht K, DasGupta DS, et al.: Myocardial infarction with topical cocaine anesthesia for nasal surgery. Arch Otolaryngol Head Neck Surg 112:988, 1986
183. el-Din AS, Mostafa SM: Severe hypertension during anaesthesia for dacryocystorhinostomy. Anaesthesia 40:787, 1985
184. Michel R, Adams AP: Acute amphetamine abuse: Problems during general anaesthesia for neurosurgery. Anaesthesia 34:1016, 1979
185. Eriksson M, Larsson G, Zetterstrom R: Amphetamine addiction and pregnancy. II: Pregnancy, delivery and the neonatal period. Sociomedical aspects. Acta Obstet Gynecol Scand 60:253, 1981
186. Guttmann L, Frankel HL, Paeslak V: Cardiac irregularities during labour in paraplegic women. Paraplegia 3:144, 1965
187. Nath M, Vivian JM, Chernny WB: Autonomic hyperreflexia in pregnancy and labor: A case report. Am J Obstet Gynecol 134:390, 1979
188. Rolbin SH, Levinson G, Shnider SM, et al.: Anesthetic considerations for myasthenia gravis and pregnancy. Anesth Analg 57:441, 1978
189. Bender S: Placenta previa and previous lower segment cesarean section. Surg Gynecol Obstet 98:625, 1954
190. Chervenak FA, Lee Y, Hendler MA, et al.: Role of attempted vaginal delivery in the management of placenta previa. Obstet Gynecol 64:798, 1984
191. Hibbard LT: Placenta previa. Am J Obstet Gynecol 104:172, 1969
192. Morgan J: Placenta previa: Report on a series of 538 cases. J Obstet Gynaecol Br Commonw 72:700, 1965
193. Abdella TN, Sibai BM, Hays JM Jr, et al.: Relationship of hypertensive disease to abruptio placentae. Obstet Gynecol 63:365, 1984
194. de Valera E: Abruptio placentae. Am J Obstet Gynecol 100:599, 1968
195. Hibbard BM, Hibbard ED: Aetiological factors in abruptio placentae. Br Med J 2:1430, 1963
196. Pritchard JA: Genesis of severe placental abruption. Am J Obstet Gynecol 108:22, 1970
197. Hurd WW, Miodovnik M, Hertzberg V, et al.: Selective management of abruptio placentae: A prospective study. Obstet Gynecol 61:467, 1983
198. Knab DR: Abruptio placentae: An assessment of the time and method of delivery. Obstet Gynecol 52:625, 1978
199. Sher G: A rational basis for the management of abruptio placentae. J Reprod Med 21:123, 1978
200. Hibbard BM, Jeffcoate TA: Abruptio placentae. Obstet Gynecol 27:155, 1966
201. Rivera-Alsina ME, Saldana LR, Maklad N, et al.: The case of ultrasound in the expectant management of abruptio placentae. Am J Obstet Gynecol 146:924, 1983
202. Fox H: Placenta accreta, 1945–1969. Obstet Gynecol Surv 27:475, 1972
203. Pasto ME, Kurtz AB, Ripkin MD, et al.: Ultrasonographic findings in placenta accreta. J Ultrasound Med 2:155, 1983
204. Schrinsky DC, Benson RC: Rupture of the pregnant uterus: A review. Obstet Gynecol Surv 33:217, 1978

205. Frutchman S, Aledort LM: Disseminated intravascular coagulation. J Am Coll Cardiol 8:159B, 1986
206. Nielsen NC: Coagulation and fibrinolysis in mothers and their newborn infants following premature separation of the placenta. Acta Obstet Gynecol Scand 49:77, 1970
207. Phillips LL, Mohager-Shojai E, Dillon TF: Coagulation studies during second trimester abortions induced by PG F₂. Am J Obstet Gynecol 119:577, 1974
208. Nossel HL: Fibrinogen proteolysis by thrombin, plasma and release in relation to disseminated intravascular coagulation. Bibl Haematologica 49:151, 1983
209. Helegren M, Egberg N, Eklind J: Blood coagulation and fibrinolytic factors and their inhibitors in critically ill patients. Intensive Care Med 10:23, 1984
210. Rand J, Fruchtman SM, Aledort L: Coagulation disorders of pregnancy. In: Cherry SH, Berkowitz R, Kase NG (eds): Medical, Surgical and Gynecological Complications of Pregnancy, 3rd ed. Baltimore: Williams & Wilkins, 1985, p 241
211. Eastman NJ, Hellman LM (eds): Williams Obstetrics, 12th ed. New York: Appleton, 1961, p 573
212. Carp HA, Mashiach S, Serr DM: Vasa previa: A major complication and its management. Obstet Gynecol 53:273, 1979
213. Bromage PR: Physiology and pharmacology of epidural analgesia: A review. Anesthesiology 28:592, 1967
214. Marx GF: Shock in the obstetric patient. Anesthesiology 26:423, 1965
215. Eckstein KL, Marx GF: Aortocaval compression and uterine displacement. Anesthesisology 40:92, 1974
216. Kerr MG, Samuel E: Studies on the inferior vena cava in late pregnancy. Br Med J 1:532, 1964
217. Greiss FC Jr, Crandell DL: Therapy for hypotension induced by spinal anesthesia during pregnancy. JAMA 191:793, 1965
218. Martin CB Jr, Gingerick B: Uteroplacental physiology. J Obstet Gynecol Neonatal Nurs 5(Suppl):16, 1976
219. Adams FH, Assali N, Cushman M, et al.: Interrelationships of maternal and fetal circulations. Pediatrics 27:627, 1961
220. Myers RE: Two patterns of perinatal brain damage and their condition of occurrence. Am J Obstet Gynecol 112:246, 1972
221. Albright GA: Cardiac arrest following regional anesthesia with etidocaine or bupivacaine. Anesthesiology 51:285, 1979
222. Rosen MA, Thigpen JW, Shnider SM, et al.: Bupivacaine-induced cardiotoxicity in hypoxic and acidotic sheep. Anesth Analg 64:1089, 1985
223. Clarkson CW, Hondeghem LM: Mechanism for bupivacaine depression of cardiac conduction: Fast block of sodium channels during the action potential with slow recovery from block during diastole. Anesthesiology 62:396, 1985
224. Kileff ME, James FM, DeWan DM, et al.: Neonatal neurobehavioral responses after epidural anesthesia for cesarean section using lidocaine and bupivacaine. Anesth Analg 63:413, 1984
225. Moore DC, Batra MS: The components of an effective test dose prior to epidural block. Anesthesiology 55:693, 1981
226. O'Brien JE, Abbey V, Hinsvark O, et al.: Metabolism and measurement of 2-chloroprocaine, an ester-type local anesthetic. J Pharm Sci 68:75, 1979
227. Kuhnert BR, Kuhnert PM, Prochaska BS, et al.: Plasma levels of 2-chloroprocaine in obstetric patients and their neonates after epidural anesthesia. Anesthesiology 53:21, 1980
228. Philipson EH, Kuhnert BR, Syracuse CD: Fetal acidosis, 2-chloroprocaine, and epidural anesthesia for cesarean section. Am J Obstet Gynecol 151:322, 1985
229. Reisner LS, Hockman BN, Plumer MH: Persistent neurologic deficit and adhesive arachnoiditis following intrathecal 2-chloroprocaine injection. Anesth Analg 59:452, 1980
230. Ravindran RS, Bond VK, Tasch MD, et al.: Prolonged neural blockade following regional analgesia with 2-chloroprocaine. Anesth Analg 59:447, 1980
231. Moore DC, Spierdijk J, Van Kleef JD, et al.: Chloroprocaine neurotoxicity: Four additional cases. Anesth Analg 61:155, 1982
232. Gissen AJ, Datta S, Lambert DH: The chloroprocaine controversy. II. Is chloroprocaine neurotoxic? Reg Anesth 9:135, 1984

233. Bromage PR, Robson JG: Concentrations of lignocaine in the blood after intravenous, intramuscular, epidural and endotracheal administration. Anaesthesia 16:461, 1961
234. Mather LE, Tucker GT, Murphy TM, et al.: The effects of adding adrenaline to etidocaine and lignocaine in extradural anaesthesia: II. Pharmacokinetics. Br J Anaesth 48:989, 1976
235. Scott DB, Jebson PR, Braid DP, et al.: Factors affecting plasma levels of lignocaine and prilocaine. Br J Anaesth 44:1040, 1972
236. Rosenfeld CR, Barton MD, Meschia G: Effects of epinephrine on distribution of blood flow in the pregnant ewe. Am J Obstet Gyncol 124:156, 1976
237. Wallis KL, Shnider SM, Hicks JS, et al.: Epidural anesthesia in the normotensive pregnant ewe: Effects on uterine blood flow and fetal acid-base status. Anesthesiology 44:481, 1976
238. Rucker MP: The action of adrenalin on the pregnant uterus. South Med J 18:412, 1925
239. Gunther RE, Bauman J: Obstetrical caudal anesthesia: I. A randomized study comparing 1% mepivacaine with 1% lidocaine plus epinephrine. Anesthesiology 31:5, 1969
240. Gunther RE, Bellville JW: Obstetrical caudal anesthesia: II. A randomized study comparing 1 per cent mepivacaine with 1 per cent mepivacaine plus epinephrine. Anesthesiology 37:288, 1972
241. Matadial L, Cibils LA: The effect of epidural anesthesia on uterine activity and blood pressure. Am J Obstet Gynecol 125:846, 1976
242. Zador G, Nilsson BA: Low dose intermittent epidural anaesthesia with lidocaine for vaginal delivery. II. Influence on labour and foetal acid-base status. Acta Obstet Gynecol Scand (Suppl) 34:17, 1974
243. Hood DD, Dewan DM, Rose JC, et al.: Maternal and fetal effects of intravenous epinephrine containing solutions in gravid ewes. Anesthesiology 59:A393, 1983
244. Datta S, Briwa J: Modified laryngoscope for endotracheal intubation of obese patients. Anesth Analg 60:120, 1981
245. Patil VU, Stehling LC, Zauder HL: An adjustable laryngoscope handle for difficult intubations. Anesthesiology 60:609, 1984
246. Spotoft H, Christensen P: Laryngeal oedema accompanying weight gain in pregnancy. Anaesthesia 36:75, 1981
247. Seager SJ, Macdonald R: Laryngeal oedema and preeclampsia. Anaesthesia 35:360, 1980
248. Millar WL: Management of a difficult airway in obstetrics. Anesthesiology 52:523, 1980
249. Buckley FP, Robinson NB, Simonowitz DA, et al.: Anaesthesia in the morbidly obese. Anaesthesia 38:840, 1983
250. Morison DH: Placental transfer of dantrolene. Anesthesiology 59:265, 1983
251. Shnider SM: Serum cholinesterase activity during pregnancy, labor and puerperium. Anesthesiology 26:335, 1965
252. Weissman DB, Ehrenwerth J: Prolonged neuromuscular blockade in a parturient associated with succinylcholine. Anesth Analg 62:444, 1983
253. Viby-Mogenson J: Correlation of succinylcholine duration of action with plasma cholinesterase activity in subjects with the genotypically normal enzyme. Anesthesiology 53:517, 1980
254. Ravindran RS, Cummins DF, Pantazis KL, et al.: Unusual aspects of low levels of pseudocholinesterase in a pregnant patient. Anesth Analg 61:953, 1982
255. Viegas O: Guest discussion. Anesth Analg 56:81, 1977
256. Usubiaga JE, La Iuppa M, Moya F, et al.: Passage of procaine hydrochloride and paraaminobenzoic acid across the human placenta. Am J Obstet Gynecol 100:918, 1968
257. Roberts RB, Shirley MA: Reducing the risk of acid aspiration during cesarean section. Anesth Analg 53:859, 1974

7. Perinatal Evaluation and Management of Premature Birth, Breech Presentation, and Multiple Gestation

Haywood L. Brown, M.D.
James H. Diaz, M.D.

188

PREMATURE BIRTH

A preterm or premature birth is a delivery prior to 37 weeks' gestation or less than 259 days from the first day of the last normal menstrual period. In the United States, the incidence of preterm delivery is approximately 9% of all births. Although better availability of prenatal care provides earlier diagnosis and treatment of preterm labor, the incidence of prematurity has remained essentially unchanged for the past three decades. In 1980, the overall preterm delivery rate was 89 per 1000 live births, with blacks having significantly more premature infants at 32 weeks' gestation or earlier (23%) than whites (16%).[1] Although prematurity accounts for only 9% of all births, it contributes to 75% of neonatal deaths and to 50% of neurologic handicaps. Recent medical advances in neonatal intensive care, however, have been responsible for the decrease in infant mortality from 20 per 1000 live births in the 1950s to fewer than 10 per 1000 in the 1980s.

Risk Factors Contributing to Preterm Delivery

Common maternal factors predisposing to preterm delivery include age 18 years and younger or 40 years and older; low socioeconomic status; nonwhite race; low prepregnancy maternal weight; maternal smoking; previous preterm birth, stillbirth, or neonatal death; threatened abortion; and previous antepartum hemorrhage.[2-4] Lack of prenatal care also correlates with a higher incidence of preterm delivery, but timing of the first prenatal visit for the current pregnancy has minimal impact on the incidence of preterm delivery.[5]

One of the most significant risk factors for preterm birth is a prior maternal history of prematurity. One previous preterm birth is associated with a 17% to 40% risk of recurrence in the next pregnancy.[2] The risk of recurrence increases with the number of preterm births and decreases with the number of previous term deliveries.[2,6] A prior history of pregnancy loss in the second trimester may also contribute to an increase in subsequent preterm births.

Although uncommon, uteroplacental malformations also predispose pregnant patients to preterm delivery. In these patients, the poorest pregnancy outcomes occur in women with unicornuate or bicornuate uteri. Another uterine anomaly, cervical incompetence or silent dilation of the cervix, is a known cause of midtrimester abortion and a contributing factor in both preterm labor and premature rupture of the membranes. Placental abnormalities including placenta previa, placental abruption, and marginal cord insertion have also been related to preterm birth.[3] Other uncommon risk factors for preterm delivery include multiple gestation, polyhydramnios, and congenitally deformed fetuses with polyhydramnios or oligohydramnios. Recently, it has been suggested that maternal genital tract infection or colonization may also play a role in initiating premature birth.[7] Finally, the mother who is delivered prematurely is likely to have had preterm labor with prematurely ruptured membranes. Besides preterm labor that cannot be stopped, other fetomaternal indications for early delivery of preterm infants include pregnancy-induced hypertension, placenta previa, placental abruption, fetal isoimmunization syndromes, and correctable congenital anomalies (e.g., hydrocephalus, obstructive uropathy; see Chapter 5).

Preterm Labor

Of premature births, 33% to 50% occur as a result of premature labor without rupture of membranes. The diagnosis of preterm labor depends upon the recognition of uterine contractions and cervical changes. The diagnosis is often difficult because many patients have regular contractions without cervical changes (false labor) that resolve spontaneously without therapy. The most widely used definition for preterm labor is six to eight contractions per hour or four contractions in 20 minutes associated with cervical changes.[8] Minimal cervical changes after initiation of therapy for preterm labor usually indicate successful pharmacologic termination of preterm labor. Therefore, early tocolytic treatment of patients with threatened preterm labor and little to no cervical change is recommended to ensure successful pharmacologic tocolysis before preterm labor advances and the fetal membranes rupture.

Management. The maternal-fetal advantages and cost savings of stopping preterm births are obvious, and a number of tocolytic treatment regimens and drugs have been recommended. Fortunately for the fetus, the earlier the gestational age is at the onset of preterm labor, the more successful early tocolytic therapy is likely to be.

Bed Rest. Strict bed rest with intravenous hydration may be the only treatments necessary to stop uterine contractions in some patients with early preterm labor. However, most patients require more specific pharmacologic therapy with tocolytic drugs like magnesium sulfate or beta-mimetics if preterm labor is to be halted long enough to permit further gestational development of a fetus who is likely to survive a later birth.

Magnesium Sulfate. High-dose magnesium sulfate therapy can inhibit myometrial contractility and stop premature uterine contractions.[9] Magnesium ions stop premature uterine contractions by antagonizing calcium ions at the muscle motor endplate, reducing calcium influx into myofibrils, and preventing effective excitation-contraction coupling in uterine smooth muscle. For effective tocolysis, magnesium sulfate should be administered intravenously in a loading dose of 4 to 6 g, followed by a maintenance infusion of 2 to 3 g/hour to maintain serum magnesium levels above the normal range. Normally increased rates of glomerular filtration in pregnancy rapidly eliminate magnesium ions in the urine (see Chapter 2). Magnesium sulfate should therefore be administered cautiously, in reduced doses, to patients with renal dysfunction or oliguria in order to avoid toxic hypermagnesemia with ventilatory depression and neuromuscular paralysis. Magnesium sulfate has few symptomatic side effects in healthy patients and is less costly than the more widely used beta-mimetic, tocolytic agents. However, pulmonary edema has been reported after high doses of magnesium sulfate administered in attempts to terminate preterm labor and prevent premature birth.[10]

Beta$_2$-Adrenergic Agents. In 1980, the U.S. Food and Drug Administration approved ritodrine as the first beta-mimetic tocolytic, and since then, the beta$_2$-mimetics have been the most widely prescribed tocolytics. Prior to 1980, other nonspecific beta-mimetics, including nebulized and subcutaneous terbutaline and oral and intravenous isoxsuprine, were used as tocolytic agents in the treatment of preterm labor. All beta-mimetic tocolytics, including ritodrine, can cause beta$_1$-mediated cardiovascular and metabolic side effects (Table 7–1). Fetomaternal side effects of beta-mimetic tocolytics include hypoglycemia, hypocalcemia, hypotension, and paralytic ileus. For effective acute tocolysis, ritodrine is administered intravenously in loading doses of 50 μg/min to 350 μg/min, followed by maintenance doses of oral ritodrine (20 mg every 4 hours) until 37 weeks' gestation, when oral therapy is stopped. Beta-mimetic tocolysis can aggravate any preexisting condition characterized by tachyarrhythmias, hemodynamic instability, or hyperglycemia, such as cardiovascular disease, hyperthyroidism, hypovolemia, antepartum hemorrhage, or diabetes mellitus. Of course, any obstetric or medical condition

Table 7–1. Maternal Changes Associated with Beta-Mimetic Tocolytics

Cardiovascular	Metabolic
Tachycardia	Hyperglycemia
Arrhythmias	Hyperinsulinemia
Palpitations	Hyperlacticacidemia
Angina pectoris	Hypokalemia
Hypotension	Ketonemia
Pulmonary edema	Lipemia

that requires early delivery, such as severe diabetes or preeclampsia, also contraindicates tocolysis and prolongation of pregnancy. Potential tocolytic agents that may arrest preterm labor through a variety of nonadrenergic mechanisms include ethanol, indomethacin, calcium channel blockers, and progestational agents.

Premature Rupture of the Membranes

Leakage of amniotic fluid through the cervix prior to the onset of labor is known as premature rupture of the membranes (PROM). PROM prior to 37 weeks' gestation increases the likelihood of preterm delivery and is an important cause of perinatal morbidity and mortality.

Diagnosis of PROM. A patient with PROM commonly gives a history of a gush of fluid from the vagina followed by continuous leakage of amniotic fluid. The diagnosis is confirmed by sterile speculum examination of the vagina, which demonstrates amniotic fluid draining from the cervix. With an alkaline pH near 7.15, amniotic fluid can be easily identified in pooled vaginal secretions by pH testing, a technique that identifies PROM with 90% to 98% accuracy.[11] Amniotic fluid can also be identified on light microscopy by its unique property of crystallization or ferning. Ferning describes the leaf-like pattern of crystallization by amniotic fluid proteins and salts seen on light microscopy following air drying of a droplet of amniotic fluid on a glass slide. Vaginal cultures for group B streptococci may be taken during vaginal speculum examination for PROM, since group B streptococci contribute significantly to neonatal sepsis and death in preterm neonates. Pooled vaginal fluids can also be assayed for phosphatidylglycerol, a surfactant precursor and an indicator of fetal lung maturity. If phosphatidylglycerol is present and labor does not occur spontaneously within 24 hours of PROM, the clinician may opt to proceed with induction of labor and delivery. Digital examination of the cervix should be avoided in preterm patients with PROM who are not in labor, in order to reduce the risks of neonatal infection and sepsis.

Etiology of PROM. Studies suggest that ultrastructural defects or chronic infections of the fetal membranes may predispose some patients to PROM.[12] Collagen content in the fetal membranes may decrease as gestational age advances, and, in cases of PROM, the collagen content may be lower than in control subjects matched for gestational age.[13] Recently, several investigators have suggested that some women are predisposed to PROM by a variety of subclinical, often asymptomatic, genital infections that weaken the membranes and lead to their rupture. Organisms associated with chronic genital infections in pregnancy and PROM include *Bacteroides fragilis* and other gram-negative anaerobes,

Neisseria gonorrhoeae, Chlamydia trachomatis, Trichomonas vaginalis, and the group B beta-hemolytic streptococci.[7]

Maternal and Fetal Risks. The greatest maternal risk of PROM is chorioamnionitis, a serious intrauterine infection that complicates PROM in 8% to 28% of cases.[14] Fetal and neonatal infectious contamination may also occur in PROM, with neonatal sepsis complicating 2% to 19% of cases.[14] When PROM occurs prior to 26 weeks, the fetus is also at risk of pulmonary hypoplasia if the amniotic fluid leak does not stop spontaneously within 1 week.

Management. The management of patients with PROM should include consideration of the risks of neonatal respiratory distress syndrome (RDS), maternal infection, and fetal or neonatal sepsis. In patients with PROM before 32 weeks' gestation, the risks of extreme prematurity and neonatal RDS outweigh the risks of maternofetal infections, and a conservative approach to management of PROM is advised for patients not in labor. Delivery should be delayed beyond 32 weeks' gestation to permit further fetal lung development and reduce the risks of neonatal RDS. In PROM prior to 32 weeks' gestation, vaginal fluid may be checked periodically for phosphatidylglycerol content. Once phosphatidylglycerol is identified in the leaking amniotic fluid, pharmacologic induction of labor may commence. If chorioamnionitis occurs during conservative management of PROM, delivery should be brought about quickly to prevent maternal chorioamnionitis and neonatal sepsis.

Delivery of the Preterm Fetus

The preterm fetus is at greater risk of intrauterine asphyxia and acidosis than is the term fetus, making continuous electronic fetal monitoring a necessary part of documenting fetal well-being during preterm labor. Abnormalities in fetal heart rate tracings should be evaluated promptly during preterm labor and, if they are recurrent and severe, the fetus should be delivered abdominally immediately unless vaginal delivery is imminent. Acidosis and asphyxia are the greatest intrauterine risks to the preterm fetus, and birth injury is the greatest risk to the preterm infant at delivery.

The optimal method of delivery for the preterm infant of very low birth weight remains controversial. For vaginal delivery, a generous episiotomy and outlet forceps are recommended to minimize the effects of resistance, pressure, and recoil on the small fetal head as it reaches the perineum. The use of outlet forceps for operative delivery of fetuses weighing less than 2000 g has been recommended in some studies to protect the fragile fetal head and reduce risks of intracranial hemorrhage.[15] However, other studies have not shown that outlet forceps protect small preterm neonates from head injury and intracranial hemorrhage.[16]

Routine cesarean delivery for the very low birth weight, preterm infant seems to have little merit because no advantage over vaginal delivery has been demonstrated once normal labor has begun.[16–18] Cesarean delivery is, however, recommended for a preterm infant engaged in a nonvertex presentation at the onset of labor.[17] During cesarean delivery of a preterm fetus, adequate skin, fascial, and uterine incisions must be made to prevent difficult abdominal delivery. The type of uterine incision (vertical or low transverse) will be dictated by the fetal presentation, the placental attachment site, and the configuration of the lower uterine segment.

Analgesia and Anesthesia for Preterm Labor and Delivery

Maternal anxiety, pain, and accompanying hyperventilation may limit uteroplacental perfusion and cause fetal acidosis and asphyxia during preterm labor. Some forms of analgesia or anesthesia may be needed in laboring patients to minimize maternal pain and its attendant risks to the fetus. Since parenteral narcotics and barbiturates have been associated with neonatal respiratory depression even after prolonged labors, their use should be minimized in the management of maternal pain during preterm labor and delivery. Continuous lumbar epidural anesthesia appears to offer more advantages and flexibility in the management of maternal pain during preterm labor and delivery than parenteral analgesics. Continuous epidural anesthesia provides uninterrupted pain relief, relaxes the pelvic floor, and decreases muscular pressure and resistance on the preterm fetal head at vaginal delivery. For cesarean section, epidural anesthesia offers similar advantages if there are no maternal or fetal contraindications to an anesthetic that requires patient cooperation and takes time to set up. General anesthetics for cesarean section are also safe for the mother and the preterm fetus unless a prolonged time from skin incision to delivery is anticipated.

Summary

Preterm labor and delivery pose risks of serious consequences for the neonate, particularly sepsis, asphyxia, birth injury, and RDS. Whenever possible, prevention of preterm delivery should be considered. Preterm labor should be diagnosed accurately and treated aggressively with tocolytics. Factors predisposing pregnant patients to preterm delivery should be identified early in pregnancy and eliminated. When preterm delivery is imminent, obstetric operations should be conducted in centers where a team approach to neonatal intensive care is immediately available.

BREECH PRESENTATION

Breech presentations occur in 3% to 4% of singleton pregnancies at term. The breech presentation is more common earlier in gestation, with an incidence of 28% at 25 to 28 weeks, 14% at 29 to 32 weeks, and 8.8% at 33 to 36 weeks.[19] The mortality from vaginal delivery of term infants with breech presentation is 3.5 times higher than the mortality from vaginal delivery of term infants with vertex presentation. If both term and preterm breech presentations are considered, the perinatal mortality rate is 5.5 times higher for vaginal breech deliveries than for vaginal vertex deliveries. This significantly increased mortality for vaginal breech delivery has resulted in more frequent operative deliveries for infants in breech presentation, whether premature or term.

Etiology

Late in the second trimester, the fetus begins to accommodate to the shape of the uterus. The uterus develops a wider upper pole to accommodate the breech and a narrower lower pole, or lower uterine segment, for the vertex. In the vertex presentation, the wider pole of the fetal breech tends to accommodate to the larger, upper part of the uterus. However, by 30 to 37 weeks' gestation in a breech presentation, the fetal head occupies the upper uterus and the breech fills the narrow lower uterine segment. As term approaches, the breech engages in the lower uterine segment and extends the vertex to fill the larger fundal portion of the uterus.

Many factors other than prematurity and fetal dimensions contribute to breech presentation. Placental implantation in the cornual-fundal angle of the uterus is associated with a 73% frequency of breech presentation.[20] Breech presentation also occurs frequently in placenta previa, multiparity, multiple gestation, polyhydramnios, and oligohydramnios, and in women with congenital uterine anomalies or uterine tumors, particularly leiomyomas. Fetal anomalies, especially hydrocephalus, anencephaly, goiter, abdominal wall defects, and flank masses, often predispose the fetus to breech presentation. Finally, breech presentation commonly recurs, probably because of unchanging pelvic and uterine dimensions and the same placental implantation sites.

Diagnosis

The posture of the fetal lower extremities and buttocks determines the type of breech presentation and the degree of difficulty of vaginal delivery. The three major categories of breech presentation are frank, complete, and incomplete or footling breech (Fig. 7–1). In frank breech presentation, the lower extremities are flexed at the hips and extended at the knees, with the feet straddling the head or vertex. In complete breech presentation, both knees are flexed rather than extended, with the fetus in a sitting position holding the feet at the level of the buttocks. In incomplete breech presentation, one or both legs are extended at the hips and enter the lower uterine segment before the buttocks. If one leg is completely extended and the other flexed, the incomplete breech presentation is referred to as a single footling breech. If both legs are extended below the buttocks, the incomplete presentation is referred to as a double footling breech. The frank breech presentation is most common at term.

Physical diagnosis of breech presentation in utero is by bimanual abdominal examination (Leopold's maneuvers), auscultation of fetal heart tones above the umbilicus, and vaginal identification of such irregular presenting parts as the ischial tuberosities, sacrum, anus, or external genitalia. As breech labor progresses, the fetal perineum becomes edematous and distorted, making differentiation of a breech from a face presentation difficult on palpation. In complete or incomplete (footling) breech presentations, vaginal diagnosis is facilitated by palpation of one or both feet at a level below the buttock. If abdominal and vaginal examinations fail to diagnose breech presentation, abdominal ultrasonography and x-ray films can confirm clinical impressions. Ultrasonography often fails to define the degree of head extension or determine the relationship of the fetal lower extremities to the fetal pelvis. When

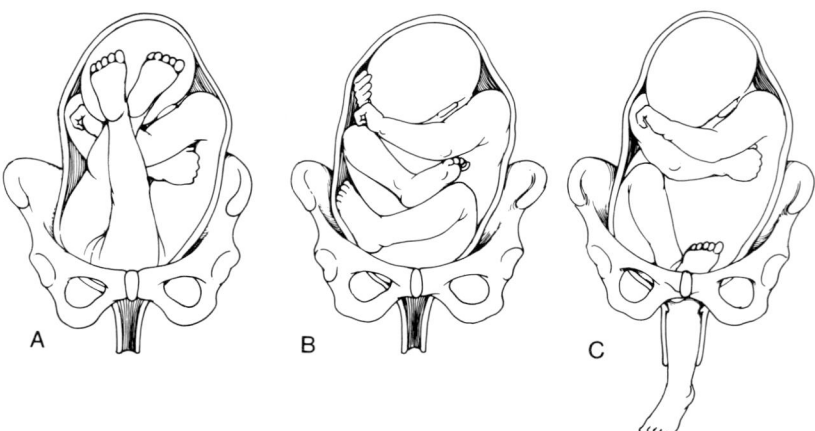

FIGURE 7–1. Types of breech presentations. *A,* Frank breech. *B,* Complete or full breech. *C,* Incomplete breech (single footling). (Modified with permission from Nursing Education Service, Ross Laboratories, Columbus, OH.)

vaginal delivery is planned in breech presentation, x-ray studies are usually necessary to determine whether the breech is frank or nonfrank and the aftercoming fetal head is flexed, erect (military), or extended.

Method of Delivery and Anesthesia

A breech fetus is at a greater risk for perinatal complications than a vertex fetus. In breech presentation, the mother also is frequently at greater risk for perinatal complications that may necessitate operative delivery by forceps or cesarean section.[21] Major perinatal factors contributing to fetal loss in breech presentation include prematurity, congenital malformations, and birth injury[22] (Table 7–2). Cesarean section is now recommended in 85% to 95% of term breech presentations because of the hazards of vaginal breech delivery.

In 1,016 vaginal breech extractions, Brenner and associates[23] reported an overall mortality rate of 25.4% compared with 2.6% for a control population of vaginal vertex deliveries. The authors also noted significantly more antepartum, intrapartum, and neonatal deaths among breech infants than among vertex presentations.[23] Apgar scores were significantly lower in breech survivors than in vertex-presenting control neonates.[23]

Occasionally, no clear advantages of abdominal over vaginal delivery can be demonstrated in breech management, especially in frank breech deliveries at term. Cesarean section is not necessary in all cases of breech presentation, but only careful clinical appraisal and diagnostic imaging can be relied on to identify cases in which vaginal delivery is appropriate.

In difficult vaginal or abdominal deliveries of breech fetuses, the organs most frequently injured are the brain, spinal cord, liver, adrenal

Table 7–2. *Fetomaternal Risks Associated with Breech Presentation and Twin Pregnancy*

Risks Associated with Breech Presentation		Risks Associated with Twin Pregnancy	
Maternal	*Fetal*	*Maternal*	*Fetal*
Cervical tears	Prematurity	Anemia	Prematurity
Vaginal lacerations	Congenital anomalies	Preeclampsia	Congenital anomalies
	Umbilical cord prolapse	Eclampsia	Abnormal presentation
	Intrapartum asphyxia	Placenta previa	Umbilical cord prolapse
	Entrapment of aftercoming head	Polyhydramnios	Birth injury (breech)
	Birth injury	Premature rupture of the membranes	Twin interlocking
	Cervical spinal cord injury	Premature labor	
	Adrenal hemorrhage		
	Clavicular fracture		
	Intracranial hemorrhage		

glands, and spleen.[24] Even in institutions with high rates of cesarean section for breech presentations, infant mortality for breech-first deliveries is still higher than in vertex-first deliveries.[25] Regardless of delivery methods, the risks to infants delivered breech first are two times higher than for infants delivered vertex first, even if premature or congenitally abnormal fetuses are excluded.

Controversy surrounds the best route of delivery for preterm breech fetuses and breech fetuses of low birth weight. The greatest risks associated with vaginal extraction of small breech infants are injury to the extremities and flanks and cervical entrapment of the aftercoming head. Unfortunately, cesarean delivery does not improve overall perinatal outcome of low birth weight or preterm breech infants, and few studies exist to support recommendations that all preterm breech infants be delivered abdominally.[26] Myers and Gleicher[26] were unable to demonstrate significant differences in outcome among preterm breech infants (30 to 37 weeks' gestation) of low birth weight (1500 to 2500 g) delivered vaginally and those delivered abdominally. Kitchen and associates[27] delivered 16% of 117 preterm (24 to 28 weeks' gestation) breech infants by cesarean section and found no significant differences in perinatal outcomes between the 16% delivered abdominally and the remaining breech population delivered vaginally. In 1977, Goldenberg and Nelson[28] reported that 33% of a population of preterm breech infants weighing less than 2000 g were delivered vaginally as frank breech presentations, and the remaining infants were delivered vaginally as complete or incomplete breech presentations. The authors suggested that preterm breech infants of low birth weight (less than 2000 g) would be more likely than larger breech infants to present for nonfrank breech deliveries.[28] Nonfrank breech presentations and vaginal extractions of nonfrank breech presentations are characterized by more numerous instances of umbilical cord prolapse and are accompanied by more perinatal mortality than frank breech presentations and frank breech vaginal extractions.[22, 29] However, in a prospective study, Gimovsky and coauthors[30] were unable to demonstrate a better outcome for nonfrank breech presentations delivered abdominally than for a control population of nonfrank breech presentations delivered vaginally.

Vaginal delivery of a fetus in breech presentation is a difficult obstetric operation. Cesarean delivery should be elected for the breech fetus if circumstances are not favorable for vaginal delivery. Candidates for vaginal delivery of a breech fetus should have careful clinical pelvic assessment with both pelvic ultrasonography and x-ray films to evaluate the presenting parts and the degree of hyperextension of the fetal head. Continuous electronic fetal heart rate monitoring is an absolute prerequisite for vaginal breech delivery.

Assisted breech delivery is the ideal mode of vaginal birth for the frank breech fetus. Assisted breech delivery allows the breech fetus to deliver spontaneously to the umbilicus without maternal pushing. The infant's lower extremities are delivered, and then the lower torso is supported by the obstetrician until the scapulas are delivered with the help of uterine contractions and maternal pushing. After delivery of the shoulders, the obstetrician applies minimal traction and slight rotation to the infant torso until each fetal arm and then the fetal neck are delivered. Piper forceps should be applied to the aftercoming fetal head to provide atraumatic head extraction from the vagina and to avoid hyperextension of the cervical spine[31] (Fig. 7–2). For assisted breech delivery, only local or pudendal block anesthesia is recommended to ensure the mother's complete participation and full pushing efforts when called for in the delivery process.

Precipitous breech delivery and total breech extraction contribute to significantly higher perinatal mortality, and these situations should be avoided in breech management. Total breech extraction by an experienced obstetrician is acceptable only in certain instances, such as a footling breech presenting in an inevitable vaginal delivery or the unanticipated discovery of a distressed second twin in a complete breech presentation. In both instances, vaginal breech delivery is difficult and may require general endotracheal anesthesia with profound neuromus-

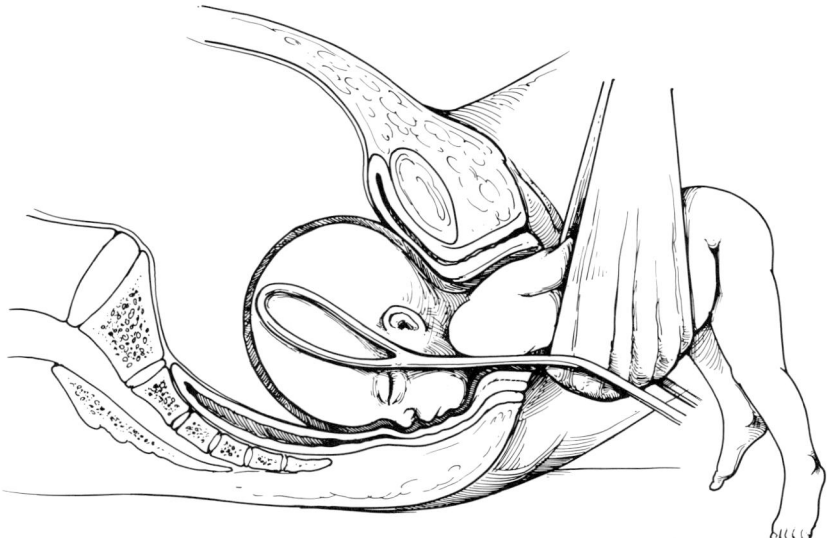

FIGURE 7–2. Delivery of aftercoming head by Piper forceps. The arms and body of the infant are suspended in a towel sling. An assistant grasps the towel or the infant's feet, or both. The operator delivers the head by flexion, keeping the handles of the Piper forceps below horizontal. (Modified from Dennen PC: Dennen's Forceps Deliveries, 3rd ed. Philadelphia: F. A. Davis © 1989.)

cular paralysis to obtain the uterine relaxation necessary to avoid maternal and fetal injury during vaginal manipulations and forceps application.

External Cephalic Version in Breech Presentation

External cephalic version is the rotation of a breech fetus to a vertex presentation by bimanual manipulation of the fetus through the maternal abdominal wall. External cephalic version is not without risk and carries a 0.9% fetal mortality and a 3% incidence of antepartum hemorrhage. External cephalic version is no longer recommended as a safe and dependable means of decreasing the incidence of breech presentation in labor.[32] Cesarean delivery continues to be the recommended method for delivery of most breeches, especially preterm or nonfrank breeches, in modern obstetric practice.

MULTIPLE GESTATION

Multiple gestation occurs with an incidence of 10 to 13 per 1000 live births, with a perinatal mortality for twins alone being four to ten times greater than for singleton births.[33-36] Twins are also at greater risk than singleton fetuses for such perinatal complications as hypoxia, asphyxia, and preterm birth (see Table 7–2). Twins are more than four times more likely than singleton fetuses to develop cerebral palsy.[37]

Complications of twin pregnancy are not limited to the fetus. A woman pregnant with twins is five times more likely to develop preeclampsia than is a woman with a singleton pregnancy. The incidence of preeclampsia in twin pregnancies is 20% to 30%.[38] Maternal iron- and folate-deficient anemias and perinatal hemorrhage are also more common in twin pregnancies than in singleton pregnancies.[39] As in breech management, the method of delivery that will secure the best perinatal outcome for twins remains controversial. Earlier diagnosis of twin pregnancy and antepartum monitoring of each fetus have certainly improved outcomes in multiple gestations.

Etiology

One-third of twin gestations arise from a single fertilized ovum or zygote that subsequently divides into two zygotes, each with the potential to develop into a separate embryo.[40] Such twin fetuses are designated as monozygotic, or identical, twins. More often, twin gestations occur from the fertilization of two separate ova by two separate sperm, resulting in dizygotic, or fraternal, twins.[40]

The frequency of monozygotic twinning is relatively constant throughout the world (one set of twins per 250 live births).[40] Unlike monozygotic twinning, dizygotic twinning is determined by race, heredity, maternal age, maternal parity, and often by the administration of fertility drugs.[40] Dizygotic twinning is more common in black patients than in white patients, with incidences of 1 in 80 pregnancies and 1 in 1000 pregnancies, respectively.[40] Dizygotic twinning is rare in Asian patients, although Asian patients have the highest incidences of conjoined twinning (see Chapter 13).[40] Women who are themselves dizygotic twins give birth to dizygotic twins with an incidence of 1 in 58 births.[40] Dizygotic twinning increases as maternal age increases, up to age 40 years.[40] The frequency of dizygotic twinning also increases as parity increases, up to seven births.[40]

In monozygotic twinning, the developmental stage at the time of division of the ovum determines placental implantation and membrane formation. If division occurs within the first 72 hours after fertilization, the two embryos will be surrounded by two amnions (diamnionic) and two chorions (dichorionic), and the placentas may be fused or separate.[41] If division occurs between day 4 and day 8 of development, the twin embryos will have two separate amnionic sacs (diamnionic) and a single chorionic membrane (monochorionic).[41] If the division occurs after day 8 of development, the twin embryos will be in a single amnionic (monoamnionic) and chorionic (monochorionic) sac.[41] If monozygotic division occurs after the eighth day of development, incomplete cleavage of the embryonic disk may occur, resulting in conjoined twins in monochorionic, monoamnionic membranes (see Chapter 13).[41] Examination of the placenta and membranes after delivery usually determines twin zygosity.[41] The rare finding of one common amnionic sac or two amnions not separated by chorion identifies monozygotic twins.[41] If two amnions are separated by chorion, the twins are probably dizygotic, but they may be monozygotic.[41] If such examinations fail to prove zygosity, evaluation of major blood groups or blood and tissue antigen typing of the twins and their parents may be required to determine zygosity.[41]

Diagnosis

The most important aspect of obstetric management of twin gestation is early diagnosis. Early diagnosis of multiple gestation allows well-planned perinatal care with better neonatal outcomes. Diagnostic ultrasound has now replaced physical and radiographic screening tests in the early diagnosis of twins. Ultrasound diagnosis of twins by the visualization of more than one gestational sac can be made as early as 6 weeks' gestation. By 8 to 10 weeks' gestation, ultrasound will identify more than one fetal heart. Thanks to screening ultrasound examinations early in pregnancy, the incidence of twin conception is now known to be greater than incidences predicted by actual delivery data.[42] Consecutive ultrasound examinations have now documented the first trimester disappearance of twin gestations, an uncommon situation now referred to as "the vanishing twin phenomenon."[43] Some instances of early first trimester bleeding have resulted in the loss of one embryo from an unrecognized twin gestation, with a gestational continuation of the surviving twin embryo.

Pregnancy Outcome

The perinatal mortality rate for monozygotic twins is 2.5 times higher than that for dizygotic twins. The fetal mortality rate for monoamnionic twins is nearly 50% and usually occurs because of intertwining of umbilical cords.[44] Major congenital malformations occur in 2.1% of twin infants compared with 1.0% of singleton infants. Malformations are more common among monozygotic, monoamnionic twins.

Abortion and intrauterine fetal demise are more likely to occur with multiple gestations than with single gestations. In twin pregnancy, one twin may die at midterm, and its calcified remains may be identified as a fetus paparyceous at the eventual delivery of the other twin. Disseminated intravascular coagulation, a sequel to missed abortion, may occur if one twin dies and remains in utero for more than 1 month.

Twins often exhibit discordant patterns of growth and development. Growth discordancy in twins may be the result of congenital abnormalities, fetal sex difference, intrauterine growth retardation, unequal placental perfusion, or twin-to-twin transfusion (luxury perfusion of one twin at the other's expense). Fetal growth retardation and premature delivery both contribute to the high incidence of low birth weights in multiple gestations. The greater the number of fetuses that develop, the more likely are growth retardation and low birth weights. Monozygotic twins are more likely to be growth retarded than are dizygotic twins. Maternal factors correlated with intrauterine growth retardation in twins include age greater than 39 years, nulliparity, parity greater than three, short stature, previous stillbirth or neonatal death, and static or decreasing weight during pregnancy.[45]

The incidence of growth retardation in one or both fetuses of a twin pregnancy is nearly 30%.[46] Serial ultrasound examinations of twin pregnancies will identify growth discrepancies in the fetuses. Normal twin growth in utero parallels singleton growth until 26 to 30 weeks' gestation. Growth retardation in twins is the second most common cause of perinatal death after preterm delivery and is responsible for 44% of all twin stillbirths.[47] Identification of intrauterine growth retardation in twin pregnancies through extensive antenatal sonographic surveillance is critical to ensure a good outcome for the twins.

As the number of fetuses in a multifetal gestation increases, both gestational duration and individual birth weights decrease. The mean duration of gestation for twins is 260 days (37 weeks) and for triplets it is 247 days (35 weeks), compared with 280 days (40 weeks) for a singleton pregnancy. Preterm labor occurs in 25% to 46% of all twin pregnancies and is more common in nulliparous patients, in monozygotic, monoamnionic twins, and in male twins. Preterm labor in twin pregnancies results from rapid expansion of intrauterine volume at a rate exceeding myometrial accommodation.

Antepartum Management

The goals of prenatal care in twin pregnancies are focused on prevention of preterm births. Preterm birth and its neonatal consequences may be prevented by liberal use of bed rest, prophylactic administration of tocolytic agents to prevent preterm labor, home uterine monitoring, and aggressive intravenous tocolysis when premature contractions develop. Frequent prenatal visits should be supplemented by ultrasonographic evaluation every 4 to 6 weeks to identify congenital anomalies or growth retardation. Antepartum fetal heart rate monitoring (nonstress testing) should begin weekly at 30 to 32 weeks; in addition to documentation of fetal movements, it provides a reliable, noninvasive means of monitoring fetal well-being in twin pregnancies. The absence of spontaneous fetal heart rate accelerations or less than two accelerations of 15 beats per minute for 15 seconds within a 10-minute period in either fetus has been correlated with poor fetal outcomes in twin pregnancies.

Management of Labor and Delivery

In most twin pregnancies, spontaneous labor usually begins at 37 to 38 weeks' gestation. If twin pregnancy lasts beyond 38 weeks, concern for fetal well-being should prompt delivery no later than at 40 weeks' gestation. As with breech delivery, the optimal mode of delivery for twin pregnancies is a controversial issue, especially in delivery of the second twin. Nationwide cesarean delivery rates for twins are now greater than 50%.[48] Indications for cesarean delivery of twins include malpresentation of either fetus, arrest of labor, fetal distress, cord accidents, maternal hypertension, placental abruption, or placenta previa.

Combined presentations are likely with twins; the incidences of types of twin presentations are listed in Table 7–3. The first twin (twin A) presents vertex in 80% of cases, and the second twin (twin B) presents vertex in 50% of cases. If either twin is in any presentation other than vertex, cord accidents and difficult deliveries may be anticipated. Cesarean delivery is recommended for any multiple gestation whenever twin A presents nonvertex. With twin A vertex and twin B nonvertex, the

Table 7–3. Incidences of Types of Twin Presentations

Twin A	Twin B	Incidence (%)
Vertex	Vertex	39
Vertex	Breech	37
Breech	Breech	10
Vertex	Transverse	8
Breech	Transverse	5
Breech	Vertex	0.25
Transverse	Transverse	0.25
Transverse	Vertex	0.25
Transverse	Breech	0.25

experience of the attending obstetrician will determine the route of delivery. Vertex-vertex twins can often be safely delivered vaginally and deserve a trial of labor before the obstetrician resorts to cesarean section. The presentation of both twins must constantly be reevaluated during labor when vaginal delivery is planned for the twins. Frequent ultrasound and x-ray examinations will confirm the clinical evaluation of presenting parts in twin pregnancies being delivered vaginally.

Of course, fetal monitoring in twin pregnancy requires individual monitors for each fetus. After rupture of the membranes, fetal monitoring may be made easier by monitoring twin A internally by fetal scalp electrode and twin B by external Doppler ultrasound.

Twin B is at greater risk than twin A, especially when twin B is malpresenting and weighs less than 1500 g.[49–51] As in vaginal breech extraction, vaginal delivery of twin B may require intrauterine manipulation during general anesthesia with profound neuromuscular relaxation. Immediate cesarean delivery of twin B is indicated if fetal distress ensues, if twin B outweighs twin A (a 40% incidence), or if labor is arrested after twin A's delivery.

Fetal entanglement or twin interlocking is a rare complication of vaginal delivery of twins (Fig. 7–3).[52] Twin interlocking has been reported in 1 of 87 vaginal twin deliveries with a breech-vertex presentation and in 1 of 817 twin deliveries overall (see Fig. 7–3).[53] In twin interlocking, the chin of breech twin A locks in the neck and chin of vertex twin B (see Fig. 7–3). Unlocking of twins during vaginal delivery is rarely successful and requires profound uterine relaxation under deep general anesthesia. If vaginal unlocking fails, immediate cesarean delivery is indicated. If the interlocked twins are immature and previable, decapitation of presenting twin A may be necessary to effect vaginal delivery of twin B and prevent unnecessary surgery or injury.

Analgesia and Anesthesia

Analgesia or anesthesia for twin delivery is often complicated by preterm or abnormal labors, pregnancy-induced hypertension, or mater-

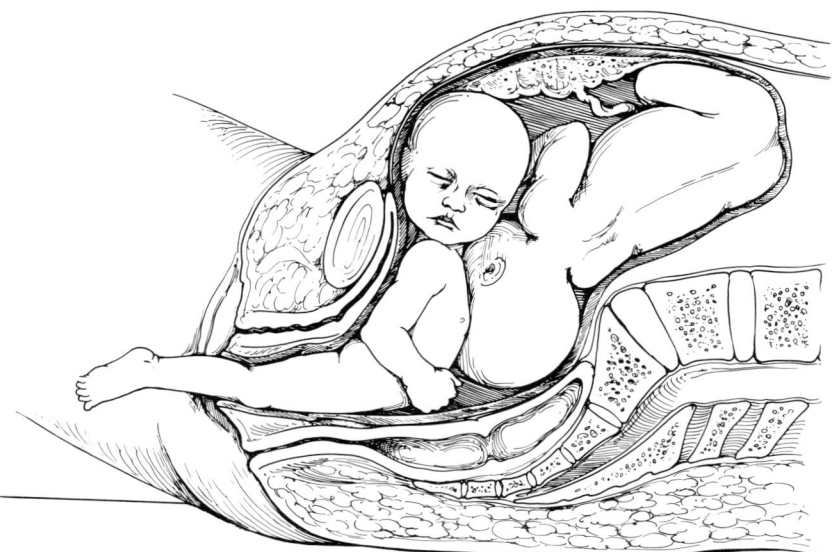

FIGURE 7–3. Fetal interlocking in twin pregnancy. (Modified from Clyne DGW: Textbook of Gynaecology and Obstetrics. London: Longmans, 1963, p 586, with permission of Churchill Livingstone.)

nal hemorrhage. Intravenous analgesia with narcotics and sedatives may be administered during twin labor in small, incremental dosages to avoid neonatal cardiopulmonary depression. In situations in which intravenous analgesics are contraindicated, pudendal nerve block with perineal local anesthetic infiltration can be administered for vaginal delivery of the twins and supplemented when necessary with nitrous oxide in oxygen. Alternatively, continuous lumbar epidural anesthesia can be administered to the laboring patient with twins and renewed to provide good anesthesia for vaginal delivery or cesarean section, if indicated. With conduction anesthesia, supine hypotension is more common in twin pregnancies than in singleton pregnancies, making labor in the left lateral decubitus position advisable. However, epidural anesthesia will not provide the immediate and profound uterine relaxation necessary for intrauterine manipulation or difficult vaginal extraction of twin B. Deep halothane anesthesia is recommended to provide the profound uterine relaxation needed for internal podalic version of a twin, usually a breech twin B. Following version, postpartal hemorrhage from halothane-induced uterine atony is likely and may require management by massive transfusion of blood products and high-dose oxytocin therapy.

Three or More Fetuses in a Multiple Gestation

Delivery in pregnancy complicated by three or more fetuses is probably best accomplished by cesarean section at or before 37 to 38 weeks' gestation. All of the problems encountered with twins are intensified by the presence of three or more fetuses.

CONCLUSIONS

The pregnant patient in labor with a preterm fetus, breech fetus, or multiple fetuses presents significant management challenges to clinicians. Obstetric delivery in such high-risk pregnancies carries significantly higher perinatal morbidity and mortality than in single, term, vertex-presenting pregnancies. In problem pregnancies such as these, the emphasis on management must be directed toward early identification of the patient at risk for preterm labor and delivery, early diagnosis of breech presentation or multiple gestation, and aggressive assessment of the breech fetus during labor, especially if a vaginal breech extraction is contemplated.

References

1. Department of Health and Human Services: Vital statistics of the U.S. 1980. Hyattsville, MD, Department of Health and Human Services, 1984
2. Fedrick J, Anderson ABM: Factors associated with spontaneous preterm birth. Br J Obstet Gynaecol 83:342, 1976
3. Papiernik E, Kaminski M: Multifactorial study of the risk of prematurity at 32 weeks of gestation. J Perinat Med 2:30, 1974
4. Myer M, Tonascia J: Maternal smoking, pregnancy complications and perinatal mortality. Am J Obstet Gynecol 128:494, 1977
5. Berkowitz G, Berkowitz R: Predicting correlates of prematurity. Contemp OB/GYN 20:183, 1982
6. Funderburk S, Guthrie D, Meldrum D: Suboptimal pregnancy outcome among women with prior abortion and premature births. Am J Obstet Gynecol 126:55, 1976
7. Minkoff H: Prematurity: Infection as an etiologic factor. Obstet Gynecol 62:137, 1983
8. Lauersen N, Merkatz I, Tejani I, et al.: Inhibition of premature labor: A multicenter comparison of ritodrine and ethanol. Am J Obstet Gynecol 127:837, 1977
9. Spisso K, Harbert G, Triagarajan S: The use of magnesium sulfate as the primary tocolytic agent to prevent premature delivery. Am J Obstet Gynecol 142:840, 1982
10. Elliott J: Magnesium sulfate as a tocolytic agent. Am J Obstet Gynecol 147:227, 1983
11. Smith R: A technique for the detection of rupture of the membranes. A review and preliminary report. Obstet Gynecol 48:172, 1976
12. Lavery J, Miller C: Deformation and creep in the human chorioamniotic sac. Am J Obstet Gynecol 134:366, 1979
13. Skinner S, Campo SG, Liggins G: Collagen content of human amniotic membranes: Effect of gestation length and premature rupture. Obstet Gynecol 57:487, 1981
14. Kitzmiller J: Preterm premature rupture of membranes. In: Fuchs F, Stubblefield PG (eds): Preterm Birth: Causes, Prevention and Management. New York: Macmillan, 1984, p 298
15. Bishop E, Israel S, Driscoe C: Obstetric influences on the premature infant's first year of development: A report from the Collaborative Study of Cerebral Palsy. Obstet Gynecol 76:628, 1965

16. Barrett J, Boehm F, Vaughn W: The effect of type of delivery on neonatal outcome in singleton infants of birthweight of 1000 grams or less. JAMA 250:625, 1983
17. Main D, Main E, Maurer M: Cesarean section versus vaginal delivery for the breech fetus weighing less than 1500 grams. Am J Obstet Gynecol 146:580, 1983
18. Olshan A, Shy K, Luthy D, et al.: Cesarean birth and neonatal mortality in very low birth weight infants. Obstet Gynecol 145:123, 1983
19. Scheer K, Nubar J: Variation of fetal presentation with gestational age. Am J Obstet Gynecol 125:269, 1976
20. Fianu S, Vaclavinkova V: The site of placental attachment as a factor in the aetiology of breech presentation. Acta Obstet Gynecol Scand 57:371, 1978
21. Collea JV, Chien C, Quilligan EJ: The randomized management of term breech presentation: A study of 208 cases. Am J Obstet Gynecol 137:235, 1980
22. Seeds S, Cefalo R: Breech delivery. Clin Obstet Gynecol 25:145, 1985
23. Brenner WE, Bruce RD, Hendricks CH: The characteristics and perils of breech presentation. Am J Obstet Gynecol 118:700, 1974
24. Tanks ES, Davis R, Holt JF, et al.: Mechanism of trauma during breech delivery. Obstet Gynecol 38:761, 1971
25. Gimovsky ML, Paul RH: Singleton breech presentation in labor. Am J Obstet Gynecol 143:733, 1982
26. Myers SA, Gleicher N: Breech delivery: Why the dilemma. Am J Obstet Gynecol 156:6, 1987
27. Kitchen W, Ford GW, Doyle LW, et al.: Cesarean section versus vaginal delivery at 24 to 28 weeks' gestation: Comparison of survival and neonatal and two year morbidity. Obstet Gynecol 66:149, 1985
28. Goldenberg RL, Nelson KG: The premature breech. Am J Obstet Gynecol 127:240, 1977
29. Karp LE, Doney JR, McCarthy J, et al.: The premature breech: Trial of labor or cesarean section? Obstet Gynecol 53:88, 1979
30. Gimovsky ML, Wallace RL, Shifrin BS, et al.: Randomized management of the nonfrank breech presentation at term: A preliminary report. Am J Obstet Gynecol 146:34, 1983
31. Dennen PC: Dennen's Forceps Deliveries, 3rd ed. Philadelphia: F. A. Davis, 1989, p 166.
32. Ferguson JE, Armstrong MA, Dyson DC: Maternal and fetal factors affecting success of antepartum external cephalic version. Obstet Gynecol 70:722, 1987
33. Powers WF: Twin pregnancy: Complications and treatment. Obstet Gynecol 42:795, 1973
34. Nylander PP: Perinatal mortality in twins. Acta Genet Med Gemell (Roma) 28:347, 1979
35. Zah'alko'va M: Perinatal and infant mortality in twins. Prog Clin Biol Res 24:115, 1978
36. Hawrylyshyn PA, Barking M, Bernstein A, et al.: Twin pregnancies—a continuing perinatal challenge. Obstet Gynecol 59:463, 1983
37. Kenny JD, Corbet AJ, Adams JM, et al.: Hyaline membrane disease and acidosis at birth in twins. Obstet Gynecol 50:710, 1977
38. Farr V: Prognosis for the babies, early and late. In: MacGillivray L, Nylander PPS, Comey G (eds): Human Multiple Reproduction. London: W. B. Saunders, 1975, p 188
39. Nylander PPS, MacGillivray I: Complications of twin pregnancy. In: MacGillivray I, Nylander PPS, Comey G (eds): Human Multiple Reproduction. London: W. B. Saunders, 1975, p 137
40. White C, Whyshak G: Inheritance in human dizygotic twinning. N Engl J Med 271:1003, 1964
41. Benirschke K, Kim CK: Multiple pregnancy. N Engl J Med 288:1276, 1973
42. Robinson HP, Caines JS: Sonor evidence of early pregnancy failure in patients with twin conceptions. Br J Obstet Gynaecol 84:22, 1977
43. Landy H, Keith L, Keith D: The vanishing twin. Acta Genet Med Gemell (Roma) 31:179, 1982
44. Benirschke K: Personal communication, 1983
45. Houlton MC, Marivate M, Philpott RH: The prediction of fetal growth retardation in twin pregnancy. Br J Obstet Gynecol 88:264, 1981
46. Houlton MCC: The Management of the Twin Fetus. Thesis, University of Natal, South Africa, 1979

47. Manlan G, Scott KE: Contribution of twin pregnancy to perinatal mortality and fetal growth retardation: Reversal of growth retardation after birth. Can Med Assoc J 118:365, 1978
48. Thompson SA, Lyons TL, Makowski E: Outcome of twin gestation at the University of Colorado Health Science Center, 1973–1983. J Reprod Med 32:328, 1987
49. Acker D, Lieberman M, Holbrook H, et al.: Delivery of the second twin. Obstet Gynecol 59:710, 1982
50. Rabinovici J, Barkal G, Reichman B, et al.: Randomized management of the second nonvertex twin: Vaginal delivery or cesarean section. Am J Obstet Gynecol 156:52, 1987
51. Barrett JM, Staggs SM, Hooydonk JE: The effect of type of delivery upon neonatal outcome in premature twins. Am J Obstet Gynecol 143:360, 1982
52. Clyne DGW: Textbook of Gynaecology and Obstetrics. London: Longmans, 1963, p 586
53. Cohen M, Kohl SG, Rosenthal AH: Fetal interlocking complicating twin gestation. Am J Obstet Gynecol 91:407, 1965

8. Resuscitation of the Neonate

Jay P. Goldsmith, M.D.
Edward H. Karotkin, M.D.

INTRODUCTION

Resuscitation, derived from the Latin *resuscitare*, means "to arouse again." In neonatology, resuscitation is indicated in several clinical

---

Sections of this chapter have been reproduced or adapted with permission from Goldsmith JP, Karotkin EH (eds): *Assisted Ventilation of the Neonate.* 2nd ed. Philadelphia: W. B. Saunders, 1988.

settings. The first indication is the emergency situation, when unexpected respiratory or cardiac arrest occurs in the delivery room, nursery, neonatal intensive care unit (NICU), or operating suite, and measures are taken to restore life. On other occasions, resuscitation is indicated in infants who have deteriorated through measurable stages of respiratory or cardiac failure. In still other instances, a new complication that is not predictable or preventable (e.g., tension pneumothorax) requires immediate intervention (e.g., tube thoracostomy) for resuscitation.

Another aspect of neonatal resuscitation includes the procedures used to assist the newly born infant in making the transition from dependent fetal to independent neonatal life. Complex changes occur in the fetus during the transition from intrauterine to extrauterine life, yet the birth process is accomplished with relative ease in most circumstances. Only 5% to 10% of infants have difficulty making this transition and require assistance in the delivery room if their chances for intact survival are to be realized. In many instances this difficulty is predictable, and data concerning gestation, labor, and delivery can be used to prepare for the resuscitation procedure. Although the mature fetus usually makes the crucial adjustments at birth without significant intervention, the preterm or asphyxiated infant may need immediate and skillfully performed lifesaving measures to make this transition. Of critical importance are expansion of the lungs, establishment of alveolar ventilation, and conversion from fetal to adult circulatory patterns so that there is direct venous return to the lungs for oxygenation.

Perinatal asphyxia is the major indication for newborn resuscitation. Perinatal asphyxia usually implies a complex combination of hypoxemia, hypercapnia, and circulatory insufficiency beginning in the fetus and continuing in the neonate that may be induced by a variety of prenatal events including abruptio placentae, meconium aspiration, and excessive blood loss. The aim of a neonatal resuscitation protocol should be the immediate reversal of hypoxemia, hypercapnia, and circulatory insufficiency so that permanent central nervous system damage or damage to other end-organs is prevented. To achieve optimal outcome, a resuscitation protocol should be directed toward (1) clearing the upper airway of secretions or meconium so that alveolar expansion can occur; (2) providing adequate arterial oxygenation and eliminating excessive carbon dioxide; (3) ensuring adequate cardiac output; (4) keeping oxygen consumption to a minimum by reducing heat loss; and (5) providing adequate energy substrates for metabolism.

This chapter reviews the pathophysiology of perinatal asphyxia and outlines the steps needed to perform successful resuscitation of newborn infants, either in the delivery room, the nursery, or the operating room.

PHYSIOLOGIC CHANGES DURING ASPHYXIA AND RESUSCITATION

Pathophysiologic changes during asphyxia in human infants are, in all likelihood, analogous to changes in animal models described by Dawes[1] and by Adamsons and associates.[2, 3] In monkey models, these investigators inserted catheters in fetal femoral vessels. At cesarean section, they also covered the neonates' heads with saline-filled bags to prevent any air entry during breathing. Umbilical cords were ligated at delivery, and approximately 30 seconds later all experimental animals exhibited gasping respirations. Between 30 seconds and 1 minute after the onset of asphyxia, the newborn animal's skin became blotchy from peripheral vasoconstriction. This lasted for approximately 1 minute and was followed by the onset of primary apnea, which also lasted for approximately 1 minute (Fig. 8–1).[1-3] During this time, the heart rate decreased to about 100 beats per minute (180 to 220 beats is normal), and there was a moderate rise in intra-arterial blood pressure. The period of primary apnea was followed by a 4- to 5-minute period of deep gasping efforts that gradually weakened before ceasing completely in the last gasp.

The last gasp heralded the onset of secondary apnea in animal models. Spontaneous respirations could not be induced by exogenous sensory stimuli during secondary apnea, and death occurred if the animal was not vigorously resuscitated. The longer the delay in initiating adequate resuscitative measures during secondary apnea, the longer the time to first gasp after resuscitation. For every 1-minute delay in resuscitation,

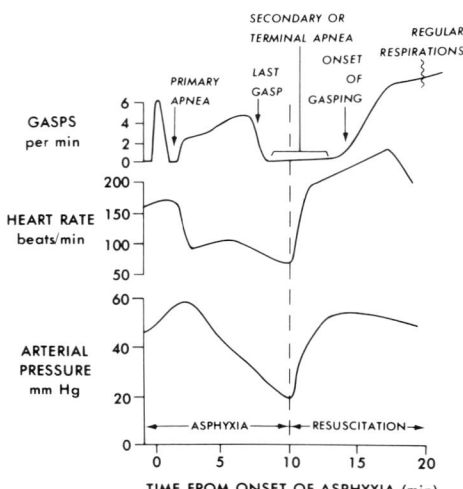

FIGURE 8–1. Changes in physiologic parameters during asphyxiation and resuscitation of the rhesus monkey fetus at birth. Rhesus monkeys were asphyxiated at birth by tying the umbilical cords while their heads were in saline-filled rubber bags. Resuscitation was by positive pressure ventilation. (Adapted with permission from Dawes GS: Foetal and Neonatal Physiology. Chicago: Year Book Medical Publishers, 1968; and Adamsons K Jr, Behrman R, Dawes GS, et al.: The treatment of acidosis with alkali and glucose during asphyxia in foetal rhesus monkeys. J Physiol 169:679, 1963; reprinted with permission from Karotkin EH, Goldsmith JP: Resuscitation. In: Goldsmith JP, Karotkin EH (eds): Assisted Ventilation of the Neonate, 2nd ed, Philadelphia: W. B. Saunders, 1988, p 71.)

the time to first gasp was increased by 2 minutes and the time to rhythmic breathing was increased by 4 minutes or more.

During total anoxia, a variety of changes occurred in the cardiovascular system, pulmonary circulation, and other tissues. These experimental changes may reflect the response of the human fetus to birth asphyxia (Table 8–1).[4] However, it should be noted that the Dawes monkey model is rarely duplicated by the human fetus or neonate. Whereas Dawes' animals were totally asphyxiated in relatively short periods (minutes), the human fetus is usually partially asphyxiated over many hours or days. Therefore, not all conclusions drawn from acutely asphyxiated animals may be applicable to chronically asphyxiated human neonates.

As a result of animal experiments, the following phenomena are believed to characterize asphyxia in the human infant. First, a sequence of events may start in utero with partial asphyxia and continue after delivery. Second, the irregular and weak gasp of the asphyxiated infant at birth may not generate sufficient intrathoracic pressure to expand the lungs. Third, neither alveolar ventilation nor pulmonary perfusion alone is sufficient to reverse the effects of birth asphyxia. Fourth, the severity and duration of asphyxia will affect multiple end-organ systems to different degrees depending upon a variety of physiologic responses to asphyxial stresses.[5] A variety of causes of neonatal asphyxia have been identified (Table 8–2).[4]

Cell injury and death are usually caused by a combination of asphyxial events. Hypoxemia is probably the least damaging aspect of perinatal

Table 8–1. Fetal Changes in Response to Asphyxia

pH	↓
P_{CO_2}	↑
P_{O_2}	↓
Lactate	↑
Plasma potassium	↑
Free fatty acid	↑
Glycerol	↑
Catecholamines	↑
Blood pressure	Transient ↑, then ↓ with prolonged asphyxia
Heart rate	Modest ↑, then ↓ with prolonged asphyxia
Umbilical blood flow	↓
Cardiac output	↓
Skin perfusion	↓
Pulmonary vascular resistance	↑
Oxygen consumption	↓
Shunting of blood through foramen ovale	↑
Glucose metabolism	Shifts from aerobic to anaerobic

From Karotkin EH, Goldsmith JP: Resuscitation. In: Goldsmith JP, Karotkin EH (eds): Assisted Ventilation of the Neonate, 2nd ed. Philadelphia: W.B. Saunders, 1988, pp 70–89. Used with permission.

Table 8–2. Causes of Neonatal Asphyxia

Cause	Pathophysiologic Effect	Examples
Drugs	Respiratory depression	Anesthetics, narcotics, alcohol, magnesium sulfate, tranquilizers
Physical/mechanical	Interruption of blood supply	Prolapsed cord, head entrapment
Hemorrhage	Hypovolemia/shock	Abruptio placentae, ruptured umbilical cord
Developmental anomalies	Cardiorespiratory insufficiency	Congenital heart disease, diaphragmatic hernia, choanal atresia
Environmental	Hypothermia	Delivered in cool environment, lack of external heat source
Postmaturity	Pneumonia, pulmonary hypertension	Meconium aspiration syndrome, persistent pulmonary hypertension of the newborn
Iatrogenic		
Excessive airway pressure generated at resuscitation	Pulmonary and cardiac embarrassment	Pulmonary air leak syndrome

Adapted from Karotkin EH, Goldsmith JP: Resuscitation. In: Goldsmith JP, Karotkin EH (eds): Assisted Ventilation of the Neonate, 2nd ed. Philadelphia: W.B. Saunders, 1988, pp 70–89. Used with permission.

asphyxia because in utero the fetus tolerates extremely low oxygen tensions well, and fetal tissue oxygenation is augmented by hypoxemia-induced leftward shifts of the oxyhemoglobin dissociation curve. Moreover, infants born with cyanotic congenital heart disease may experience profound hypoxemia for days without developing metabolic acidosis or converting to anaerobic metabolism. Recent experiences with cyanotic cardiac patients prior to extracorporeal membrane oxygenation (ECMO) support the hypothesis that neonates can survive prolonged hypoxemia.[6] Neonates with arterial oxygen tensions as low as 10 to 20 torr have been maintained in alkalotic conditions (pH greater than 7.50) prior to ECMO cannulation for 12 to 24 hours and have survived such profound hypokalemia with excellent neurologic outcomes.

Metabolic acidosis seems to be a much more specific marker of tissue asphyxia. Metabolic acidosis results in cellular swelling and wall breakdown, enhanced capillary permeability, and leakage of cytosolic enzymes into tissues. Ischemic damage results from diminished tissue perfusion, triggers anaerobic metabolism in end-organs, and results in extracellular accumulation of lactic and pyruvic acids. Areas most distal to major arteries are the most susceptible to ischemic injuries. In addition, recent evidence implicates the generation of oxygen-derived free radicals by the reperfusion process as major factors in postischemic tissue injury.[7] Future research in the prevention and management of reperfusion injuries may significantly alter our present methods of cardiopulmonary resuscitation, especially in neonates.

PREPARATIONS FOR NEONATAL RESUSCITATION

Three principal factors necessary for successful neonatal resuscitation include (1) anticipation of such incidents; (2) preparation of a treatment area, equipment, drugs, and personnel; and (3) an organized response to the emergency when it occurs.

Anticipation

Although most cardiorespiratory arrests in the nursery or operating room are not anticipated, the delivery of a baby requiring resuscitation may often be predicted. Traditionally, pediatricians attended "high-risk" deliveries, especially cesarean sections. However, with modern surgical obstetrics, a cesarean birth of a term infant is usually a benign event.

Many other conditions should alert the obstetrician to the need for pediatric assistance at delivery. The term "high-risk pregnancy" does not necessarily indicate or predict the need for resuscitation of the infant at birth. This classification of high-risk pregnancies is quite broad (Table 8–3),[8] and only a small percentage of these pregnancies will involve perinatal asphyxia. The American Academy of Pediatrics and the American College of Obstetricians and Gynecologists have published guidelines stating that each institution should develop a list of maternal and fetal complications that require the presence in the delivery room of an individual qualified in newborn resuscitation.[9] Cesarean delivery is included in the sample list contained in the guidelines.[9] However, a recent review by Press and colleagues[10] on cesarean delivery of full-term infants noted that resuscitative interventions in the delivery room for *repeat* cesarean delivery were rare (one tracheal intubation required in 111 deliveries), whereas interventions for urgent cesarean deliveries for fetal distress were common (24 intubations required in 66 deliveries). Moreover, these same investigators noted that the rate of tracheal intubation in the repeat cesarean group was lower than for term infants born vaginally in their hospital. Thus, a graded response to the high-risk delivery seems appropriate, and traditional hospital policies for mandatory pediatric attendance at certain types of deliveries (e.g., repeat cesarean sections) may have to be reviewed.

In any event, the true high-risk pregnancy resulting in a high-risk delivery may be anticipated in most cases. Under certain circumstances, and if time allows, the mother may be transferred to a tertiary care center where the infant may be delivered under optimal conditions.

Table 8–3. *Criteria for Identification of High-Risk Pregnancy*

The Patient	Medical History	Previous Pregnancy History	Pregnancy-Related Medical Conditions (Past or Present)
Teenage (age <16 years at conception)	Hypertension	Grand multiparity	Toxemia
Elderly (age >40 years at conception)	Renal disease	Previous surgical delivery	Bleeding after 12 weeks' gestation
Underweight or overweight (>2 SD from mean when compared with standard chart appropriate for race and/or ethnic group)	Diabetes	Previous prolonged labor (>24 hours)	Multiple pregnancy (present)
Low socioeconomic status	Cancer	Previous fetal loss	Abnormal presentation or position of fetus (present)
	Thyroid disease	Previous live premature infant	Polyhydramnios/oligohydramnios
	Cardiovascular disease	Previous infant death in first week of life	General anesthesia during pregnancy
	Pulmonary disease	Previous "damaged" infant (birth trauma, cerebral palsy, mental retardation, etc.)	Administration of certain drugs to mother (propylthiouracil)
	Rh sensitization		Anemia (Hgb <8 g/dl)
	Tuberculosis		Indifference to health needs (multiple missed appointments, failure to follow recommendations)
	Lupus erythematosus		Abruptio placentae
	Mental retardation		Placenta previa
	Alcohol or other drug abuse		Blood group isoimmunization
	Major psychoses		Prolapsed cord
	Neurologic disease		Forceps other than low elective
	Severe anemia (sickle cell, thalassemia)		Chorioamnionitis
	Surgery in pregnancy		Prematurity
			Abnormal fetal monitoring tracing
			Scalp pH <7.25
			Meconium-stained fluid
			Intrauterine growth retardation (<2 SD below mean)
			Immature lecithin-sphingomyelin (L/S) ratio
			Hydrops fetalis
			Potentially life-threatening anomalies detected prenatally
			Large for gestational age (LGA) (>2 SD above mean)
			Uterine anomaly
			Multiple abortions

Adapted from Fisher DE, Paton JB: Resuscitation of the newborn infant. In: Klaus MH, Fanaroff AA (eds): Care of the High-Risk Neonate, 2nd ed. Philadelphia, W. B. Saunders, 1979. Used with permission. SD = Standard deviation.

However, advanced labor and imminent delivery may preclude transfer of the mother to avoid delivery in transit. Often telephone consultation or request for a neonatal transport before delivery is worthwhile.

Pregnancies identified as high-risk require special management and intensive monitoring during gestation, labor, and delivery. Fisher and Paton[8] divide monitoring of the high-risk pregnancy into the following four phases:

1. Evaluation of the fetal placental unit during gestation
2. Estimation of fetal growth
3. Evaluation of fetal maturity, especially pulmonary maturity
4. Acute monitoring of the fetus during labor and delivery

While the first three observations may be helpful in anticipating a high-risk delivery (e.g., immature pulmonary maturity studies), they are beyond the scope of this chapter. The fourth monitoring technique, however, will be discussed briefly.

Fetal Monitoring

Many obstetricians feel that all pregnancies become high-risk once labor begins. Although this may be an overstatement, it nevertheless highlights the important contribution made by intrapartum deaths to overall perinatal mortality.[11] With the availability of new methods for monitoring the fetus in labor (e.g., electronic monitoring and fetal scalp pH sampling), controversy remains over whether these techniques should be applied universally to all deliveries.[12] Some studies show no difference in perinatal outcome with or without electronic monitoring in the patients.[13, 14] Moreover, as the use of electronic monitoring has become more widespread, the rate of cesarean deliveries has increased.[15, 16] Although data are inconclusive, many clinicians feel that the increase in the number of cesarean sections is due to overzealous interpretation of electronic monitoring traces.[17]

Most authorities agree that mothers who have any high-risk criteria (Table 8–3)[8] should have electronic fetal monitoring during labor and that outcomes in this group can be improved with appropriate applications of fetal monitoring.[12] Using modern instrumentation, labor can be monitored continuously by evaluation of intrauterine pressure and fetal heart rate. Many physicians find electronic monitoring superior to intermittent counting of fetal heart tones by stethoscope and evaluation of intrauterine pressure by palpation. Stethoscopic evaluation cannot detect beat-to-beat variability of the fetal heart rate and may also miss significant rate changes during a contraction, when heart tones are least audible. Moreover, intermittent stethoscopic evaluation of the fetal heart rate in high-risk patients should be made every 15 minutes during the active phase of the first stage of labor and every 5 minutes during the second stage of labor.[18]

Figure 8–2[19] demonstrates the three most common types of fetal heart rate changes associated with uterine contractions. Three types of decelerations are identified and named according to their time relationship to the contractions.[19] Although type I (early) decelerations are usually benign, type II (late) or type III (variable) decelerations are commonly associated with uteroplacental insufficiency and may indicate fetal distress.

The interpretation of electronic fetal monitoring tracings is very complex. Often the fetal heart pattern may be difficult to interpret or may be ambiguous.[20] If the cervix is dilated several centimeters, fetal scalp blood may be sampled for acid-base status. Blood is collected from

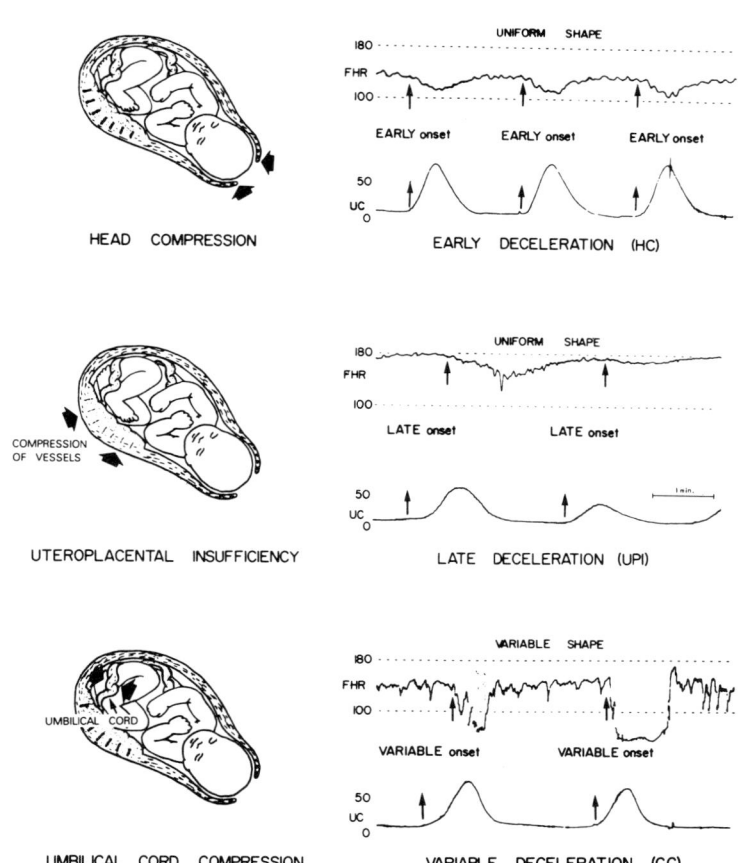

FIGURE 8–2. Three fetal heart rate deceleration patterns of clinical significance. (From Hon EH: An Atlas of Fetal Heart Rate Patterns. New Haven: Harty Press, 1968.)

a scalp incision in a long, heparinized capillary tube and evaluated for pH. A fetal blood pH of less than 7.15 in the presence of normal maternal blood pH is strong evidence of fetal asphyxia.[21] However, the information provided by electronic monitoring and fetal scalp sampling is not the only data used in evaluating the complete medical picture of the fetus during labor. Many observers feel that the rise in the rate of cesarean sections is due to overreliance on these rather isolated parameters of fetal well-being.[22]

After fetal distress is identified by meconium staining of amniotic fluid, abnormal fetal heart rate pattern, or low fetal pH, attention should be directed toward the treatment of the fetus in utero while preparation is under way for delivery. Administration of oxygen to the mother is one of the few effective methods of treating acute fetal distress. The mother should also be repositioned on her left side to relieve aortocaval compression by the gravid uterus and mechanical compression of the umbilical cord by the presenting part.[23] Aortocaval compression decreases venous return, reducing cardiac output and uterine blood flow. Intravenous tocolytic agents may be indicated to stop or limit the intensity of hypertonic uterine contractions and thus improve uteroplacental perfusion. If these simple measures fail to restore fetal homeostasis, immediate abdominal delivery should be considered to ensure a normal neonatal outcome.

Immediate Preparation

Preparation for neonatal resuscitation occurs in two stages. The first stage begins days, weeks, or months before the emergency, and the second stage occurs immediately before the high-risk delivery. During the first stage of preparation, an area in or near the delivery room is designated as resuscitation space. Provision is made for adequate space, ample heat (radiant warmer), blended oxygen supply, and suction. Resuscitation equipment (Table 8–4)[4] and drugs (Table 8–5)[4] are obtained, identified, placed in a resuscitation cart, or hung on a pegboard near the radiant warmer for easy access.[24] A resuscitation protocol should be written that identifies procedures to be followed and personnel responsibilities during an emergency. In hospitals in which actual resuscitations are infrequent, a periodic resuscitation drill may be necessary to maintain the skills and reiterate the duties of the team.

The second stage of preparation occurs only when a neonatal resuscitation can be predicted in a high-risk parturient. With adequate warning, the neonatal resuscitation team can be present in the delivery room to assume immediate care of the neonate. The resuscitation director should review the mother's chart, looking for clues in the perinatal history that could indicate birth asphyxia, such as administration of narcotic analgesics

Table 8–4. *Resuscitation Equipment*

1. Overhead warmer	17. Syringes
2. Cardiac monitor	a. Three 3-ml syringes
3. Monitor wires and pads	b. Six tuberculine syringes
4. Blood pressure monitor (zeroed and ready)	c. Three 5-ml syringes
	d. Three 10-ml syringes
5. Statham transducer (zeroed and ready)	18. Red-top tubes (2), blood culture bottles (2), and purple-top tubes (2)
6. Bag and mask (masks of varying sizes)	19. Hematocrit tubes (4)
	20. Chemstrips
7. Endotracheal tubes (2.5–4.0 mm internal diameter) uncuffed	21. Blood available
	22. Blood filter
8. Laryngoscope handle and blades (Miller 0 and 1)	23. Extension sets (2)
	24. Needles
9. Stethoscope	a. Two No. 18
10. Warm blankets	b. Two No. 23 butterfly
11. Umbilical catheter tray	c. Two No. 25 butterfly
12. Stopcocks (5)	25. Centrifuge (hematocrit)
13. Heparinized saline	26. Clipboard with respiratory sheet and nurse's notes
14. Regular saline	
15. D_5W and $D_{10}W$	
16. Sterile water	

From Karotkin EH, Goldsmith JP: Resuscitation. In: Goldsmith JP, Karotkin EH (eds): Assisted Ventilation of the Neonate, 2nd ed. Philadelphia: W.B. Saunders, 1988, pp 70–89. Used with permission.

during labor. Some mothers may be taking depressant drugs that also affect the fetus, such as sedatives or tranquilizers, without the knowledge of their health care providers. Meanwhile, the temperature in the delivery room and resuscitation area can be raised, equipment can be organized, and medications can be drawn up and made ready for rapid intravenous administration. The laryngoscope light source should be checked and the oxygen supply turned on so that once the infant is delivered, the essentials needed for the resuscitation are ready, operational, and close at hand.

Personnel

The most important aspect of resuscitation is competent personnel available to respond immediately to any emergency. If a high-risk delivery is anticipated, such personnel can be called in. Smith[25] aptly describes an individual properly prepared to lead a neonatal resuscitation as having "the diagnostic competence of a pediatrician and an internist, the technical skills of an anesthesiologist and a surgeon, and the organizational ability of a gang boss." As he also notes, these talents are rarely found in one person. Fortunately, not every high-risk delivery requires all of these skills. Personnel attending a high-risk delivery should be experienced in infant orotracheal intubation, assisted ventilation, cardiopulmonary resuscitation, and insertion of umbilical vascular catheters.[26]

Table 8–5. Drugs Used for Neonatal Resuscitation

Drug	Indication	Dose	Route	Response	Complication
Atropine	Bradycardia	0.01–0.03 mg/kg	IV, IT, SQ	↑ Heart rate	↓ Cardiac output, tachycardia
Epinephrine	Flat line ECG, intractable bradycardia	1 ml/kg of 1:10,000 solution	IV, IT	Convert flat line to rhythm	Hypertension, ventricular fibrillation
Sodium bicarbonate	Metabolic acidosis	2–3 mEq/kg	IV	↑ pH	IVH, acidosis if not ventilated
Naloxone	Maternal narcotic depression	0.01–0.1 mg/kg	IV, IM	↑ Breathing; ↑ tone and improve perfusion	Acute withdrawal if mother addicted
Whole blood	Shock, hypotension, blood loss	10–20 ml/kg	IV	↑ BP, ↑ tone, improve perfusion	Fluid overload
Dextrose	Hypoglycemia	0.5–1 g/kg	IV	Normalization of blood glucose	Rebound hypoglycemia
Albumin	Decreased perfusion, hypotension	10–15 ml/kg of 5% solution	IV	↑ BP, improve perfusion	Fluid overload
Dopamine	Hypotension, ↓ perfusion	5–15 μg/kg/min	IV	↑ BP ↑ Perfusion	Skin slough, renal shutdown

BP = blood pressure; IM = intramuscular; IT = intratracheal; IV = intravenous; IVH = intraventricular hemorrhage; SQ = subcutaneous
Adapted from Karotkin EH, Goldsmith JP: Resuscitation. In: Goldsmith JP, Karotkin EH (eds): Assisted Ventilation of the Neonate, 2nd ed. Philadelphia: W.B. Saunders, 1988, pp 70–89. Used with permission.

Neonatal resuscitation requires a full-team approach with specific tasks assigned to certain team members. Generally, two skilled clinicians and one or two assistants are necessary for a smooth, efficient neonatal resuscitation.

CONDUCT OF NEONATAL RESUSCITATION

The three steps in an appropriate initial resuscitation response are evaluation, diagnosis, and treatment.

Initial Evaluation

The initial evaluation of a depressed infant is essential to avoid treatment mistakes in an emergency situation. For newly born infants, the Apgar scoring system[27] may be helpful in assessing the infant's general condition, but in most cases of neonatal asphyxia resuscitation commences before assignment of the 1-minute Apgar score (Table 8–6).[28] Most infants with 1-minute Apgar scores of less than 3 will require vigorous resuscitative efforts. Apgar scores may be difficult to assign in premature infants, whose normal muscular tone and reflex irritability are significantly lower than in term infants. The Apgar score was originally devised as a means of evaluating the newborn for multisystem depression requiring resuscitation. The score is not a retrospective report card on the effects of labor and delivery on the neonate or a predictor of neonatal neurologic outcome. In fact, Nelson and Ellenberg[29] have shown that 1-minute Apgar scores are poor prognosticators of future

Table 8–6. *Apgar Evaluation of the Newborn Infant*

Sign	Score 0	Score 1	Score 2
Heart rate	Absent	Below 100	Over 100
Respiratory effort	Absent	Slow, irregular	Good, crying
Muscle tone	Limp	Some flexion of extremities	Active motion
Response to catheter in nostril (tested after oropharynx is clear)	No response	Grimace	Cough or sneeze
Color	Blue, pale	Body pink, extremities blue	Completely pink

Modified from Apgar V: Proposal for method of evaluation of newborn infant. Anesth Analg 32: 260, 1953. In: Behrman RE, Vaughan VC: Nelson's Textbook of Pediatrics, 13th ed. Philadelphia, W.B. Saunders, 1987. Used with permission.

Sixty seconds after the complete birth of the infant (disregarding the cord and placenta) the five objective signs above are evaluated, and each is given a score of 0, 1, or 2. A total score of 10 indicates an infant in the best possible condition. The score should be repeated at 5 minutes of age and every 5 minutes thereafter until score is >7.

mental retardation or cerebral palsy. Despite a recent *Lancet* editorial urging abandonment of the Apgar score as outmoded,[30] most neonatologists still find the simple score a valuable teaching aid and diagnostic tool.[31] Besides birth asphyxia, low Apgar scores may result from maternal cardiodepressant drugs or anesthetics, fetal systemic diseases, fetal vasovagal reactions, and major congenital anomalies (see Chapter 4).

Initial evaluation of the severely depressed premature neonate for future viability and intact neurologic outcome is also an important part of neonatal resuscitation. An infant of less than 24 weeks' gestational age and less than 500 g in birth weight or an infant with multiple major congenital anomalies incompatible with prolonged life may not be a candidate for vigorous resuscitation at birth. As always, initial evaluation before neonatal resuscitation is also essential to rule out a possible mechanical failure (e.g., a detached electrocardiograph lead) before external cardiac massage commences.

Diagnosis

Another important requirement for successful neonatal resuscitation is accurate initial diagnosis. Although treatment of neonatal cardiorespiratory failure must be immediate, every step of therapy should be based on accurate historical and clinical information, initial evaluation, and initial physical diagnosis. Procedures that may be lifesaving in one situation, such as needle thoracostomy in tension pneumothorax, may be harmful in another clinically similar situation, such as diaphragmatic hernia (see Chapter 12).

Although there are many causes of neonatal asphyxia and cardiac arrest, several aspects of prenatal history and physical diagnosis should guide the clinician's responses to neonatal cardiorespiratory arrest. The differential diagnosis can often be narrowed considerably and depends on a number of criteria, including location of cardiorespiratory arrest (delivery room, nursery, operating suite, or NICU), age at delivery (preterm or term), and ventilatory performance (spontaneous or assisted ventilation) prior to the arrest.

Cord blood gas levels at birth may assist and often direct the neonatologist in resuscitating the depressed newly born infant in the delivery room. A section of umbilical cord is clamped by the obstetrician within 30 seconds after delivery for sampling of pH, $PaCO_2$, and base deficit. Results, often available within minutes, will inform the resuscitation team of the acid-base status of their infant patient and direct appropriate resuscitative therapy. Frequently, initial cord blood gases do not correlate with the 1-minute Apgar scores.[32] Additionally, constant relationships have not been demonstrated among the most common measures of fetal distress (fetal heart rate abnormality, poor Apgar score, or abnormal cord blood gas values) and subsequent long-term neurologic disabilities. The cord blood gas may, however, alert the physician to possible fetal distress and the potential need for cardiopulmonary resuscitation.

Degree of asphyxia is best evaluated by analysis of arterial blood gases. Blood gas analysis, however, may fail to reflect the full extent of tissue asphyxia that occurs when blood flow to organs is reduced by low cardiac output, peripheral blood pooling, and tissue lacticacidemia. Restoration of adequate circulating blood volume will help to adjust the pH toward normal as pooled and acidic blood is returned to the central circulation for oxygenation and redistribution. The longer the duration of asphyxia, the more abnormal the blood gas values will be and the longer it will take to reverse these acid-base derangements.

In the NICU or operating room, an infant being mechanically ventilated has an onset and clinical presentation of cardiorespiratory arrest quite different from newborn cardiopulmonary depression. Frequently, technical complications (e.g., misplaced endotracheal tubes, pulmonary air leaks) cause respiratory arrest in mechanically ventilated patients. Restoring effective alveolar ventilation by reintubating the trachea or decompressing a pneumothorax will also restore hemodynamic stability in such cases.

Treatment: General

At birth, the newly born infant should be placed quickly in a radiant warmer in or adjacent to the delivery room. A severely asphyxiated infant should not be transported to a remote nursery because this wastes valuable resuscitation time and subjects the unstable infant to cold stress. Before beginning the resuscitation, the infant should be dried completely, and any wet blankets or wrappings should be removed. The airway should be cleared by gentle suctioning through the nose and mouth to remove mucus, amniotic fluid, or meconium. Suctioning should take no longer than 10 to 15 seconds. Vigorous or prolonged suctioning may produce a vagal reflex with bradycardia, apnea, or both.[33] The immediate goals of neonatal resuscitation are (1) to provide adequate blood oxygen-carrying capacity;[33] (2) to establish and maintain optimal cerebral blood flow; (3) to minimize cerebral anaerobic metabolic activity, fluid shifts, and serum electrolyte abnormalities; and (4) to provide adequate energy substrates for aerobic metabolism. A simple resuscitation outline for neonatal cardiopulmonary arrest is presented in Figure 8–3.[34]

Oronasal and tracheal suctioning may be performed with a DeLee suction trap or with mechanical wall suction or directly through an endotracheal tube. Direct mouth-to-tube suction is not recommended because of recent increases in perinatally transmitted viruses. If wall

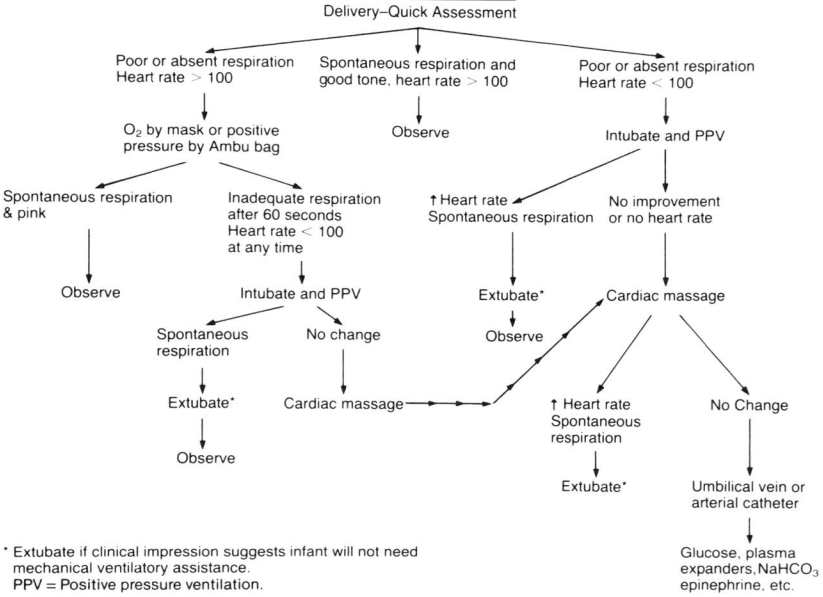

RESUSCITATION OUTLINE
Delivery–Quick Assessment

* Extubate if clinical impression suggests infant will not need
  mechanical ventilatory assistance.
PPV = Positive pressure ventilation.

FIGURE 8–3. Resuscitation outline. Steps: (1) quick physical assessment; (2) maintain head-down position; (3) suction upper airway with DeLee or mechanical suction; (4) dry with towel and place under radiant heater. (Outline adapted from Schreiner RL: Neonatology for the Pediatrician. Indianapolis: Medical Educational Resources Program, Indiana University School of Medicine, 1978, p 187; reprinted with permission from Karotkin EH, Goldsmith JP: Resuscitation. In: Goldsmith JP, Karotkin EH (eds): Assisted Ventilation of the Neonate, 2nd ed. Philadelphia: W. B. Saunders, 1988, p 81.)

suction is used, excessive negative pressure should be avoided because of the possibility of mucosal suction trauma in the upper airway. Oronasal or tracheal suctioning alone may provide the infant with enough noxious stimulation to breathe, and further resuscitative measures may not be needed.

Treatment: Mild to Moderate Neonatal Depression

Apgar scores between 3 and 6 at 1 minute are indicative of mild to moderate neonatal depression. Tracheal suctioning, flicking of the heels, and vigorously drying the trunk with towels often stimulate breathing in mildly to moderately depressed near-term and term infants. Neonates responding to these limited measures generally can be assumed to have been mildly depressed from primary apnea. Further resuscitative efforts may be necessary in more moderately depressed neonates.

Oxygen should be administered to moderately depressed neonates by placing a face mask close to the nose and mouth without providing positive pressure. If the respiratory pattern is still slow and irregular and the heart rate is less than 100 beats per minute, positive-pressure bag-and-mask ventilation should be initiated. The heart rate is the best indicator of the success of initial resuscitative efforts. Persistent bradycardia generally indicates inadequate reversal of hypoxemia, hypercarbia, or acidosis. Vagolysis with intravenously administered atropine increases the heart rate immediately but may give the clinician a false sense of successful resuscitation despite lingering acidosis; therefore, atropine is not recommended as a first-line drug in infant cardiopulmonary resuscitation (CPR).[35]

An oropharyngeal airway may be inserted to help ensure a patent upper airway during bag-and-mask ventilation. An orogastric tube can be passed to relieve any gastric distention from bag-and-mask ventilation and to empty the stomach of its contents, which could be aspirated. The proper face mask should fit securely over the nose and mouth but still allow a minimal air leak to prevent barotrauma and carbon dioxide (CO_2) accumulation. A second member of the resuscitation team should assess the adequacy of ventilation by listening for bilateral breath sounds at the apices and in the axillae. A visual count of a stable heart rate also indicates effective alveolar ventilation. The heart rate can be counted by direct auscultation over the infant's precordium or by gently palpating the neonate's umbilical cord for pulsations of the umbilical artery. A sniffing or neutral position of the infant's head without cervical extension will help to maintain a patent upper airway, permit effective bag-and-mask ventilation, and reduce the possibility of gastric insufflation and resulting distention (Fig. 8–4).

Controlled ventilation may be initiated by bag and mask or by bag and endotracheal tube. Bag-and-mask ventilation is commonly used first, especially by less experienced resuscitators, but its use still requires skill and frequent practice. To ventilate the infant patient effectively by bag

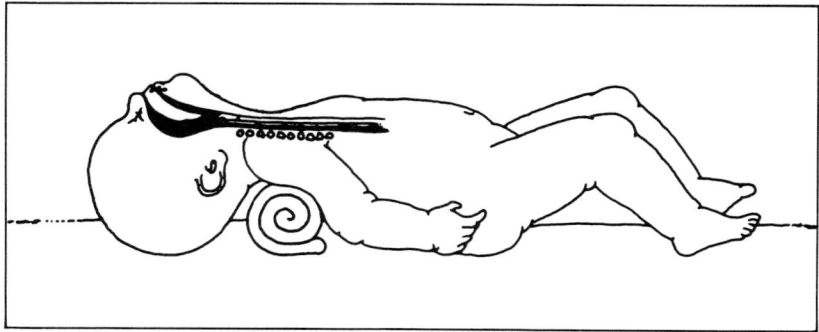

FIGURE 8–4. Sniffing position for bag-and-mask ventilation or endotracheal intubation.

and mask, the following criteria must be satisfied: (1) appropriate equipment available, (2) proper seal between mask and face, (3) delivery of 100% oxygen, and (4) proper monitoring of ventilatory rates and pressures.

Controlled ventilation with 100% oxygen at a rate of 60 to 80 breaths per minute should be delivered by a rebreathing bag (Mapleson C) with an easily adjustable pressure-relief valve that can be inserted between the face mask or endotracheal tube and the rebreathing bag. An in-line manometer to monitor the delivered inspired pressures and prevent barotrauma is recommended (see Chapter 11, Fig. 11–2).[36]

A second choice of rebreathing bag is the Infant Hope self-inflating bag, which has a pressure-relief valve that releases at 40 cm H_2O peak inspired pressure. Two serious disadvantages of the Infant Hope bag are an inspired oxygen limit of 40% and an inspired pressure limit of 40 cm H_2O. These disadvantages make the Infant Hope bag unsuitable for controlled ventilation in extremely cyanotic babies with very stiff lungs from pulmonary edema or hyaline membrane disease (Table 8–7).[37]

Bag-and-mask ventilation with 100% oxygen will initiate a first gasp in

Table 8–7. Neonatal Manual Resuscitators

Types	Self-inflating (Ambu E_2, Laerdol, Infant Hope, Penion Infant)	Anesthesia (Mapleson C)
Operator	Little experience needed	Experience needed to adjust gas flow and pressure valves
O_2-Air Source	None required	O_2-air source required
Positive FiO_2 delivery	Unable to exceed 40%–60% unless reservoir system added. With reservoir, 85%–95%, unless rapid rate of bpm then less	Will deliver any FiO_2
	No O_2 delivery between or with spontaneous breathing (except Laerdol)	O_2 delivery between and with spontaneous breathing
Ventilated pressures	Pressure relief valve set to open at 35–40 cm H_2O. Inspiratory pressures difficult to assess	Will deliver any inspiratory pressure
Comments	Good for transport or CPR when resuscitation with room air or <40% FiO_2 is indicated	Accuracy of ventilatory control and simplicity of apparatus make this system a versatile and valuable tool
	Difficult to obtain adequate "feel" of ventilation volume delivered and lung compliance	Easy to judge ventilation volume and lung compliance. Should be used with in-line manometer to avoid delivery of excessive pressures

Adapted from Nugent J, Matthews BJ, Goldsmith JP: Pulmonary care. In: Goldsmith JP, Karotkin EH (eds): Assisted Ventilation of the Neonate, 2nd ed. Philadelphia: W.B. Saunders, 1988, pp 90–106. Used with permission.

bpm = breaths per minute; CPR = cardiopulmonary resuscitation.

approximately 85% of patients and has proved to be an acceptable and efficient way to resuscitate the mildly or moderately asphyxiated infant.[38] By comparing bag-and-mask ventilation with endotracheal ventilation of asphyxiated term newborns, Milner and coworkers[38] concluded that bag-and-mask ventilation was relatively inefficient and exchanged less than one-third of the tidal volume during transtracheal intubation for controlled ventilation. Despite these findings, all babies resuscitated in the study by bag-and-mask ventilation began spontaneous breathing within 4 minutes of birth. The authors concluded that successful resuscitation depends on successful stimulation of independent respiratory efforts by any means. With mild to moderate respiratory depression at birth, bag-and-mask ventilation may be enough to stimulate spontaneous ventilation. With severe respiratory depression at birth, it is unlikely that the infant will be able to initiate and sustain ventilation, and tracheal intubation for controlled ventilation is recommended. Moreover, when prolonged controlled ventilation is necessary following resuscitation, tracheal intubation is recommended as a secure and dependable artificial airway.

Treatment: Severe Neonatal Depression

Apgar scores of 0 to 2 at 1 minute indicate severe neonatal depression. In the severely depressed infant with low Apgar scores, or in an infant whose heart rate does not increase after 8 to 10 breaths by bag and mask, immediate endotracheal intubation for controlled ventilation is indicated. The size of the endotracheal tube selected may be determined by the infant's weight and gestational age (Table 8–8).[37]

The largest caliber endotracheal tube that fits the nasal septum or vocal cords and that also allows some air leak at 20 to 30 cm H_2O peak inspiratory pressures should be chosen. Endotracheal tubes of the largest possible caliber will facilitate suctioning, occlude less, and not generate excessive intratracheal pressures during mechanical ventilation. A good rule of thumb is that the *external* diameter of the tube divided by the gestational age of the infant should not be greater than 0.1.[39]

Table 8–8. *Guidelines for Choosing Size of Endotracheal Tube (Neonatal)*

Weight of Infant (grams)	Size (ID in mm)
<1,000	2.5
1,000–2,000	3.0
2,000–4,000	3.5
>4,000	4.0

Adapted from Nugent J, Matthews BJ, Goldsmith JP: Pulmonary care. In: Goldsmith JP, Karotkin ED (eds): Assisted Ventilation of the Neonate, 2nd ed. Philadelphia: W.B. Saunders, 1988, pp 90–106. Used with permission.
ID = internal diameter.

Whether the tube should be inserted transnasally or orally is a matter of time available and personal preference. If rapid tracheal intubation is indicated, orotracheal intubation can be performed faster than nasotracheal intubation. Once the baby is stabilized, the orotracheal tube may be removed and a nasotracheal tube inserted. The nasal route may offer better tube stabilization for long-term ventilation but has been associated with injury to the nasal septum if the tube is left in place for long periods.[40] In addition, postextubation atelectasis after prolonged mechanical ventilation occurs more frequently after nasotracheal intubation, probably as a result of decreased nasal air flow through edematous nares in nose-breathing infants (see Table 8–9).[40] The tip of the endotracheal tube should be located between the epiglottis and the carina. This distance may be approximated by measuring 20% of the infant's length if the endotracheal tube is inserted transnasally, and this same distance less 2 cm is used if the tube is inserted orally. Tochen[41] has suggested that accurate tube placement can be achieved using birth weight and his simple formula, "the rule of 7–8–9." Tochen's rule states that an orotracheal tube is inserted to 7 cm at the mouth for an infant weighing 1 kg, 8 cm for an infant weighing 2 kg, and 9 cm for an infant weighing 3 kg. The rule of 7–8–9 is not applicable in infants with hypoplastic mandibles (i.e., Pierre Robin syndrome) or short necks (i.e., Turner syndrome).

Interposing a pressure manometer in the circuit is often helpful in assessing the initial pressures required to inflate the lungs (see Chapter 11, Fig. 11–2).[36] Although starting pressures are usually between 20 and 30 cm H_2O, such inflation pressures may be insufficient to expand stiff and atelectatic lungs in some infants with severe respiratory distress

***Table 8–9.** Problems in Newborn Infants with Oral and Nasal Endotracheal Tubes*

Common problems
    Postextubation atelectasis—more common with nasal endotracheal tubes
    Pneumonia/sepsis
    Accidental extubation
    Intubation of mainstem bronchus
    Occlusion of tube from thickened secretions
    Tracheal erosion
    Pharyngeal, esophageal, tracheal perforation
    Subglottic stenosis
Problems unique to nasal endotracheal tubes
    Nasal septal erosion
    Stricture of the nasal vestibule
Problems unique to oral endotracheal tubes
    Palatal grooving
    Interference with subsequent primary dentition

From Spitzer AR, Fox WW: The use of oral versus nasal endotracheal tubes in newborn infants. J Calif Perinat Assoc 4:32, 1984. Reprinted by permission of Appleton & Lange, Inc.

syndrome or neonatal pneumonia. In such cases, inspired pressures that exceed 40 cm H_2O may be required to provide adequate ventilation at increased risks of pulmonary barotrauma. Moreover, the initial ventilatory breaths for an asphyxiated term newborn may require up to 60 cm H_2O positive inspired pressure. The inspiratory phase of ventilation should be slightly less in time than the expiratory phase or 35% to 40% of the ventilatory cycle. The lowest effective inspiratory pressures should be maintained during mechanical ventilation to reduce the risks of pulmonary barotrauma, hyperventilation, or both. Optimal inspired pressures can be determined by matching peak pressures to maximum chest excursion and end-inspired breath sounds.

Treatment: Volume Expansion/Biochemical Resuscitation

In most instances, pulmonary resuscitation alone is sufficient to establish some spontaneous respiratory efforts. However, once effective ventilation is achieved, major resuscitative efforts should be redirected toward achieving cardiovascular and metabolic stability. Systemic blood pressure, pulmonary blood flow, and myocardial contractility should be restored. To accomplish this, more than one resuscitator is often needed, with one skilled operator to manage controlled ventilation and another to insert umbilical catheters, restore circulatory volume, and administer drug therapy.

When vascular access is delayed or unreliable in emergency situations, the endotracheal tube provides a rapid and reliable route for administration of epinephrine, atropine, and lidocaine only.[42] The endotracheal dose of these drugs is double the recommended intravenous dose. In desperate situations, intraosseous infusions of inotropes may be used.[43] Spinal intraosseous needles are now manufactured for infants and should be available on the resuscitation cart or tray.

Techniques for placing umbilical catheters are described in major neonatal texts.[44] An umbilical artery catheter is preferred over an umbilical vein catheter because of the added information it provides (i.e., blood gas samples and intra-arterial blood pressures). Precious resuscitation time should not be wasted, however, with repeated attempts at difficult arterial cannulations. The umbilical vein is much larger and easier to cannulate quickly.

If the umbilical vein is catheterized, rapid intravenous administration of hypertonic solutions, like sodium bicarbonate or normal saline, could cause liver damage. Until their location can be confirmed radiographically, umbilical venous catheters should be inserted to a depth of less than 5 cm (beneath the liver) or more than 10 cm (through the ductus venosus and into the inferior vena cava) for slow infusion therapy.

Once a vascular access is secured, hemodynamic resuscitation and correction of metabolic acidosis may proceed. Restoration of acid-base balance decreases pulmonary vascular resistance, restores cardiac output, and improves tissue oxygenation and muscular tone. In addition, increased brain tolerance of hypoxemia may result from normalizing pH.

Drugs commonly used during neonatal resuscitation, with their doses, routes of administration, expected response, and complications, are listed in Table 8–5.[4] Posting such a list near the infant resuscitation area provides a helpful dosage reminder during a resuscitation crisis.

Sodium bicarbonate therapy for metabolic acidosis remains controversial. A positive correlation may exist between the administration of sodium bicarbonate to infants weighing less than 2000 g and the subsequent development of intraventricular hemorrhage (IVH).[45] Causative factors of IVH may include the rapidity of bicarbonate administration, acutely increased plasma osmolarity, hypernatremia from sodium loading (serum sodium greater than 150 mEq/L), and increased intracranial volumes and pressures.[45] However, other studies do not confirm the association of sodium bicarbonate administration in premature neonates with IVH.[46, 47] The actual causes of IVH in neonates continue to be investigated. Current guidelines for sodium bicarbonate administration include the following: (1) do not administer buffer in the absence of adequate ventilation; (2) do not administer buffer in concentrations greater than 0.5 mEq/kg/min; and (3) use buffer sparingly in extremely premature infants (< 2000 g) who are at increased risk of IVH.

Other volume expanders may substitute for and limit bicarbonate use in preterm infants weighing less than 2000 g. Volume expansion alone may correct metabolic acidosis without the need for buffer administration. Ballard and colleagues[48] reported that nearly 60% of preterm infants asphyxiated in utero are volume deficient at birth. These infants may have normal mean arterial pressures because of acidosis-directed peripheral vasoconstriction. If possible, accurate arterial blood pressure should be monitored during resuscitation of such infants by transducing umbilical artery pressures or detecting brachial or femoral artery pressures by Doppler or Dinamap. As noted, blood pressures may be misleading, and hypovolemia with normal blood pressure may be suspected by irregularities in activity, color, capillary refill, and pulse volume.

Clinical entities other than prematurity may give rise to hypovolemia and shock, including multiple gestation, prolapsed umbilical cord, or hemorrhagic shock from abruptio placentae or placenta previa.[49] When indicated, volume expansion may proceed with the following fluids, in order of preference:

1. Fresh whole blood, 10 to 20 ml/kg (heparinized from placenta)
2. Fresh whole adult blood, 10 to 20 ml/kg (typed and cross-matched with the mother before delivery)

3. Fresh O negative, low-titer blood, 10 to 20 ml/kg (less than 72 hours old)
4. Fresh frozen plasma, 10 to 20 ml/kg
5. Albumin (5% salt poor) or human albumin 5% (Albuminar), 10 to 15 ml/kg
6. Ringer's lactate, 10 to 20 ml/kg
7. Normal saline, 10 to 20 ml/kg

The best fluid replacement for hypovolemic shock in the delivery room remains controversial. Although placental blood is theoretically an ideal replacement for fetal blood loss, its collection and administration are associated with many potential hazards, particularly infection, embolization, and coagulopathy. To reduce such risks, the placental blood must be aspirated aseptically from the umbilical vein prior to placental separation, adding 1 unit of heparin per milliliter of placental blood. This procedure is not approved by present blood banking regulations.[50] Albumin has also been questioned as an effective agent for use in premature infants. Although a slight rise in blood pressure is noted with its use, there may be an impairment of oxygenation if continuous distending pressure is not being used.[51] In addition, all low molecular weight fluids may seep through damaged pulmonary capillaries and into the interstitial lung space, causing pulmonary edema within 4 to 8 hours.

All resuscitative fluids should be administered slowly, especially to premature infants of less than 34 weeks' gestational age, who are susceptible to germinal matrix hemorrhages. With circulatory volume restored, blood gas determinations will aid in further management of the birth-asphyxiated infant. If the infant is normovolemic with significant metabolic acidosis, dilute sodium bicarbonate therapy (2 to 4 mEq/kg) is indicated. The amount of buffer required to correct base deficits greater than −5 may be calculated by the following equation:

$$\text{Bicarbonate required (mEq)} = 0.3 \text{ (weight in kilograms)}$$

Bicarbonate infusion should be extremely slow (no faster than 1 ml/kg/min), with care taken to avoid administering more than 10 mEq/kg/24 hours to any infant (see Table 8–5).[4]

SPECIAL PROBLEMS IN NEONATAL RESUSCITATION

Severe Bradycardia

If the heart rate remains depressed after effective alveolar ventilation is restored and pulmonary barotrauma is excluded as the cause, external cardiac massage by one of two effective methods may be indicated.

With standard technique, the infant should be placed on a firm surface and adequate compressive force supplied by depressing the middle one-third of the sternum 1 to 2 cm with the index and middle fingers of one hand.[52] Todres and Rogers[53] have suggested an alternative method of neonatal external cardiac massage. These authors advise encircling the infant's chest with both hands and compressing the midsternum 100 to 120 times per minute with both thumbs. A lung inflation should be provided between every two or three sternal compressions (Fig. 8–5).[53]

Recent anatomic studies indicate that the infant heart lies under the lower third of the sternum.[54] Guidelines for infant external cardiac massage over the midsternum may need revision in light of this anatomic finding. Compression of the lower third of the sternum may damage abdominal viscera, especially the liver.[52] Although many texts advocate specific ratios of cardiac compressions to lung inflations (e.g., three compressions to one inflation), such ratios may be less crucial in neonates. In fact, animal studies of simultaneous ventilation and cardiac compression in cardiac arrest suggest that the flaccid heart is merely a conduit for blood and not a reservoir or a pump.[55, 56] Adult studies using lower extremity or abdominal binding with military antishock trousers suggest that simultaneous lung inflation and external cardiac compression will

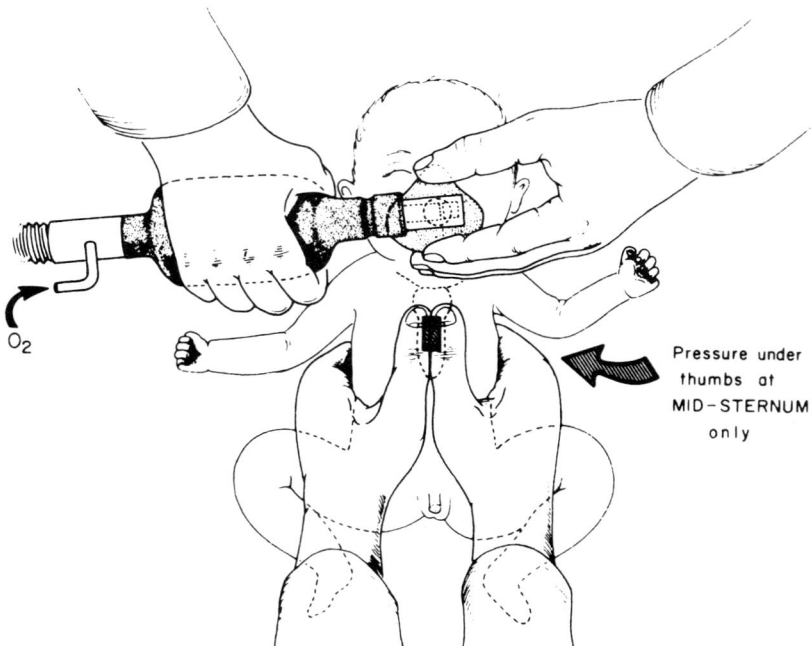

O_2

Pressure under
thumbs at
MID–STERNUM
only

FIGURE 8–5. Diagram of the two-handed method of cardiac massage. Note how both hands encircle the chest and how both thumbs are used for cardiac compression. (From Todres ID, Rogers MC: Methods of external cardiac massage in the newborn infant. J Pediatr 86:781, 1975.)

squeeze blood out of the thorax and into the circulation more efficiently than conventional CPR. Such a new process of CPR may be augmented with continuous epinephrine infusions.[57] While this new type of CPR is not currently a recommended method, a renaissance of CPR research may dramatically change conventional techniques over the next decade.

External cardiac massage may be stopped once a regular heartbeat and adequate peripheral pulses are restored. If metabolic acidosis exists despite normovolemia, diluted sodium bicarbonate (2 to 4 mEq/kg/min) may be administered. Sodium bicarbonate may be diluted in equal parts with D_5W or sterile water. Acid-base balance must be restored with buffer if epinephrine therapy is to be effective.

Epinephrine therapy is indicated if asystole or bradycardia persists after 1 minute of external cardiac massage. A dose of 0.2 ml/kg of a 1 to 10,000 dilution of epinephrine is injected intravenously or instilled into the trachea. Calcium therapy (calcium gluconate, 100 to 200 mg/kg) may also increase myocardial contractility by improving ventricular conduction velocity during cardiac arrest.

Ventricular Fibrillation

Ventricular fibrillation is seldom encountered during neonatal resuscitation in the delivery room. Nevertheless, provisions should be made for electrical cardioversion in the delivery room, NICU, or operating suite. External defibrillation can be achieved with an appropriate electrical shock (2 watt-sec/kg initially; 3 to 5 watt-sec/kg in subsequent shocks) applied through paddles of appropriate size to skin surfaces protected from burns with conductive jelly or pads.

Meconium Aspiration

If meconium is present in the amniotic fluid, the infant's upper airway should be suctioned carefully as soon as the head is delivered and once again prior to initiating positive pressure ventilation by bag and mask or bag and endotracheal tube.[58] The DeLee catheter suction is more efficient than the bulb syringe for aspirating meconium from the nose and oropharynx for several reasons, including (1) two aspirating ports on the suction catheter versus one on the bulb syringe; (2) continuous suctioning provided by the catheter versus intermittent bulb suctioning; and (3) suction force of 130 mmHg by catheter versus 70 mmHg by bulb syringe.[59]

After delivery, the meconium-stained infant is handed to the pediatrician, who performs further suctioning by direct tracheal aspiration and endotracheal intubation if indicated before the infant makes inspiratory efforts and aspirates more meconium. Tracheal suctioning of meconium is repeated until the trachea is clear. If the infant becomes bradycardic, suctioning should be stopped until the heart rate is restored. Recent studies indicate, however, that direct tracheal suctioning of meconium-stained neonates with 1-minute Apgar scores of 8 or greater is unnecessary and may even lead to increased incidence of morbidity.[60]

Saline lavage of tracheal meconium is controversial and should be reserved for infants who have aspirated thick meconium that cannot be removed by direct tracheal suctioning. Infants with significant meconium aspiration in utero will require vigorous resuscitation at birth and are at risk for a variety of complications, including meconium aspiration pneumonia, respiratory failure, persistent pulmonary hypertension, and pulmonary barotrauma syndromes. Accordingly, such patients should be monitored closely in the postpartum period with frequent blood pressure and blood gas measurements and periodic chest x-ray films.

Circulatory Shock

The infant resuscitator must be prepared to reexpand intravascular volume quickly with a variety of solutions in the event of severe hypotension and hypovolemia at birth. If acute blood loss has occurred, volume replacement is best accomplished by administration of whole blood. When shock persists despite adequate intravascular volume expansion, an intravenous inotrope (e.g., dopamine, 5 to 15 µg/kg/min) may be indicated to restore myocardial contractility and organ perfusion.

Pneumothorax

With tension pneumothorax, immediate lung reexpansion is an essential part of successful neonatal resuscitation. Emergency reexpansion of the collapsed lung may be performed by inserting a scalp vein needle with an attached aspirating syringe into the second intercostal space for temporary air evacuation until tube thoracostomy for closed chest drainage is performed.

Congenital Upper Airway Obstruction

If bilateral choanal atresia prevents nose breathing, an oropharyngeal airway or oral endotracheal tube should be inserted before neonatal resuscitation begins, to prevent the tongue from occluding the upper airway and preventing effective mouth breathing.

Most children with defects of the tongue and mandible (e.g., Pierre Robin syndrome) will maintain a patent upper airway after oral airway insertion or prone positioning. When resuscitation is required in severely depressed infants with these conditions, endotracheal intubation is recommended to provide a secure and reliable artificial airway in the supine position.

Narcotic-Induced Neuromuscular Depression

The neonate may be severely depressed because of maternal narcotics administered during labor or unsuspected maternal drug abuse. Neonates who remain limp and fail to initiate spontaneous breathing after effective ventilation has been restored may have narcotic overdose. In such cases, intravenous or intramuscular naloxone, 0.01 to 0.1 mg/kg, will provide dramatic but short-lived reversal of narcotic-induced respiratory depression within minutes.[61] Naloxone doses may have to be repeated if symptoms of narcotic depression recur. Recently, the Drug Committee of the American Academy of Pediatrics has recommended that neonatal naloxone be provided in doses of 0.1 to 0.4 mg/ml to limit excessive fluid volumes with multidose therapy.[61]

POSTRESUSCITATION PROCEDURES

After resuscitation and stabilization, the infant should undergo a complete physical examination to detect congenital anomalies that may have contributed to birth asphyxia. Persistent cyanosis with adequate ventilation and normal blood pH may suggest congenital heart defects or persistent pulmonary hypertension of the newborn. An orogastric tube should be passed into the stomach to relieve gaseous distention, remove gastric secretions, reduce aspiration risks, and improve diaphragmatic excursions.

All tubes and monitoring devices should be fastened securely. If long-term ventilation is anticipated, an orotracheal tube may be replaced with a nasotracheal tube and secured. If transport is necessary, a transport incubator with a portable electrocardiograph monitor facilitates movement of the infant from the delivery room or operating room to the NICU without heat loss or interruption of intensive care. All specimens taken during the resuscitation (i.e., cultures, gastric aspirates, and blood samples) should be delivered to the laboratory promptly. All notes made during the procedure should become part of the patient's permanent record. Before the transfer process begins, the NICU should be alerted so that preparation can be made to accommodate the infant.

A SAMPLE PROTOCOL FOR NEONATAL RESUSCITATION

The following protocol for neonatal resuscitation is used at our institution for team resuscitation of severely depressed neonates at delivery.

Procedure

Newborn intensive care in the delivery room.

Purpose

To prepare for the delivery of an extremely small or possibly as-phyxiated infant and to stabilize the baby as quickly as possible. This task requires appropriate equipment, manpower, and readiness in the delivery room in order to facilitate the immediate and orderly resuscitation of the newborn at high risk.

Candidate

Infants at extremely high risk will be candidates for this protocol (Table 8–10).[4]

Initiation

1. All infants deemed at high risk for needing resuscitation will be so identified on the high-risk slip when processed in the delivery suite. In these cases, the attending neonatologist or fellow will be notified that a neonatal resuscitation is pending.

2. The obstetrician will attempt to give the nursery staff 1 hour notification before delivery for equipment to be prepared in the delivery room.

3. Any pregnancy that does not meet the criteria but that is deemed sufficiently high-risk by the attending obstetrician or neonatal house staff will require evaluation by the attending physician, neonatologist, or fellow before the procedure is initiated.

Personnel

Physicians. The attending pediatrician, neonatologist, or fellow will participate in and supervise all neonatal resuscitations. An additional house officer will also be present for the delivery and resuscitation.

Nursery. One or more nurses skilled in nursery intensive care will set

Table 8–10. Attendance at High-Risk Delivery (Full-Team Resuscitation)

1. Prematurity (less than 34 weeks' gestation or predicted weight less than 1800 g)
2. Immature L/S ratio (less than 1.8:1)
3. Infant of diabetic mother (class C or worse)
4. Suspected severe hypovolemia secondary to abruptio placentae or placenta previa
5. Severe preeclampsia or eclampsia
6. Predicted severe asphyxia by electronic fetal monitoring and/or fetal pH
7. Rh sensitization with predicted anemia and/or prematurity
8. Other (at discretion of obstetrician)

From Karotkin EH, Goldsmith JP: Resuscitation. In: Goldsmith JP, Karotkin EH (eds): Assisted Ventilation of the Neonate, 2nd ed. Philadelphia: W.B. Saunders, 1988, pp 70–89. Used with permission.

up the equipment before the delivery and assist in the resuscitation. An additional obstetric nurse will assist in the resuscitation.

Ancillary Personnel. The respiratory therapy department and the pulmonary function laboratory will have personnel on immediate standby. If considered necessary by the attending pediatrician, neonatologist, or fellow, these personnel will be in surgical clothing and standing by in the delivery room.

Equipment and Drugs

The following equipment will be set up and operational in the delivery room (see Tables 8–4 and 8–5):[4]

1. Radiant warmer
2. Electrocardiographic equipment with leads attached
3. Pulse oximeter
4. Blood pressure transducer and monitor (calibrated and ready)
5. Centrifuge with hematocrit tubes, hematocrit reader, optical densitometer, and blood glucose strips
6. IV solutions—$D_{10}W$, 500 ml—with tubing filled and ready for use (no additives)
7. Syringes
   a. Three 3-ml syringes
   b. Three 5-ml syringes
   c. Three tuberculine syringes heparinized and labeled for blood gases (0.01 ml heparin)
   d. Three tuberculine syringes plain
   e. Three 10-ml syringes
8. Umbilical catheter tray with two catheters filled and ready for insertion; one catheter heparinized, one with sterile water only
9. Laryngoscope with 0-1 Miller blades, appropriate endotracheal tubes, adaptors, oxygen tubing, rebreathing bag, and appropriate masks
10. Suction equipment with appropriate-sized suction catheters for endotracheal tube suction and soft catheters for mouth suction
11. Laboratory tubes for CBC, platelets, prothrombin time (PT), partial thromboplastin time (PTT); and culture bottles for blood, skin, and urine
12. Povidone-iodine (Betadine), tincture of benzoin, ½-inch and 1-inch paper and cloth tape, scissors, and wrapping bandages for securing infant and all tubes prior to movement

The following fluids and drugs will be available for immediate use:

1. Blood: One 50-ml unit of recently drawn, packed red cells, preferably less than 72 hours old, typed against the mother. If this is unavailable,

any O negative, low-titer packed cells less than 3 days old will suffice. Blood should be in the obstetric unit when the patient goes into the delivery room.

2. Albumin: One vial of 20 ml (5% salt poor).
3. Sodium bicarbonate and D_5W: 10 ml of each will be drawn and placed together in a 20-ml syringe and labeled.
4. All other drugs listed in the emergency list (see Table 8–5)[4] will be available in the delivery room.

Personnel Responsibilities

Head Nurse. The head nurse will initiate the procedure by notifying the attending pediatrician, neonatologist, and/or fellow, altering work assignments to free nurses to prepare the equipment (this may require an additional nurse to be called in from home), and ordering the blood. The head nurse will then be responsible for coordinating the course of action in the delivery room and notifying the pulmonary function laboratory and respiratory therapy department.

Neonatologist and/or Fellow. The neonatologist and/or fellow will review the case with the obstetric staff and coordinate efforts with the head nurses to ensure that all preparations are under way. During the resuscitation, the neonatologist will manage the ventilatory resuscitation at the head of the radiant warmer, including tracheal intubation and controlled ventilation.

House Officer. The house officer will be responsible for inserting catheters, drawing laboratory tests, and administering drugs. He will coordinate with the neonatologist and/or fellow the overall care of the infant.

Nurses. One nurse will set up the equipment, check oxygen and resuscitation equipment, calibrate blood pressure transducers, check all drugs, and ready the catheter tray. During the resuscitation, nurses will assist with all medications, determine the hematocrit and serum glucose, and note all drugs given, vital signs, and times. A second nurse (float nurse) will act as record keeper (charting drugs, vital signs, Apgar scores, and procedures) and messenger (e.g., taking blood gases to the laboratory). NICU nursing notes will be started and kept by the float nurse from the moment of delivery.

Course of Action

1. The infant will be delivered and moved immediately to the radiant warmer.

2. While the infant is being dried and suctioned with a bulb syringe and/or DeLee suction, an Apgar assessment will be made.

3. If deemed necessary, ventilation will begin immediately and the nurse will place restraints on the infant's arms and legs and attach ECG leads.

4. A section of umbilical cord will be double clamped and passed off the delivery table to the float nurse, who will draw 0.3 ml of blood from the umbilical artery into a heparinized TB syringe and send this sample to the blood gas laboratory for immediate analysis.

5. If immediate vascular access is required, the house officer will insert a peripheral or umbilical venous catheter and give the necessary drugs immediately. An umbilical artery catheter will then be inserted and systemic blood pressures obtained.

6. After the vascular catheters are secured, blood gas samples and appropriate laboratory tests will be obtained.

7. The infant will remain in the delivery room or resuscitation area until stabilized. The senior physician will determine when the infant can be moved safely to the intensive care nursery and will order equipment to be readied in the nursery (e.g., radiant warmer, ventilator, x-ray machine).

References

1. Dawes GS: Foetal and Neonatal Physiology. Chicago: Year Book Medical Publishers, 1968
2. Adamsons K Jr, Behrman R, Dawes GS, et al.: The treatment of acidosis with alkali and glucose during asphyxia in foetal rhesus monkeys. J Physiol 169:679, 1963
3. Adamsons K Jr, Behrman R, Dawes GS, et al.: Resuscitation by positive pressure ventilation and Tris-hydroxymethylamniomethane of rhesus monkeys asphyxiated at birth. J Pediatr 65:807, 1964
4. Karotkin EH, Goldsmith JP: Resuscitation. In: Goldsmith JP, Karotkin EH (eds): Assisted Ventilation of the Neonate, 2nd ed. Philadelphia: W. B. Saunders, 1988, pp 70–89
5. Perlman JM: Systemic abnormalities in term infants following perinatal asphyxia: Relevance to long-term neurologic outcome. Clin Perinatol 16:475, 1989
6. Towne BH, Lott IT, Hickes DA, et al.: Long-term follow-up of infants and children treated with extracorporeal membrane oxygenation (ECMO): A preliminary report. J Pediatr Surg 20:410, 1985
7. McCord JM: Oxygen-derived free radicals in postischemic tissue injury. N Engl J Med 312:159, 1985
8. Fisher DE, Paton JB: Resuscitation of the newborn infant. In: Klaus MH, Fanaroff AA (eds): Care of the High-Risk Neonate, 2nd ed. Philadelphia: W. B. Saunders, 1979, pp 23–44
9. Brann AW Jr, Cefalo RC (eds): Guidelines for Perinatal Care. Evanston, IL: American Academy of Pediatrics and the American College of Obstetricians and Gynecologists, 1983, pp 67, 260–261
10. Press S, Tellechea C, Pregen S: Cesarean delivery of full-term infants: Identification of those at high risk for requiring resuscitation. J Pediatr 106:477, 1985
11. Lilien AA: Term intrapartum fetal death. Am J Obstet Gynecol 107:595, 1970
12. Zuspan FP, Quilligan EJ, Iams JD, et al.: NICHD Consensus Development Task Force Report: Predictors of intrapartum fetal distress—the role of electronic fetal monitoring. J Pediatr 95:1026, 1979
13. Kelso IM, Parsons RJ, Lawrence GF, et al.: An assessment of continuous fetal heart rate monitoring in labor—a randomized trial. Am J Obstet Gynecol 131:526, 1978
14. Neutra RR, Fienberg SE, Greenland S, et al.: Effect of fetal monitoring on neonatal death rates. N Engl J Med 299:325, 1978

15. Queenan JT: There's no substitute for experience, but sometimes you wish there were (editorial). Contemp OB/GYN, 28:7, 1986
16. Bottoms SF, Rosen MG, Sokol RJ: The increase in cesarean birth rate. N Engl J Med 302:559, 1980
17. Haverkamp AD, Thompson HE, McFee JG, et al.: The evaluation of continuous fetal heart rate monitoring in high risk pregnancy. Am J Obstet Gynecol 125:310, 1976
18. Frigoletto FD, Little GA (eds): Guidelines for Perinatal Care, 2nd ed. Evanston, IL: American Academy of Pediatrics and American College of Obstetricians and Gynecologists, 1988, p 67
19. Hon EH: An Atlas of Fetal Heart Rate Patterns. New Haven, CT: Harty Press, 1968
20. Goodlin RC: History of fetal monitoring. Am J Obstet Gynecol 133:323, 1979
21. Beard RW, Morris ED, Clayton SG: pH of foetal capillary blood as an indicator of the condition of the foetus. J Obstet Gynaecol Br Commonwealth 74:812, 1967
22. Quilligan EJ: Making inroads against the c-section rate. Contemp OB/GYN, 21:221, 1983
23. Seeds AE: Adverse effects on the fetus of acute events in labor. Pediatr Clin North Am 17:811, 1970
24. Clark JM, Brown ZA, Jung AL: Resuscitation equipment board for nurseries and delivery rooms. JAMA 236:2427, 1976
25. Smith RM: Diagnosis and treatment—the critically ill child: Respiratory arrest and its sequelae. Pediatrics 46:108, 1970
26. Brann AW, Cefalo RC: Committee on fetus and newborn: Care of the newborn in the delivery room. Pediatrics 64:970, 1979
27. Apgar V: Proposal for method of evaluation of newborn infant. Anesth Analg 32:260, 1953
28. Vaughan VC: Nelson's Textbook of Pediatrics, 11th ed. Philadelphia: W. B. Saunders, 1979, p 393
29. Nelson KB, Ellenberg JH: Neonatal signs as predictors of cerebral palsy. Pediatrics 64:225, 1979
30. Editorial: Is the Apgar score outmoded? Lancet 1:591, 1989
31. Martin GI, Holgaren JE, Quilligan EJ, et al.: Point-counterpoint: The Apgar score revisited. J Perinatol 9:338, 1989
32. Fields LM, Entman SS, Boehm FH: Correlation of the one-minute Apgar score and the pH value of umbilical arterial blood. South Med J 76:1477, 1983
33. Cordero L Jr, Hon EH: Neonatal bradycardia following nasopharyngeal stimulation. J Pediatr 78:441, 1971
34. Schreiner RL: Neonatology for the Pediatrician. Medical Educational Resources Program, Indianapolis, Indiana University School of Medicine, 1978, p 187
35. Bloom RS, Cropky C: Textbook of Neonatal Resuscitation. American Heart Association and American Academy of Pediatrics, 1988
36. Diaz JH: Tension pneumoperitoneum-pneumothorax during repair of congenital diaphragmatic hernia. Anesth Analg 66:577, 1987
37. Nugent J, Matthews BJ, Goldsmith JP: Pulmonary care. In: Goldsmith JP, Karotkin EH (eds): Assisted Ventilation of the Neonate, 2nd ed. Philadelphia: W. B. Saunders, 1988, pp 90–106
38. Milner AD, Vyas H, Hopkin IE: Efficacy of facemask resuscitation at birth. Br Med J 289:1563, 1984
39. Sherman JM, Nelson H: Decreased incidence of subglottic stenosis using an "appropriate-sized" endotracheal tube in neonates. Pediatr Pulmonol 6:183, 1989
40. Spitzer AR, Fox WW: The use of oral versus nasal endotracheal tubes in newborn infants. J Calif Perinat Assoc 4:32, 1984
41. Tochen ML: Orotracheal intubation in the newborn infant: A method for determining depth of tube insertion. J Pediatr 95:1050, 1979
42. Powers RD, Donowitz LG: Endotracheal administration of emergency medications. South Med J 77:340, 1984
43. Orlowski JP: Editorial: My kingdom for an intravenous line. Am J Dis Child 138:803, 1984
44. MacDonald MG: Umbilical-artery catheterization. In: Fletcher MA, MacDonald MG, Avery GB (eds): Atlas of Procedures in Neonatology. Philadelphia: J. B. Lippincott, 1983, pp 130–145
45. Simmons MA, Adcock EW, Bard H, et al.: Hypernatremia and intracranial hemorrhage in neonates. N Engl J Med 291:6, 1974

46. Anderson J, Bain AD, Brown J, et al.: Hyaline membrane disease, alkaline buffer treatment, and cerebral intraventricular hemorrhage. Lancet 1:117, 1979
47. Volpe JJ: Neonatal periventricular hemorrhage: Past, present, and future. J Pediatr 92:693, 1978
48. Ballard RA, Kitterman JR, Phibbs RH, et al.: Observations on hypovolemia in the newborn (abstract). Clin Res 20:278, 1972
49. Paxson CL Jr: Neonatal shock in the first postnatal day. Am J Dis Child 132:509, 1978
50. Oberman HA (ed): Standards for Blood Banks and Transfusion Services, 7th ed. Washington, DC: American Association of Blood Banks, 1974
51. Barr PA, Bailey PR, Sumners J, et al.: Relation between arterial blood pressure and blood volume and effect of infused albumin in sick preterm infants. Pediatrics 60:282, 1977
52. 1985 Standards of cardiopulmonary resuscitation and emergency cardiac care, Part VI. Neonatal advanced life support. JAMA 255:2969, 1986
53. Todres ID, Rogers MC: Methods of external cardiac massage in the newborn infant. J Pediatr 86:781, 1975
54. Finholt DA, Kettrick RG, Wagner HR, et al.: The heart is under the lower third of the sternum. Am J Dis Child 140:646, 1986
55. Weisfeldt ML, Chandra N: Physiology of cardiopulmonary resuscitation. Annu Rev Med 32:435, 1981
56. Chandra N, Rudikoff M, Weisfeldt ML: Simultaneous chest compression and ventilation at high airway pressure during cardiopulmonary resuscitation. Lancet 1:175, 1980
57. Koehler RC, Michael JR, Guerci AD, et al.: Beneficial effect of epinephrine infusion on cerebral myocardial blood flows during CPR. Ann Emerg Med 14:744, 1985
58. Carson BS, Losey RW, Bowes WA Jr, et al.: Combined obstetric and pediatric approach to prevent meconium aspiration syndrome. Am J Obstet Gynecol 126:712, 1976
59. Gage JE, Taeusch HW Jr, Treves S, et al.: Suctioning of the upper airway meconium in newborn infants. JAMA 246:2590, 1981
60. Linder N, Aranda JV, Tsur M, et al.: Need for endotracheal intubation and suction in meconium-stained neonates. J Pediatr 112:613, 1988
61. Committee on Drugs, American Academy of Pediatrics: Emergency drug doses for infants and children and naloxone use in newborns: Clarification. Pediatrics 83:803, 1989

9. The Neonatal Effects of Anesthetic Agents and Techniques

Jay P. Goldsmith, M.D.
Andrea L. Starrett, M.D.

INTRODUCTION

The risks and benefits of obstetric anesthesia and analgesia have often been debated. Drugs have been used to alleviate pain during labor and delivery since 1853, when Queen Victoria inhaled chloroform during the birth of Prince Leopold. Today the vast majority of women receive some

242

form of anesthesia or analgesia during labor. In one survey of mothers delivered vaginally,[1] only 8% received no pain-relieving therapy. Epidural anesthesia was the most frequent form of pain control (50%), followed by narcotic analgesics (26%). Despite current recommendations by women's groups for natural childbirth and by physicians for regional anesthesia, narcotics are still widely used for pain relief during labor in the United States today.[2]

The type of anesthetic and amount of analgesic used in the pain management of labor and delivery have profound implications for the neonate. Analgesic administration during labor and delivery should be based on maternal perception of pain, effectiveness of ancillary analgesic techniques (psychoanalgesia, whirlpool baths, breathing exercises), and the cardiopulmonary status of the mother and fetus.

Neonatal morbidity and mortality may result from maternal anesthetic catastrophes or from direct or indirect effects of various anesthetics or analgesics administered. Additionally, interactions between indirect effects of anesthetics and various perinatal illnesses may produce severe consequences not seen in healthy pregnancies. Even the judicious use of modern anesthetics may result in subtle neurobehavioral changes in the neonate with possible long-term consequences.

This chapter reviews the hemodynamic and neurobehavioral effects of obstetric anesthetics and analgesics on the neonate. The effects of frequently used obstetric anesthetics and analgesics are emphasized, and some past misadventures in obstetric anesthesia are recalled. Chapters 2, 4, 6, and 7 provide a more complete review of the technical aspects of administration of obstetric anesthetics, standards of anesthetic care, and maternal complications.

EVALUATION OF THE NEWBORN

Traditional methods of evaluating the newborn have recently been questioned by many investigators. Apgar scoring, while indicating the need for resuscitation, is not a valid method for determining the degree of asphyxia and does not correlate with umbilical cord blood gas analysis.[3, 4]

Neonatal shock is not easily identified by blood pressure but rather by a constellation of clinical features including decreased arterial pulses, tachycardia, tachypnea, poor capillary refill, mottled skin, cool extremities, metabolic acidosis, and oliguria. Initial hemodynamic assessment of the newborn depends on many clinical signs and laboratory values and must be performed rapidly in the depressed neonate by experienced personnel to avoid end-organ asphyxial damage.

Delivery Room Assessment

The quantitative assessment designed by anesthesiologist Virginia Apgar to determine a newborn's need for resuscitation is the most widely used first measurement to evaluate the well-being of the newborn. The Apgar score is based on five simple parameters that give the observer an indirect measurement of newborn hemodynamic status (see Table 8–6 in Chapter 8).[5] Each individual parameter is scored from 0 to 2 by a nonbiased observer 1 minute and 5 minutes after delivery. Generally, a score of 7 or greater indicates a hemodynamically stable infant not in need of active resuscitation. A score of 4 to 7 indicates mild to moderate difficulty in making the transition from intrauterine to extrauterine life. A score of 3 or less indicates a need for immediate resuscitation, including positive-pressure ventilation with 100% oxygen and cardiovascular resuscitation (see Chapter 8).

Dr. Apgar devised this score in 1953 as a simple means to quickly evaluate the newborn's need for active resuscitation. At that time, many infants were delivered during profound maternal analgesia or general anesthesia and needed rapid and effective resuscitation. Unfortunately, low Apgar scores have been misinterpreted as being synonymous with perinatal asphyxia.[6] The causes of low Apgar scores are diverse and are listed in Table 8–2.

A much better indicator of the hemodynamic status of the newborn is an umbilical cord arterial blood gas analysis, although neither cord blood gas analysis nor Apgar score correlates well with neurologic outcome.[7] The cord blood sample should be obtained from a section of the umbilical cord that has been double-clamped within 30 seconds of delivery. A pH of greater than 7.20 is considered normal, since the stresses of labor cause mild acidosis even in a healthy fetus. Several investigators have shown very poor correlation between cord blood gas analysis and the 1-minute Apgar score.[3, 4, 8] Many authorities now recommend routine measurements of cord blood gases at delivery to identify all acidotic infants.

Interestingly, neonates obviously sedated by maternal drugs may have normal cord gas studies at delivery, especially if the mother is hemodynamically stable. Once the cord has been severed, however, sedative levels will rise in the neonate, leading to respiratory depression and potential asphyxia if appropriate treatment is not given. However, if an anesthetic administered during labor reduces uteroplacental perfusion (e.g., maternal hypotension after epidural administration), the fetus may be chronically asphyxiated and delivered subsequently with poor cord blood gas studies.

Electronic fetal monitoring (EFM) has been advocated as a means of monitoring effects of obstetric anesthetics on the fetus. The interpretation of EFM may, however, be confused by systemic analgesics that decrease fetal heart rate variability[9] and make accurate diagnosis difficult.

Additional perinatal factors that may exacerbate drug-induced asphyxia include interruption of adequate umbilical blood flow, failure of adequate gas exchange across the placenta, and inability of the fetus to tolerate the intensity of labor. Sedatives taken by the mother without the advice or knowledge of the obstetrician may further exacerbate newborn depression and confuse the etiology. Any infant who is unexpectedly depressed at birth should be evaluated by toxicology screening for maternal drug abuse.

Hemodynamic Assessment

Direct intra-arterial measurement of blood pressure in the umbilical artery is the most accurate method of determining blood pressure in the neonate.[10] Central aortic pressure measurements through an umbilical artery catheter are more reliable than peripheral blood pressures, direct or indirect. Indirect measurement by Doppler or ultrasonic sphygmomanometry may also be used but is less reliable in the depressed neonate because of peripheral hypoperfusion. Clinical manifestations of neonatal shock are often present before significant blood pressure reductions are noted, especially if such measurements are made peripherally.[11] Frequently, the signs of poor peripheral perfusion, including intense vasoconstriction, prolonged capillary refill, and pallid and cold extremities, are apparent in the delivery room before the indirect blood pressure is taken or direct arterial access is accomplished.

Technical problems and the skill of the treating personnel are, of course, important factors in the reliability of blood pressure measurements in the newborn.

Accurate intra-arterial monitoring depends on the site of cannulation, the size and composition of the arterial catheter, the position of the monitored extremity, and the presence of air bubbles or blood clots in the transducing system.[12] Small-bore Teflon catheters often produce poor arterial waveforms that are not reflective of umbilical artery pressure. A 5.0 French, Argyle catheter in an umbilical artery will give better pressure readings than a 3.5 French catheter, but the former is not appropriate in infants with birth weights less than 1250 g. Accurate intra-arterial monitoring also depends on the absence of air bubbles in the transducing system, since air bubbles, unlike fluids, are easily compressed, dampen pulsatile waveforms, and do not transmit accurate pressure oscillations to the transducer. In addition, blood clots in the fluid-filled transducing system or on the catheter tip will dampen pulsatile waves, causing the dicrotic notch to disappear and giving spuriously low readings of arterial blood pressure. The entire monitoring system should be leak-proof and bubble-free. The tubing connecting the strain gauge transducer to the patient should be noncompliant and have a lumen equal to or larger than the intra-arterial catheter, to avoid artifacts in pulsed wave transmissions.

Flush techniques, palpation, auscultation, and Doppler detection of arterial pressure are acceptable alternatives to intra-arterial measurements but are less accurate and are user dependent.[13] The size of the bladder (not the cuff) and the interpretation of the pitch, quality, and intensity of the Karotkoff sounds may make these techniques less than reliable in inexperienced hands. The flush method is unreliable during severe hypotension, severe anemia, edema of the extremities, and marked hypothermia.

Normal values for neonatal blood pressure are shown in Table 11–2.[14] Aortic pressures increase in direct relationship to birth weight. For example, at 1000 g, the average systolic pressure is 46 mmHg, the average diastolic pressure is 25 mmHg, and mean pressure is 32 mmHg. For each 100-g increase above 1000 g there is an incremental increase of 1 mmHg in blood pressure.

Many factors affect arterial pressure measurements at birth, including maternal cardiovascular (e.g., toxemia) and endocrine (e.g., diabetes mellitus) disorders, method of delivery, timing of cord clamping, fetomaternal hemorrhage, and birth asphyxia. Infants delivered by cesarean section or breech extraction have lower systemic arterial pressures than vertex infants delivered vaginally.[15]

Shock and hypotension are the cardinal presenting signs of significant perinatal asphyxia. Decreased arterial pressure, metabolic acidosis, poor cardiac output, and wet lungs are often associated with perinatal asphyxia. Asphyxiated infants who fail to take a good initial breath at birth may leave up to 20% of their available blood volume in the umbilical cord and placenta and thus may be hypovolemic as well as asphyxiated. However, hypocarbia from overaggressive ventilation may elevate intrathoracic pressure and limit venous return, producing systemic hypotension even when blood volumes are normal. Adequate oxygenation, positive-pressure ventilation, and correction of respiratory and metabolic acidosis are the initial corrective steps in managing newborn shock. Intravascular volume expansion and early administration of inotropic agents may also be necessary. Infants depressed by narcotics may respond to naloxone.

Occasionally hypertension may be an early response to asphyxia, especially with primary apnea. Clinical signs of peripheral vasoconstriction and blood gas analysis indicating metabolic acidosis will often guide the clinician to the correct diagnosis and management. Repetitive measurements of acid-base status, arterial access for direct pressure measurements, and occasionally central venous cannulation for filling pressure measurements may be necessary to adequately treat the hemodynamically unstable and asphyxiated newborn. Once the newborn is stabilized, a thorough evaluation for causative factors can proceed, searching for treatable conditions including sepsis, drug overdose, perinatal asphyxia, metabolic derangements, and hypovolemia from fetomaternal or twin-to-twin transfusions or umbilical cord accidents.

Neurobehavioral Assessment

The widespread use of obstetric anesthesia and analgesia has led to concern about the effects of these drugs on the neurologic status and behavior of the neonate. Gross neurologic effects have been described only with neonatal local anesthetic intoxication syndromes. However, high doses of narcotic analgesics, particularly meperidine, have been associated with neonatal respiratory depression and altered muscle tone. More subtle depressant effects of anesthetics and analgesics may alter the neonate's behavior and ability to adapt to an extrauterine environment by affecting the state of alertness, feeding habits, and maternal-infant bonding.[16, 17] These concerns led to studies evaluating the neonatal neurologic and behavioral effects of obstetric anesthesia and analgesia.[18–20]

Although various physiologic measures can be used to assess the neurologic integrity and behavioral capacities of the newborn, the most commonly used neurologic assessment is clinical examination. Neurologic examination of the newborn assesses cranial nerve function, muscle tone, spontaneous movement, deep tendon reflexes, elicited reflexes, and automatic response patterns. Behavioral assessment of the newborn examines the infant's state of alertness, regulation of state, response to meaningful environmental stimuli (orientation), response to intrusive stimuli (habituation), and ability to generate complex behaviors that elicit or reinforce caretaker behavior.[21] Philosophically, the behavioral assessment recognizes that the neonate is an integrated organism capable of reacting in an adaptive fashion to events in his environment.

The various systems of neurologic and behavioral assessment of the newborn have been devised for and standardized on healthy, full-term infants. The systems most commonly used are the Neonatal Behavioral Assessment Scale (NBAS) developed by Brazelton,[22] the Early Neonatal Neurobehavioral Scale (ENNS) developed by Scanlon and coworkers,[23] and the Neonatal Adaptive Capacity Scale (NACS) developed by Amiel-Tison and coworkers.[24]

The NBAS[22] was formulated to codify the behavior of the neonate during observation of his responses to specific environmental stimuli. It records the infant's responses to 28 behavioral items and 18 elicited behaviors, primarily reflex and muscle tone assessments, and thus combines both behavioral and neurologic assessments. Throughout the examination, the infant's state of alertness is carefully controlled to ensure optimal responses and allow the best response to be recorded. The behavioral responses are commonly analyzed in seven a priori clusters of infant functioning-habituation, orientation, motor performance, range of state, autonomic regulation, and reflexes. Cluster scores can be analyzed statistically and have been used to compare infants' behavior in a wide variety of research situations.

The drawbacks of this examination are the extended amount of time necessary to examine individual infants (30 minutes or longer) and the need for highly trained examiners to maintain interrater reliability. The examination is reliable from the first day of life to 1 month of age. Because of these drawbacks and the need for a standardized assessment of infant behavior in the period immediately after birth, other, shorter, methods of neonatal neurobehavioral assessment have been devised.

The two most commonly used abbreviated assessments of infant behavior following obstetric medication are the ENNS[23] and the NACS.[24] The scoring systems of the ENNS and NACS are simpler than that of the NBAS, and they require much less time to administer (less than 10 minutes). All three examinations have a high rate of interrater reliability among experienced examiners. The ENNS places greater emphasis on habituation to external stimuli than does the NACS, which emphasizes evaluation of active and passive muscle tone. Neither the ENNS nor the NACS clearly evaluates the neonate's state of being and its regulation, integrated behaviors that would seem to be most affected by drugs that depress the sensorium. However, the ENNS records these states prior to administration of individual test items.

Table 9–1 presents a comparison of the various neonatal behaviors elicited or rated by the NBAS, ENNS, and NCAS. Of the 52 possible behaviors observed, only six are common to all three scales. The ENNS and the NACS share only these six items; both the ENNS and NCAS have many items in common with the NBAS (ENNS has 12 of 16; NCAS has 15 of 20). Although two studies[24, 25] rate neonatal performance on simultaneously administered ENNS and NCAS scales, there are no statistical comparisons between the two tests. There are no studies correlating infant behavior on the ENNS or NACS with the NBAS. There is extensive literature documenting the stability of infant behavior on the NBAS and its relationship to maternal behavior and perceptions of the infant in the first month of life. There are no studies relating ENNS and NCAS to later infant or maternal behavior. Thus, the NBAS provides the most complete assessments of the neonate's behavior, while the ENNS and NACS screen for more gross distortions of certain neonatal behaviors. All studies using these three instruments have been performed on full-term, essentially healthy newborns. No information is

Table 9–1. *Comparison of Neonatal Behaviors in Three Neurobehavioral Scales*

	NBAS [1]	ENNS [2]	NACS [3]
Response decrement to light	X	X	X
Response decrement to rattle	X		
Response decrement to bell	X	X	X
Response decrement to tactile stimulation	X	X	
Response decrement to Moro		X	
Orientation—inanimate visual	X		
Orientation—inanimate auditory	X	X	
Orientation—inanimate visual and auditory	X		
Orientation—animate visual	X		
Orientation—animate auditory	X		
Orientation—animate visual and auditory	X		
Alertness	X	X	X
General tonus	X	X	
Motor maturity	X		X
Pull-to-sit	X	X	X
Cuddliness	X		
Defensive movements	X		
Consolability	X		X
Peak excitement	X		
Irritability	X		
Activity	X		
Tremulousness	X		
Lability of skin color	X		
Lability of states	X		
Self-quieting activity	X		
Hand-to-mouth facility	X		
Smiles	X		
Plantar grasp	X		
Hand grasp	X		X
Ankle clonus	X		
Babinski	X		
Supporting reaction	X		X
Automatic walking	X		X
Placing	X	X	
Incurvation	X		
Crawling	X		
Glabella tap	X		
Tonic deviation of eyes	X		
Nystagmus	X		
Tonic neck reflex	X		
Moro	X	X	X
Rooting	X	X	
Sucking	X	X	X
Resistance in passive movement—arms	X		X
Resistance in passive movement—legs	X		X
Recoil arms	X	X	X
Recoil legs	X		X
Tone ventral suspension		X	
Traction lifting			X
Withdrawal pin prick		X	
Blink to light			X
Startle to bell			X
Quality of cry			X
OVERALL		X	

[1]Brazelton TB, 1984
[2]Amiel-Tison et al., 1982
[3]Scanlon et al., 1974

available in this regard concerning the neurobehavioral effects of maternal anesthesia/analgesia on premature or compromised full-term infants.

MATERNAL ANESTHETIC CATASTROPHES AND NEONATAL OUTCOMES

The selection of obstetric anesthesia for the mother depends on perceived maternal need, physician's preference, emergent nature of the delivery, medical condition of the mother, and absence of potential complications. Regional anesthesia permits the mother to participate in childbirth. However, general anesthesia is often indicated for urgent cesarean section in cases of acute fetal distress. Spinal anesthesia can be administered rapidly but may be contraindicated for delivery in cases of significant maternal hemorrhage with hypovolemia.

During the late 1970s and early 1980s, Albright reported 44 cases of maternal cardiac arrest following intravascular injection of 0.75% bupivacaine during epidural anesthesia for cesarean section.[26] Maternal cardiopulmonary resuscitation was difficult and complicated by severe metabolic acidosis. Neonatal outcome was poor, especially in the event of delayed delivery. Bupivacaine 0.75% is no longer recommended for obstetric epidural anesthesia. After an appropriate test dose to rule out intravascular placement of the epidural catheter, a number of alternative local anesthetics are now available for continuous epidural anesthesia for labor and either vaginal or abdominal delivery. These include 0.5% bupivacaine, 0.25% bupivacaine, 2.0% lidocaine, 1.5% lidocaine, 3.0% chloroprocaine, and 2.0% chloroprocaine.

Maternal cardiopulmonary collapse from any cause will significantly reduce uteroplacental perfusion, resulting in fetal asphyxia. Maternal systolic blood pressure less than 80 mmHg will result in fetal bradycardia[27] within 5 minutes. Since fetal cardiac output is highly rate dependent, prolonged fetal bradycardia can result in significant fetal tissue ischemia.

During general anesthesia, maternal cardiovascular collapse may occur from respiratory or circulatory failure. Respiratory failure may result from esophageal intubation, inadequate inspired oxygen concentration, pulmonary aspiration, pulmonary edema, or upper airway loss during seizures. Circulatory failure may result from hypovolemic shock, high sympathetic blocks, intravascular local anesthetics, or overdoses of inspired anesthetics or intravenous analgesics.

The common denominator of a maternal anesthetic or medical catastrophe on the fetus is maternal shock leading to decreased placental perfusion, neonatal depression, asphyxia, and neonatal shock. A skilled resuscitation team should be present in these situations to effectively help the depressed neonate make the transition from intrauterine to extrauterine life. It is likely that the infant will be significantly depressed at birth, manifesting signs and symptoms of acute shock. The provision of O-negative blood in the delivery room may be extremely helpful in the resuscitation if the blood bank is given adequate warning. Although not approved by the American Association of Blood Banks, the administration of placental blood or walking donor blood heparinized with 1 unit of heparin per milliliter of blood and drawn under sterile conditions is an extremely rapid method of treating neonatal hypovolemic shock in the delivery room. Further resuscitation techniques are discussed in Chapter 8.

Umbilical cord blood gas analysis will rapidly give the resuscitation team an idea of the severity of the hypoxic insult and direct subsequent resuscitation. Moreover, the resuscitation team should be familiar with the physiologic limitations of the neonate's response to shock (see Chapter 11) and proceed accordingly. Perinatal asphyxia may affect multiple organ systems, and recognition of different needs during and following resuscitation is crucial for a successful outcome (Table 9–2).[28]

NEONATAL EFFECTS OF REGIONAL ANESTHETICS

Regional anesthesia should not prevent effective maternal ventilation and oxygenation if blood pressure is maintained and motor level of the block is limited. Local anesthetic-induced seizures from intravascular injection generally respond to oxygenation and antiseizure therapy

Table 9–2. Organ Involvement in Perinatal Asphyxial Injury

System	Condition
Pulmonary	Persistent pulmonary hypertension; persistent fetal circulation; respiratory distress syndrome; meconium aspiration
Cardiovascular	Myocardial dysfunction; decreased circulating blood volume
Renal	Acute renal failure; acute tubular necrosis; acute corticomedullary necrosis
Metabolic	Water and electrolyte imbalance; acidosis; hypoglycemia; hypocalcemia
Gastrointestinal	Stress ulcers: necrotizing enterocolitis; hepatic injury; elevated bilirubin; hyperammonemia; elevated transaminases
Hematologic	Thrombocytopenia; neutropenia; disseminated intravascular coagulation
Central Nervous System	Cerebral edema; seizures; inappropriate antidiuretic hormone; intracranial hemorrhage; hypothalamic injury; hypopituitarism

From Perrotta LA, Campbell D. Perinatal Asphyxia: Pediatric Emergency Casebook. New York: World Health Commentaries, 1984, p 12, with permission.

without devastating sequelae. However, the past experiences with 0.75% bupivacaine–induced seizures leading to 30 reported maternal deaths appear to contradict this general rule.[26] In addition, anecdotal data support the occurrence of fetal asphyxia from intrauterine hyperactivity or uterine artery spasm following maternal recovery from bupivacaine-induced seizures. Abboud and colleagues[29] compared the effects of commonly used epidural drugs in normotensive mothers and found a higher incidence of late decelerations (8 of 42 patients) with bupivacaine than with either lidocaine (3 of 47 patients) or chloroprocaine (0 of 34 patients), although neonatal outcome was excellent in all groups.

Severe maternal hypotension after epidural anesthesia may be due to high spinal or epidural block. The etiology of such hypotension may be helpful in determining specific treatment. A total spinal block may occur within minutes of local anesthetic injection, resulting in apnea, dilation of the pupils, hypotension, and unconsciousness. High epidural blocks have more variable onsets with milder motor blocks and more easily treated hypotension.

Mothers experiencing respiratory distress, hypotension, or unexplained fetal distress during regional anesthesia should be placed in a left lateral position, given intravenous crystalloids for volume expansion, and administered supplemental oxygen. Ephedrine sulfate, 5 to 10 mg intravenously, should be administered to maintain systolic blood pressure above 100 mmHg. While affecting prompt return of blood pressure in the mother, ephedrine therapy for maternal hypotension has been questioned because ephedrine may enter the fetal circulation and contribute to persistent pulmonary hypertension of the newborn. Severe uterine hypoperfusion from maternal hypotension, however, may also produce fetal asphyxia, which in itself will lead to pulmonary hypertension. In the absence of uteroplacental insufficiency, it is often better to stabilize the mother hemodynamically, restore uteroplacental perfusion, and resuscitate a stressed fetus in utero than to deliver an asphyxiated infant emergently.

INDIRECT EFFECTS OF ANESTHETICS ON NEWBORNS

Narcotics may decrease uterine activity and slow the progress of labor, depending on the dose and timing of administration during labor. Uterine contractions will be inhibited and cervical dilatation will be slowed by the administration of opiates during the latent phase of the first stage of labor. However, if narcotics are given in smaller doses during the active phase of labor, uterine activity is not usually affected, and the speed of labor may actually increase. Reducing maternal anxiety and discomfort early in labor will often enhance the progress of labor by decreasing endogenous catecholamine release with its significant tocolytic effects.

Narcotics may also alter the fetal heart rate pattern when administered during labor. Kariniemi and Ämmälä[30] noted a decrease in both short-term and long-term fetal heart rate variability after *intramuscular* meperidine, with maximum effect achieved 40 minutes after injection and gradual return to baseline 60 minutes after the injection. Petrie and colleagues[9] observed significant variability reduction within 10 minutes of *intravenous* meperidine, with maximum reduction occurring 25 minutes after injection. Similar effects on fetal heart rate variability have been noted with morphine, alphaprodine, hydroxyzine, and promethazine. Mechanisms for loss of beat-to-beat variability following fetal exposure to narcotics and sedatives may be due to direct depression of the fetal central nervous system and/or myocardium.

Sinusoidal fetal heart rate patterns have been observed following maternal analgesics, especially alphaprodine, butorphenol, and meperidine. Sinusoidal patterns also occur in critically ill fetuses with anemia, chronic hypoxia, or Rh isoimmunization. Unfortunately, there are no accepted criteria to distinguish narcotic-produced sinusoidal fetal heart rate patterns from similar patterns produced by hemodynamic instability in critically ill fetuses.

If administered in early labor, regional anesthetics, like parenteral analgesics, may inhibit uterine contractions. Epinephrine-containing solutions may also aggravate this tocolytic effect. The total duration of labor, however, does not seem to be prolonged by regional anesthetics, and oxytocin administration may overcome the tocolytic effects of regional or parenteral analgesics administered during the first stage of labor.

Previous studies of patients laboring without anesthesia have demonstrated a progressive fetal acidosis during the second stage of labor.[31] In the absence of complications, mothers receiving epidural anesthetics have better fetal acid-base status than those undergoing painful labors without anesthesia.[32] Several reports, however, have indicated a higher incidence of fetal bradycardia in those mothers receiving epidural anesthesia.[33] However, these anesthetics were administered without prehydration or the maintenance of a lateral laboring position. Also, several early studies on epidural anesthesia indicated an increased need for outlet forceps delivery.[34]

Decreased placental perfusion may be an indirect effect of maternally administered anesthetics. Peripheral vasodilation from sympathetic blockade may result in profound hypotension. Without prehydration, epidural anesthesia can cause sympathetic blockade with visceral pooling of blood, systemic hypotension, and diminished uterine blood flow. All patients receiving major regional anesthetic blocks (i.e., epidural and spinal blocks) should be prehydrated intravenously with 1 liter of nondextrose-containing fluids and maintained in a lateral position with uterine displacement for labor or cesarean section. Pregnancies complicated by chronic uteroplacental insufficiency are at greater risk of compromised uterine blood flow from sympathetic blocks with resulting fetal bradycardia and possible fetal asphyxia.

Uterine hypotonia and uterine artery vasospasm have been reported following paracervical block, vasopressor administration (ephedrine), or intravascular injection of local anesthetics.[35] Endogenous catecholamine release may also promote uterine artery vasoconstriction, resulting in decreased placental perfusion. Metabolic acidosis and hypovolemia will reduce uteroplacental perfusion through reductions in cardiac output and circulating blood volume.

Controversy regarding the appropriate use of vasopressors in obstetrics has been fueled by skepticism toward the extrapolation of animal data to humans, since the uterine vessels in sheep and other laboratory animals have innervation different from that in humans. Marx and colleagues[36] demonstrated no adverse effects on the fetus following intravenous ephedrine treatment of spinal-induced hypotension. However, in the face of prolonged hypotension, ephedrine did not prevent fetal acidosis and depression. Grant and colleagues[37] demonstrated that ephedrine (5 mg) and phenylephrine (100 µg) are equally effective in acutely restoring blood pressure after hypotension from epidurals. There were no differences in Apgar scores or umbilical cord blood gas analyses between the treatment groups.

The addition of epinephrine to local anesthetic solutions for epidural anesthesia is also controversial, since some studies have suggested a decrease in uterine blood flow following the use of epinephrine-containing local anesthetic solutions.[38] However, no human clinical studies have demonstrated adverse effects on neonates or decreases in intravillous blood flow when epinephrine-containing local anesthetics have been administered epidurally. Once again, animal and human studies differ in their conclusions.

DIRECT EFFECTS OF ANESTHETICS ON NEWBORNS

Neonatal morbidity and mortality may result from the direct passage of analgesics or anesthetics across the placenta, producing time-related and dose-related neonatal cardiorespiratory depression. The placental transfer of drugs is potentiated by fetal hypoxia and acidosis. Additionally, the fetal and neonatal cardiorespiratory depressant effects of maternally administered drugs are enhanced by the infant's inefficient renal excretion, deficiency of hepatic microsomal enzymes, and increased permeability of the blood–brain barrier. Premature infants will accumulate an even higher concentration of maternally administered drugs because of the more profound deficiencies in the factors mentioned and the drug-concentrating effects of a smaller fetal volume of distribution.

The most obvious effect of narcotic analgesic administration during labor is neonatal respiratory depression. Maternally administered narcotics may decrease the newborn's respiratory minute volume, producing hypoxemia, hypercarbia, respiratory acidosis, and an altered ventilatory response to carbon dioxide. Hypoxemia and respiratory acidosis will potentiate the fetal cardiodepressant effects of the narcotics and may result in rapid fetal cardiovascular collapse.

Delayed onset of sustained respirations and low 1-minute and 5-minute Apgar scores are observed more frequently in infants of mothers receiving narcotics during labor than in mothers not receiving narcotic analgesics during labor. Neonatal cardiorespiratory depression is less likely to occur if maternal narcotics are administered intramuscularly less than 1 hour or more than 6 hours before delivery. Maximal cardiorespiratory depressant effects of maternal intramuscular analgesics on newborns will occur with maternal administration 2 to 3 hours before delivery. Although meperidine has been studied the most, morphine and alphaprodine may have 10 times the cardiorespiratory depressant effects of meperidine on the neonate.[2]

Medications given in small incremental doses may be valuable adjuncts to the management of labor pain. Drugs given by rapid intravenous injection at the beginning of a uterine contraction have less placental transfer to the fetus. The maximal safe dosage for each analgesic drug in labor has not been established. Infants with normal acid-base status at birth may still require ventilatory support postpartum if their mothers have been heavily medicated with narcotics and sedatives. Naloxone may be administered to the mother to antagonize both the maternal and fetal respiratory depressant effects of narcotics. In practice, however, naloxone is usually administered only to the newborn in a dose of 0.1 mg/kg body weight intramuscularly or intravenously. This dose may be repeated in 3 to 5 minutes if there is no response. After intravenous administration, the narcotic antagonizing effects of naloxone last 1 to 2 hours. Thus, if the mother has been given long-acting narcotics such as morphine or alphaprodine, neonatal respiratory depression from long-acting narcotics may recur within 2 to 3 hours, and the newborn's naloxone dose may have to be repeated. Naloxone should not be used in narcotic addicts or in their infants, since it may precipitate acute withdrawal symptoms.

Unless the fetus is severely hypoxic and acidotic, the placental transfer of local anesthetics does not usually cause significant perinatal depression. Studies indicate that the hemodynamically stable fetus can tolerate extremely high levels of both lidocaine and mepivacaine.[39, 40] In an asphyxiated fetus, however, much lower levels of local anesthetics may cause fetal bradycardia and trigger seizures because of ion trapping of alkalotic local anesthetics in an acidotic fetus.

Direct fetal scalp injection of local anesthetics during caudal, pudendal, or paracervical blocks will result in acute fetal and neonatal cardiorespiratory depression with bradycardia, hypoventilation, hypotonia, apnea, and seizures.[41] Without an accurate history, it is often difficult to distinguish this constellation of symptoms from other causes, particularly asphyxia. Mydriasis and loss of oculocephalic and pupillary light reflexes in the first 6 hours of life are unusual in the asphyxiated fetus and suggest fetal scalp injection of massive doses of local anesthetics. Needle marks on the infant's scalp may help in the early diagnosis of local anesthetic scalp injections and direct early appropriate treatment. Earlier reports of poor neonatal outcome and death following fetal local anesthetic overdose and toxicity have now been superseded by more encouraging results of treatment.[42] Traditional support with ventilation, oxygenation, and anticonvulsants has been augmented by forced diuresis, gastric lavage, and occasionally exchange transfusion or hemofiltration to promote excretion or capture of local anesthetics and their active metabolites.

NEUROBEHAVIORAL EFFECTS OF ANESTHETICS ON NEWBORNS

There is extensive literature evaluating the effects of drugs on the neurobehavior of neonates. However, interpretation of this scientific data is hampered by various methodologic problems, including nonstandardized drug doses, routes of administration, and dose to delivery times. In addition, confounding obstetric variables (parity, gravidity, length of labor, method of delivery), pharmacologic variables (umbilical cord drug and metabolite levels), and methods of statistical analysis have also confused the interpretation of neurobehavioral studies.[43-45] Finally, studies by psychologists and others interested in neonatal behavior have often focused on behavioral patterns following mixed maternal anesthetic and analgesic administrations and are thus difficult to interpret. Only those neurobehavioral studies with adequate controls will be reviewed here to serve as a guide for the clinician in making an accurate diagnosis and selecting proper therapy.

Neonatal Behavioral Assessment Scale Studies

Early NBAS studies assessing the neurobehavioral effects of maternal analgesia and anesthesia were difficult to interpret because of mixed study groups, inconsistent scoring, and interexaminer variability. Maternal analgesia with parenteral narcotics and sedatives was related to poor scores in motor behavior.[46, 47] Regional blocks and local anesthetics affected both motor maturity and irritability scores.[45] Other studies found no effects of maternal analgesia or regional anesthesia on NBAS performance.[48, 49]

Later controlled studies on neurobehavioral effects of obstetric analgesia with meperidine[50] found that meperidine affected performance on the regulation of state and reflex cluster scores on day 1 of life but not on day 3. A comparison of infants of mothers who received epidural anesthesia with bupivacaine, analgesia with meperidine, or no drugs during labor and vaginal delivery demonstrated no significant differences in performance on the NBAS on days 1, 7, 21, and 42 of life.[51] However, higher cord blood levels of meperidine or bupivacaine and higher total doses of bupivacaine were correlated with poorer performance on the NBAS.[52, 53]

In a comparison of epidural anesthesia and no anesthesia for vaginal delivery, local anesthetic effects were seen on motor, state control, and autonomic cluster scores of the NBAS on the first day of life, but not by day 5 or at 1 month of age.[54] Mothers from the epidural group found their newborns more difficult to care for and were observed to handle their infants less affectionately during feeding. Use of bupivacaine rather than chlorprocaine during cesarean section under epidural anesthesia was associated with better performance on the orientation cluster scores at 5 hours and at 3 days of age.[55] Both local anesthetic groups improved with age in range of state, habituation, motor, autonomic regulation, and orientation cluster scores, but the chloroprocaine group showed no improvement in the range of state score. In a comparison of epidural anesthesia for vaginal or cesarean delivery, use of chloroprocaine was associated with better performance than lidocaine on the motor cluster score at 5 hours of age and autonomic regulation at 3 days of age. Performance in all cluster scores improved with age, and maternal obstetric variables had more significant effects on neonatal behavior at 3 days of age than did choice of local anesthetic.[56]

Early Neonatal Neurobehavioral Scale Studies

Using the ENNS, infants of mothers receiving meperidine for labor and delivery analgesia showed significantly poorer behavioral responses on both the first and second days of life[57] than infants of mothers receiving epidural, general, or local infiltration anesthesia for labor and delivery. Drug effects on the neonates were incremental and worsened as meperidine doses increased from 50 mg to 150 mg. No difference was noted between the neurobehavioral effects of meperidine and a butorphanol non-narcotic analgesic.[58] A variety of local anesthetics, including 0.25% bupivacaine, 0.5% lidocaine, 0.5% bupivacaine, 1.5% mepivacaine, and 2% chloroprocaine, have shown minimal to no differential neurobehavioral effects when used for pudendal[59] or paracervical blocks.[60–62]

Epidural anesthesia with lidocaine and mepivacaine has produced altered neonatal performance scores in muscle tone, rooting, sucking, and pin-prick response at 2 and 8 hours of life, in comparison with controls who received no regional anesthetics for vaginal delivery.[23] Epidural anesthesia was said by Scanlon to produce an infant who was "floppy but alert."[23] Later studies have failed to confirm this finding in infants exposed to epidural analgesia with 0.25% bupivacaine;[63, 64] 0.5% bupivacaine, 2% chloroprocaine, or 1% lidocaine;[29] or 1.5% lidocaine with epinephrine.[65]

Epidural anesthesia for cesarean section using 0.5% or 0.75% bupivacaine, 2% lidocaine, and 3% chloroprocaine[66–68] was not associated with significant differences in neonatal behavior at 2 to 4 hours or 24 hours of age on the ENNS. Infants of mothers who underwent general anesthesia for vaginal delivery,[69] however, showed minor differences in some behaviors on the ENNS at 1 day (rooting, pin-prick, and sound responses) and 2 days (pin-prick response decrement, alerting to sound) compared with infants of mothers who received epidural anesthesia with chloroprocaine. General anesthesia with ketamine–nitrous oxide and thiopental–nitrous oxide for cesarean section produced no significant neonatal neurobehavioral effects on the first day of life. These general anesthetics were, however, associated with more behavioral effects by the second day of life than was spinal anesthesia with tetracaine[70] for cesarean section. No differential effects could be demonstrated among various general anesthetic agents in studies comparing ketamine–nitrous oxide and thiopental–nitrous oxide[69] and nitrous oxide in combination with halothane or enflurane.[71]

Neonatal Adaptive Capacity Scale Studies

The NCAS has been used less extensively than the ENNS and the NBAS in assessing the effects of obstetric anesthesia on neonates. In comparing epidural analgesia with 1.5% lidocaine and 0.5% bupivacaine with and without epinephrine[65, 72] during labor and vaginal delivery, no difference was seen on NCAS scores at 15 minutes, 2 hours, and 24 hours of age.[29] Groups of infants receiving general anesthesia with nitrous oxide–oxygen and enflurane–oxygen showed no difference on the NCAS at 2 and 24 hours of age.[25] In comparing three groups of cesarean-delivered infants of mothers receiving general anesthesia with nitrous oxide, oxygen, and 0.5% enflurane; epidural with 3% 2-chloroprocaine or 2% lidocaine; or spinal anesthesia with 1% lidocaine, only those infants exposed to general anesthesia showed less optimal performance on some NCAS items (elbow recoil, palmar traction, and automatic walking) at 15 minutes but not at 24 hours of age.[73]

CONCLUSIONS

In summary, infants of mothers receiving narcotic analgesia and epidural anesthesia have performed less well on the first day of life in a variety of neonatal behavioral measures that reflect muscle tone, alertness, and motor behavior than infants of mothers who received no anesthesia or analgesia for labor and delivery. Effects on behavior are transient and are not seen after 3 days of age. There appears to be no advantage to selecting specific local anesthestic agents to limit neonatal neurobehavioral effects. Infants of mothers receiving general anesthesia for delivery have performed less well on neurobehavioral tests on the first day of life than infants of mothers receiving epidural anesthesia or spinal anesthesia. As with epidural blocks, there is no apparent advantage to selecting specific local anesthetic agents for spinal blocks.

The neonatal neurobehavioral effects of obstetric anesthesia and analgesia are transient and probably resolve during the early neonatal period. Drug effects have rarely been reported after the first 24 hours of life. Although there is potential for transient neurobehavioral effects to alter early maternal-infant interaction, there is no current evidence of long-term deleterious effects. Considering the many influences on the normal infant's development, concern about the short-term neonatal effects of obstetric analgesia or anesthesia in an otherwise healthy newborn may be unwarranted.

References

1. Morgan B, Bulpitt CJ, Clifton P, et al.: Effectiveness of pain relief in labour: Survey of 1000 mothers. Br Med J 285:689, 1982
2. Spielman FJ: Systemic analgesics during labor. Clin Obstet Gynecol 30:495, 1987
3. Sykes GS, Johnson P, Ashworth F, et al.: Do Apgar scores indicate asphyxia? Lancet 1:494, 1982
4. Poland RL, Erenberg A, Freeman JM, et al.: Use and abuse of the Apgar score. Pediatrics 78(6):1148, 1986
5. Apgar V: Proposal for new method of evaluation of the newborn infant. Anesth Analg 32:260, 1953
6. Giacoia GP: Low Apgar scores and birth asphyxia: Misconceptions that promote undeserved negligence suits. Postgrad Med 84(2):77, 1988
7. Khazin AF, Hon EH, Quilligan EJ: Biochemical studies of the fetus. III. Fetal base and Apgar scores. Obstet Gynecol 34:592, 1969
8. Fields LM, Entman SS, Boehm FH: Correlation of the one minute Apgar score and the pH value of umbilical arterial blood. South Med J 76:1477, 1983
9. Petrie RH, Yeh S-Y, Murata Y, et al.: The effects of drugs on fetal heart rate variability. Am J Obstet Gynecol 130:294, 1978
10. Cabal LA, Siassi B, Hodgman JE: Neonatal cardiovascular and pulmonary monitoring.

In: Thibeault DW, Gregory GA (eds): Neonatal Pulmonary Care, 2nd ed. Norwalk, CT: Appleton-Century-Crofts, 1986, pp 321–347

11. Paxson CL Jr: Neonatal shock in the first postnatal day. Am J Dis Child 132:509, 1978

12. Nugent J: Intra-arterial blood pressure monitoring in the neonate. J Obstet Gynecol Neonatal Nurs 11(5):281, 1982

13. Dweck HS, Reynolds DW, Cassady G: Indirect blood pressure measurements in newborns. Am J Dis Child 127:492, 1974

14. Veramold HT, Kitterman JA, Phibbs RH, et al.: Aortic blood pressure during the first 12 hours of life in infants with birth weight 610–4,220 grams. Pediatrics 67:607, 1981

15. Holland WW, Young IM: Neonatal blood pressure in relation to maturity, mode of delivery, and condition at birth. Br Med J 2:1331, 1956

16. Brazelton TB: Psychophysiologic reactions of the neonate. I. The value of observation of the neonate. J Pediatr 58(4):508, 1961

17. Brazelton TB: Psychophysiologic reactions of the neonate. II. Effect of maternal medication on the neonate and his behavior. J Pediatr 58:513, 1961

18. American Academy of Pediatrics Committee on Drugs: Effect of medication during labor and delivery on infant outcome. Pediatrics 62:402, 1978

19. U.S. Department of Health, Education, and Welfare, Public Health Service, Food and Drug Administration: Guidelines for the clinical evaluation of local anesthetics. HEW(FDA) 78–3053, Rockville, MD, September 1977

20. U.S. Department of Health, Education, and Welfare, Public Health Service, Food and Drug Administration: Guidelines for the clinical evaluation of general anesthetics. HEW(FDA) 78–3052, Rockville, MD, September 1977

21. Tronick E: The neonatal behavioral assessment scale as a biomarker of the effects of environmental agents on the newborn. Environ Health Perspect 74:185, 1987

22. Brazelton TB: Neonatal Behavioral Assessment Scale. Clinics in Developmental Medicine, No. 88. Philadelphia: J.B. Lippincott, 1984

23. Scanlon JW, Brown WU Jr, Weiss JB, et al.: Neurobehavioral responses of newborn infants after maternal epidural anesthesia. Anesthesiology 40:121, 1974

24. Amiel-Tison C, Barrier G, Shnider SM, et al.: A new neurologic and adaptive capacity scoring system for evaluating obstetric medications in full-term newborns. Anesthesiology 56:340, 1982

25. Stefani SJ, Hughes SC, Shnider SM, et al.: Neonatal neurobehavioral effects of inhalation analgesia for vaginal delivery. Anesthesiology 56:351, 1982

26. Albright GA: What is the place of bupivacaine in obstetric epidural analgesia? Can Anaesth Soc J 32:392, 1985

27. Hingson RA, Hellman LM: Anesthesia for Obstetrics. Philadelphia: J.B. Lippincott, 1956

28. Perrotta LA, Campbell D: Perinatal Asphyxia: Pediatric Emergency Casebook. New York: World Health Commentaries, 1984, p 12

29. Abboud TK, Khoo SS, Miller F, et al.: Maternal, fetal, and neonatal responses after epidural anesthesia with bupivacaine, 2-chloroprocaine, or lidocaine. Anesth Analg 61(8):638, 1982

30. Kariniemi V, Ämmälä P: Effects of intramuscular pethidine on fetal heart rate variability during labor. Br J Obstet Gynaecol 88:718, 1981

31. Pearson JF, Davies P: The effect of continuous lumbar epidural analgesia on maternal acid-base balance and arterial lactate concentration during the second stage of labour. J Obstet Gynaecol Br Commonwealth 80:225, 1973

32. Pearson JF, Davies P: The effect of continuous lumbar epidural analgesia on the acid-base status of maternal arterial blood during the first stage of labour. J Obstet Gynaecol Br Commonwealth 80:218, 1973

33. Wingate MB, Wingate L, Iffy L, et al.: The effect of epidural analgesia upon fetal and neonatal status. Am J Obstet Gynecol 119:1101, 1974

34. Bailey PW, Howard FA: Epidural anesthesia and forceps delivery: Laying a bogey. Anesthesia 38:282, 1983

35. Albright GA: Effects of anesthesia on the fetus and neonate. In: Stevenson DK, Sunshine P (eds): Fetal and Neonatal Brain Injury. Toronto: B.C. Decker, 1989, p 53

36. Marx GF, Cosmi EV, Wollman SB: Biochemical status and clinical condition of mother and infant at cesarean section. Anesth Analg 48:986, 1969

37. Grant GJ, Ramanathan S, Turndorf H: Maternal hemodynamic effects of ephedrine and phenylephrine (Abstract). Anesth Analg 66:573, 1987
38. Marx GF: Cardiotoxicity of local anesthetics—the plot thickens. Anesthesiology 60:3, 1984
39. Morishima HO, Adamson K: Placental clearance of mepivacaine following administration to the guinea pig fetus. Anesthesiology 28:343, 1967
40. Morishima HO, Heymann MA, Rudolph AM, et al.: Toxicity of lidocaine in the fetal and newborn lamb and its relationship to asphyxia. Am J Obstet Gynecol 112:72, 1972
41. Dodson WE: Neonatal drug intoxication: Local anesthetics. Pediatr Clin North Am 23:399, 1976
42. Hillman LS, Hillman RE, Dodson WE: Diagnosis, treatment, and follow-up of neonatal mepivacaine intoxication secondary to paracervical and pudendal blocks during labor. J Pediatr 95:472, 1979
43. Kuhnert BR, Linn PL, Kuhnert PM: Obstetric medication and neonatal behavior. Current controversies. Clin Perinatol 12(2):423, 1985
44. Scanlon JW: Effects of obstetric anesthesia and analgesia on the newborn: A select, annotated bibliography for the clinician. Clin Obstet Gynecol 24(2):649, 1981
45. Brackbill Y: Obstetrical medication and infant behavior. In: Osofsky J (ed): Handbook of Infant Development. New York: Wiley, 1979
46. Standley K, Soule AB III, Copans SA, et al.: Local-regional anesthesia during childbirth: Effect on newborn behaviors. Science 186:634, 1974
47. Brazelton TB, Tryphonopoulou Y, Lester BM: A comparative study of the behavior of Greek neonates. Pediatrics 63(2):279, 1979
48. Tronick E, Wise S, Als H, et al.: Regional obstetric anesthesia and newborn behavior: Effect over the first ten days of life. Pediatrics 58(1):94, 1976
49. Horowitz FD, Ashton J, Culp R, et al.: The effects of obstetrical medication on the behavior of Israeli newborn infants and some comparisons with Uruguayan and American infants. Child Dev 48(4):1607, 1977
50. Kuhnert BR, Linn PL, Kennard MJ, et al.: Effects of low doses of meperidine on neonatal behavior. Anesth Analg 64(3):335, 1985
51. Liberman BA, Rosenblatt DB, Belsey EM, et al.: The effects of maternally administered pethidine or epidural bupivacaine on the fetus and the newborn. Br J Obstet Gynaecol 86:598, 1979
52. Rosenblatt DB, Belsey EM, Lieberman BA, et al.: The influence of maternal analgesia on neonatal behaviour. II. Epidural bupivacaine. Br J Obstet Gynaecol 88(4):40, 1981
53. Belsey EM, Rosenblatt DB, Leiberman BA, et al.: The influence of maternal analgesia on neonatal behaviour. 1. Pethidine. Br J Obstet Gynaecol 88:398, 1981
54. Murray AD, Dolby RM, Nation RL, et al.: Effects of epidural anesthesia on newborns and their mothers. Child Dev 52:71, 1981
55. Kuhnert BR, Kennard MJ, Lenn PL: Neonatal neurobehavior after epidural anesthesia for cesarean section: A comparison of bupivacaine and chloroprocaine. Anesth Analg 67(1):64, 1988
56. Kuhnert BR, Harrison MJ, Lenn PL, et al.: Effects of maternal epidural anesthesia on neonatal behavior. Anesth Analg 63:301, 1984
57. Hodgkinson R, Bhatt M, Wang CN: Double-blind comparison of the neurobehaviour of neonates following the administration of different doses of meperidine to the mother. Can Anaesth Soc J 25(5):405, 1978
58. Hodgkinson R, Huff RW, Hayashi RH, et al.: Double-blind comparison of maternal analgesia and neonate neurobehavior following intravenous butorphanol and meperidine. J Int Med Res 7:224, 1979
59. Merkow AJ, McGuinness GA, Erenberg A, et al.: The neonatal neurobehavioral effects of bupivacaine, mepivacaine, and 2–chloroprocaine used for pudendal block. Anesthesiology 52(4):309, 1980
60. Meis PJ, Reisner LS, Payne TF, et al.: Bupivacaine paracervical block. Effects on the fetus and neonate. Obstet Gynecol 52(5):545, 1978
61. Nesheim BI, Lindbaek E, Storm-Mathisen I, et al.: Neurobehavioral response of infants after paracervical block during labour. Acta Obstet Gynecol Scand 58(1):41, 1979
62. Kangas-Saarela T, Joupilla R, Puolakka J, et al.: The effects of bupivacaine paracervical

block on the neurobehavioral responses of newborn infants. Acta Anesthesiol Scand 32:566, 1988

63. Corke BC: Neurobehavioral responses of the newborn. The effects of maternal analgesia. Anesthesia 32(6):539, 1977

64. Kangas-Saarela T, Koivisto M, Joupilla R, et al.: Comparison of the effects of general and epidural anesthesia for cesarean section on the neurobehavioral responses of the newborn infants. Acta Anesthesiol Scand 33:313, 1989

65. Abboud TK, David S, Nagappala S, et al.: Maternal, fetal, and neonatal effects of lidocaine with and without epinephrine for epidural anesthesia in obstetrics. Anesth Analg 63:973, 1984

66. McGuinness GA, Merkow AJ, Kennedy RL, et al.: Epidural anesthesia with bupivacaine for cesarean section: Neonatal blood levels and neurobehavioral responses. Anesthesiology 49(4):270, 1978

67. Abboud TK, Kim KC, Noueihed R, et al.: Epidural bupivacaine, chloroprocaine, or lidocaine for cesarean section—maternal and neonatal effects. Anesth Analg 62(10):914, 1983

68. Kileff ME, James FM, Dewan DM, et al.: Neonatal neurobehavioral responses after epidural anesthesia for cesarean section using lidocaine and bupivacaine. Anesth Analg 63(4):413, 1984

69. Hodgkinson R, Marx GF, Kim SS, et al.: Neonatal neurobehavioral tests following vaginal delivery under ketamine, thiopental, and extradural anesthesia. Anesth Analg 56(4):548, 1977

70. Hodgkinson R, Bhatt M, Kim SS, et al.: Neonatal neurobehavioral tests following cesarean section under general and spinal anesthesia. Am J Obstet Gynecol 132(6):670, 1978

71. Abboud TK, Kim SH, Henrekson EH, et al.: Comparative maternal and neonatal effects of halothane and enflurane for cesarean section. Acta Anesthesiol Scand 29:663, 1985

72. Abboud TK, Sheik-ol-Eslam A, Yanagi T, et al.: Safety and efficacy of epinephrine added to bupivacaine for lumbar epidural analgesia in obstetrics. Anesth Analg 64(6):585, 1985

73. Abboud TK, Nagappala S, Murakawa K, et al.: Comparison of the effects of general and regional anesthesia for cesarean section on neonatal neurologic and adaptive capacity scores. Anesth Analg 64(10):996, 1985

10. Neonatal Physiologic Adaptations and Their Anesthetic Implications

Robert H. Friesen, M.D.

INTRODUCTION

Perioperative management of the neonate is a unique and challenging undertaking for the anesthesiologist. During the first few postnatal weeks, the infant undergoes remarkable physiologic changes to adapt to extrauterine life. Perianesthetic risk is high. Anesthetic problems can arise quickly and may precipitate significant morbidity more rapidly than in older patients. Rackow and colleagues reported that the incidence of anesthetic-related cardiac arrest in infants under 1 year of age was more than three times that of older children.[1] Over a decade later, Smith reported that perioperative deaths occurred five times more frequently in infants 0 to 1 year of age than in children 1 to 10 years of age.[2] Of the infants 0 to 1 year of age suffering perianesthetic cardiac arrest or death, neonates have made up the greatest number of patients.[2-3a] The neonate's high risk, physiologic differences from older infants and children, and small size demand meticulous attention to detail. In this chapter, neonatal physiology and its implications for anesthetic management are discussed.

RESPIRATORY SYSTEM

Lung Development

Lung development begins during the embryonic period, is incomplete at birth, and continues throughout childhood. Surfactant is produced by type II alveolar cells beginning at about 24 weeks of gestation. Surfactant production is accelerated by high glucocorticoid levels during stress, so that about one-half of preterm neonates weighing 1000 g exhibit alveolar pressure–volume stability.[4] Alveolar and pulmonary capillary development is such that gas exchange can occur after 26 to 28 weeks of gestation. Alveolar epithelial cells increase in number and decrease in thickness after birth. Interalveolar communications (pores of Kohn) are scarce at birth and develop during childhood. The number of alveoli, with accompanying capillary network, increases about tenfold between birth and adulthood.[4]

Ventilatory Function

The lung is relatively noncompliant at birth, having alveoli that are collapsed or fluid filled. The pressure required for the neonate's first breath to overcome the surface tension is high, ranging from -10 to -70 cm H_2O. While functional residual capacity (FRC) appears to stabilize within the first hour after birth, lung compliance and vital capacity increase significantly during the first days of life and are stable at 1 week of age.[5]

After this initial period of stabilization, the neonate continues to have several disadvantages in ventilatory function when compared with the young adult. Lung compliance remains lower because of a lack of elastic fibers. Closing capacity approximates or exceeds the supine FRC of the lung (Fig. 10–1).[6, 7] Contraction of the diaphragm is less efficient because of its horizontal rather than oblique angle of insertion to the chest wall.[8] The diaphragm and intercostal muscles are more susceptible to fatigue because of a low percentage of type I (slow twitch, high oxidative) muscle fibers during the first few months of life.[8, 9] The neonate's rib cage is cartilaginous, rather than bony, and its elasticity gives the chest wall a tendency to collapse.

In an infant who is awake, intercostal muscle tone stabilizes the chest wall, opposing the tendency to collapse and supporting diaphragmatic function. Muscle relaxants have obvious effects on diaphragmatic and chest wall muscle tone and therefore on ventilatory function. Intercostal muscle function is also profoundly impaired by halothane.[10] This impairment causes reductions of tidal volume and FRC, which result in loss of oxygen storage capacity in the lung, closure of small airways, and decreased alveolar minute ventilation. The spontaneously breathing infant attempts to compensate by increasing respiratory rate, but fatigue, increased physiologic dead space, and depression of the ventilatory response to CO_2 by halothane[10] prevent restoration of minute alveolar ventilation. The lack of interalveolar communications may increase the risk of atelectasis in the face of small airway closure.[4] Thus, the neonate is at increased risk of perianesthetic hypercarbia, hypoxia, and atelectasis.

Problems with ventilation do, in fact, play major roles in anesthetic-related morbidity and mortality in infants. Salem and colleagues,[11] in their study of factors contributing to infant cardiac arrest during anes-

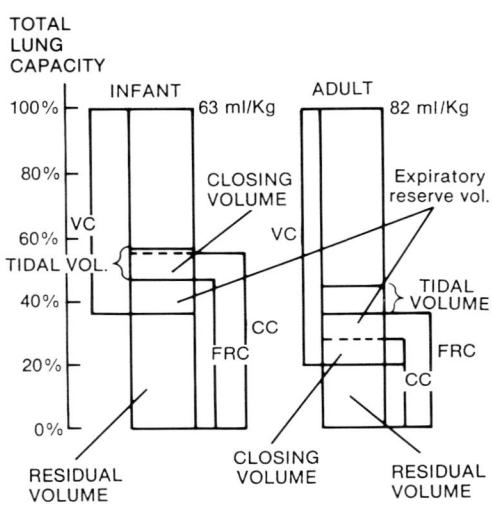

FIGURE 10–1. Lung volumes in the neonate and the adult. The neonate's closing capacity approximates tidal volume. (From Nelson NM: Respiration and circulation after birth. In: Smith CA, Nelson NM (eds): The Physiology of the Newborn Infant, 4th ed, 1976, p 207. Courtesy of Charles C Thomas, Publisher, Springfield, Illinois.)

thesia, determined that hypoventilation or loss of the airway were present in nearly one-half of such occurrences. Earlier studies by other investigators reported similar findings.[1, 3]

The anesthesiologist can take several steps to minimize the risk of ventilatory problems. First, ventilation must be supported in all neonates during anesthesia. This support may be in the form of continuous positive airway pressure (CPAP) during spontaneous ventilation, positive-pressure inspiratory assistance during spontaneous ventilation, or controlled ventilation. Such ventilatory support will help maintain tidal volume, minute volume, and FRC, and will oppose small airway closure and atelectasis.

The airway must be securely maintained during all anesthetics in neonates. Loss of the airway contributed significantly to the incidence of cardiac arrest in the study by Salem and associates.[11] Tracheal intubation provides a secure airway and facilitates ventilatory support and, as a general rule, should be provided during all neonatal anesthetics.

Vigilant monitoring of oxygenation and ventilation should be carried out both intraoperatively and postoperatively. Visual inspection of chest excursion and continuous auscultation of breath sounds through a precordial or esophageal stethoscope are basic necessities. Pulse oximetry, providing continuous, reliable, noninvasive measurement of arterial oxygen saturation, has become a standard of care to be applied to every patient. Capnometry is a desirable monitor that has been shown to provide early warning of ventilatory complications during anesthesia in pediatric patients,[12] but it is less reliable in neonates because of their very small tidal volumes. Capnometry is more accurate in infants if gas samples are obtained from the distal end of the tracheal tube rather than from a more proximal site.[13] Respiratory rate must be monitored postoperatively to detect apnea.

The Preterm Neonate

Although the stress of premature birth stimulates surfactant production, the lungs of the preterm neonate are less mature at birth than are those of the term neonate. Respiratory distress syndrome (RDS) occurs in up to 60% of preterm neonates.[14] About 20% of neonates surviving severe RDS develop bronchopulmonary dysplasia (BPD),[15] resulting in pulmonary dysfunction that persists throughout infancy.[16] Thus, preoperative and postoperative respiratory failure and requirement for mechanical ventilatory support are common.

Pulmonary interstitial emphysema, in which air leaks from the alveolus into the interstitium of the lung, can develop in patients with severe RDS. This condition can worsen when high inspiratory pressures are required and can lead to pneumothorax, pneumomediastinum, or pneumopericardium.[17] Airway pressure should be monitored by the anesthesiologist so that required inflation pressures are not exceeded (see Fig. 11–2).

Apnea, probably caused by immature control of respiration and often associated with bradycardia and hypoxemia, is a common problem in preterm neonates. Postanesthetic apnea occurs frequently in these patients and should be anticipated by proper monitoring and the routine use of postoperative mechanical ventilation following almost any operation during the neonatal period. Postanesthetic apnea continues to be a potential problem in premature babies surviving beyond the neonatal period until 44 to 55 weeks of postconceptual age.[18–20] Until that age, the former preterm neonate should be monitored for apnea for at least 12 hours following anesthesia.

CARDIOVASCULAR SYSTEM

Fetal Circulation

The fetal circulation is depicted in Figure 10–2. During fetal life, most oxygenated blood from the placenta flows through the ductus venosus into the inferior vena cava and thence into the right atrium. About one-half of this blood flows directly into the left side of the heart through the foramen ovale, resulting in relatively highly oxygenated blood flowing to the head through the ascending aorta. The remaining right atrial blood, including desaturated superior vena caval blood, flows into the right ventricle and out the main pulmonary artery. Because of high pulmonary vascular resistance, most blood in the main pulmonary artery

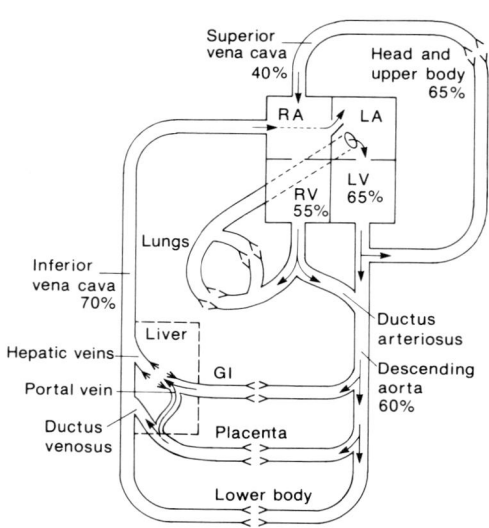

FIGURE 10–2. Diagram of the fetal circulation. The numbers indicate percent oxygen saturation at different points in the circuit. (From Avery ME, Fletcher BD, Williams RG: The Lung and Its Disorders in the Newborn Infant. Philadelphia: W.B. Saunders, 1981, pp 37–47. Reprinted with permission.)

bypasses the lungs and flows through the ductus arteriosus into the descending aorta, where it joins oxygenated blood from the aortic arch. About one-half of the descending aortic blood returns to the placenta through the low-resistance umbilical arteries.

Dramatic changes in this circulatory pattern occur at birth. Inflation of the lungs and oxygenation associated with the onset of breathing cause a rapid reduction of pulmonary vascular resistance and an increase in pulmonary blood flow. Clamping of the umbilical cord results in a sudden increase in systemic vascular resistance and a loss of placental blood return to the right atrium. These changes combine to cause an increase in left atrial pressure, which closes the foramen ovale. The increase in Po_2 causes vasoconstriction of the ductus arteriosus by an incompletely understood mechanism.

These changes are not completed immediately and remain reversible for some time after birth. Some right-to-left atrial shunting through the foramen ovale may persist in the normal neonate. Fluctuations in Po_2 may result in shunting through a patent ductus arteriosus. This is particularly true in the preterm neonate, in whom the ductus is less responsive to oxygen. Although pulmonary vascular resistance falls markedly at birth, it does not decrease to normal childhood levels until about 4 months of age.[21] The neonatal pulmonary vasculature remains highly reactive to vasoconstrictive stimuli. Thus, a hypoxic episode at birth or during the perianesthetic period can lead to a life-threatening cycle of pulmonary vasoconstriction and hypoxemia known as persistent pulmonary hypertension of the newborn (PPHN).

The Heart

The heart is not fully developed at birth. The fetal and neonatal mammalian heart, when compared with that of the adult, has fewer contractile elements, immature sympathetic innervation, lower norepinephrine stores, and poorer compliance and contractility (Fig. 10–3).[22, 23] The potential for increasing stroke volume is limited by the low compliance of the ventricles, so cardiac output is necessarily highly dependent on heart rate.

This immaturity is accompanied by increased sensitivity to the cardiovascular depressant effects of anesthetics. This has been demonstrated in laboratory studies comparing the cardiovascular responses of neonatal and adult mammals to halothane (Fig. 10–4) and other inhaled anesthetics.[24–26a] Clinical studies also have shown that halothane and isoflurane cause significant bradycardia and hypotension in neonates[27–29] and young infants.[30, 31] By the fifth month of age, this sensitivity to halothane diminishes,[27] perhaps indicating that functional myocardial maturation is near completion at this age. Atropine supports cardiac output by main-

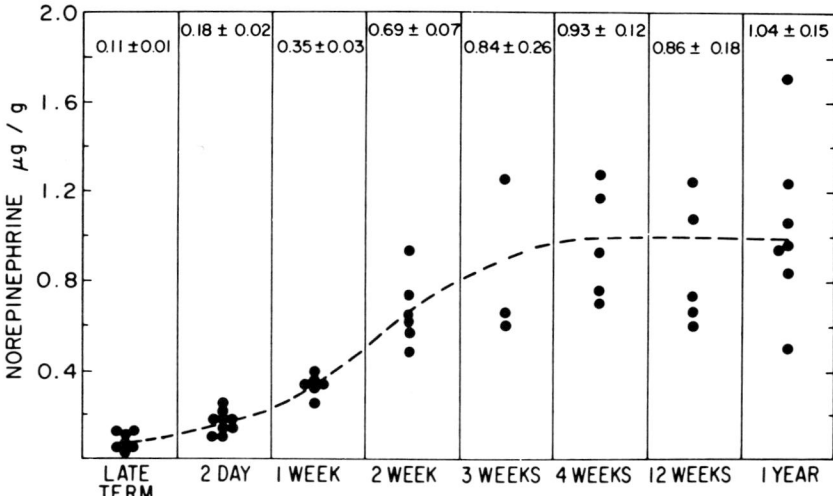

FIGURE 10–3. Norepinephrine levels in the developing rabbit myocardium are indicative of the maturation of sympathetic innervation. (From Friedman WF, Pool PE, Jacobowitz D, Seagren SC, Braunwald E: Sympathetic innervation of the developing rabbit heart: Biochemical and histochemical comparisons of fetal, neonatal, and adult myocardium. Circ Res 23:25–32, 1968. Reprinted by permission of the American Heart Association, Inc.)

taining heart rate, attenuates the cardiovascular depression caused by halothane in infants,[30, 32, 33] and prevents vagal reflexes in response to noxious stimuli. Therefore, administration of atropine, 0.02 mg/kg intravenously at induction, is an important component of anesthetic management of the neonate.

In contrast to inhaled anesthetics, fentanyl and ketamine have mild cardiovascular effects in the neonate[29, 34, 35] and, when administered along with atropine and pancuronium, are the anesthetics of choice for the very ill or preterm neonate. Hypovolemia can be a problem in neonates who have been treated for patent ductus arteriosus with fluid restriction or who have high fluid losses associated with bowel obstruction, necrotizing enterocolitis, or other disease states. A preanesthetic intravenous fluid infusion of 10 ml/kg of a balanced salt solution can contribute to cardiovascular stability intraoperatively.

NEUROLOGIC SYSTEM

Anesthetic Requirement

Although the neonate is neurophysiologically immature in some respects, there is no question that pain is perceived and that anesthesia is required for surgical procedures. The neonate's physical response to pain

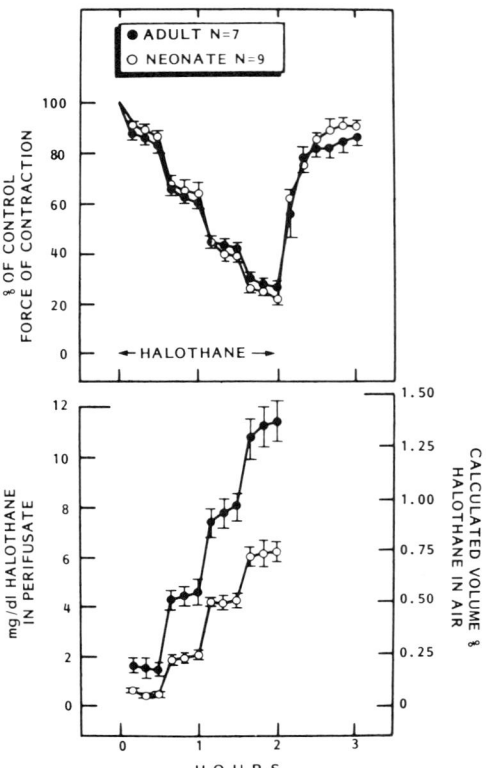

FIGURE 10–4. Only half as much halothane is required to depress myocardial contractility in the neonatal rat as in the adult rat. (From Rao CC, Boyer MS, Krishna G, Paradise RR: Increased sensitivity of the isometric contraction of the neonatal isolated rat atria to halothane, isoflurane, and enflurane. Anesthesiology 64:13–18, 1986. Reprinted with permission.)

is appropriately and specifically present even at 28 weeks of conceptual age.[36] Pain also elicits the physiologic responses of tachycardia, hypertension, PO_2 fluctuation, sweating, and release of catecholamines, corticosteroids, and other stress indicators.[37] These stress responses can be massive in the neonate and may, in fact, impair clinical outcome by causing hyperglycemia, catabolism, and perioperative autonomic instability.[37, 38] Studies of both preterm and term neonates demonstrate that anesthetic administration attenuates or abolishes physiologic and stress responses to surgical stimulation and may reduce perioperative morbidity.[37–40]

Anesthetic requirement is less in neonates than in older infants and children. Studies of the minimum alveolar concentration (MAC) of volatile anesthetics conclude that the MAC of halothane in term neonates is 0.87%[41] and that the MAC of isoflurane is 1.6% in term neonates[42] and 1.28% in preterm neonates.[43] Intravenous fentanyl, 10 μg/kg, is adequate to block the cardiovascular, hormonal, and metabolic responses to surgical incision in both term and preterm neonates.[38, 40] Nitrous oxide, a traditional anesthetic of choice for neonates, is inadequate by itself.[38] Because significant hypotension can occur during administration of sub-MAC doses of halothane or isoflurane in preterm neonates[29] or sick term neonates, the use of fentanyl, ketamine, or combinations of fentanyl and low-dose halothane or isoflurane may be preferable.

Intracranial Hemorrhage

Intraventricular and periventricular hemorrhage are leading causes of morbidity in preterm neonates, occurring in 40% to 60% of neonates younger than 34 weeks of gestation, usually during the first few days of postnatal life.[44, 45] The etiology of intracranial hemorrhage appears to be related to cerebral blood flow (CBF) fluctuations in patients with immature subependymal blood vessels and impaired CBF autoregulation.[46] Many clinical factors affecting CBF are associated with the development of intracranial hemorrhage, including severe respiratory distress (hypoxia, hypercarbia, acidosis, mechanical ventilation), blood pressure fluctuations, and rapid intravenous colloid administration.

Because these factors can be present in preterm neonates requiring anesthesia and because of the high incidence of intracranial hemorrhage in preterm neonates, it is not surprising that anecdotal reports have linked intracranial hemorrhage with the perianesthetic period. However, studies suggest that the perianesthetic period is not one of greater risk for the development or progression of intracranial hemorrhage,[47, 48] although an investigation of a large number of very premature neonates less than 4 days old has yet to be done. Administration of halothane, isoflurane, or ketamine does not increase intracranial pressure in preterm neonates[49] as it does in adults.

It is possible that the common practice of tracheal intubation in neonates who are awake increases the risk of intracranial hemorrhage. A marked increase in intracranial pressure was shown to accompany awake intubation of preterm neonates but was not observed when intubation took place during general anesthesia and muscle relaxation with pancuronium (Fig. 10–5).[50] This situation is analogous to that of a study of preterm neonates with RDS who required mechanical ventilation. Wide fluctuations in CBF velocity, presumably due to fluctuations in intrathoracic pressure, were observed in neonates breathing out of synchrony with their ventilators; muscle relaxation with pancuronium eliminated the CBF fluctuations and reduced the incidence and severity of intracranial hemorrhage.[51] Therefore, the anesthesiologist should generally perform tracheal intubation of the neonate following induction of anesthesia and paralysis, reserving awake intubation for situations in which it is specifically indicated, such as the difficult airway, the moribund or unstable patient, and gastric or bowel obstruction.

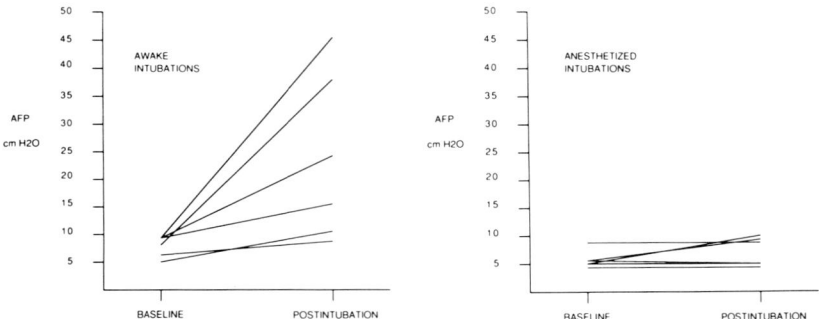

FIGURE 10–5. The marked increase in anterior fontanel pressure occurring during tracheal intubation of the awake neonate can be prevented by anesthesia and paralysis. (From Friesen RH, Honda AT, Thieme RE: Changes in anterior fontanel pressure in preterm neonates during tracheal intubation. Anesth Analg 66:874–878, 1987. Reprinted with permission from the International Anesthesia Research Society.)

Neuromuscular Transmission

The neuromuscular junction is immature for the first 2 months after birth. Neonates exhibit slower contraction time, impaired train-of-four responses, tetanic fade, post-tetanic exhaustion, and lower tetanus-to-twitch ratios when compared with older children.[52] As a result, neonates are more sensitive to nondepolarizing muscle relaxants, requiring significantly lower plasma concentrations to achieve equivalent depression of twitch height.[53] The neonate's greater extracellular fluid volume creates a greater volume of distribution of the drug, causing actual initial dose requirements to vary little with age. Subsequent doses of most nondepolarizing muscle relaxants should be lower than initial doses and are required at longer intervals in neonates because of slower elimination.[53] Because nerve stimulation will not reliably indicate reversal of neuromuscular blockade in neonates, voluntary leg lift, shown to correlate with a maximum inspiratory force of -32 cm H_2O, has been advocated as a sensitive indicator of satisfactory reversal.[54]

Retinopathy of Prematurity

Pathologic alterations in the development of the vasculature of the immature neonate's retina result in retinopathy of prematurity (retrolental fibroplasia). The very premature neonate is at greatest risk of developing this disorder. Its etiology, although incompletely understood, is multifactorial,[55] but oxygen therapy is believed to play an important role and is a factor that can be controlled to some extent by the anesthesiologist. Ventilation of preterm neonates with an air/oxygen mixture that maintains PaO_2 between 50 and 80 mmHg[56] or SaO_2 between 88% and 92% is recommended to minimize the risk of retinopathy of prematurity. This guideline should be adhered to until 38 to 44 weeks of conceptual age, when the retinal vasculature matures.[57]

METABOLISM

Temperature Regulation

Heat loss takes place by the mechanisms of radiation, conduction, convection, and evaporation and occurs at the body surface or through the airway. Heat is lost readily by the neonate, whose small mass and high ratio of body surface area to mass facilitates loss by radiation. The neonate responds to cold by attempting to conserve heat through cutaneous vasoconstriction and by increasing heat production. While the sympathetically mediated vasoconstrictive response to cold is active in neonates, its effectiveness is limited by poor tissue insulation provided by their thin layer of subcutaneous fat and skin.[58]

Heat production occurs by shivering and nonshivering thermogenesis. Although neonates can shiver in response to cold, they more commonly accomplish shivering thermogenesis by a generalized increase in motor activity.[59] Nonshivering thermogenesis is the production of heat by increased metabolic activity, chiefly combustion of fatty acids and glucose.[60] It is stimulated by norepinephrine and occurs in several sites, including brown adipose tissue, which is rich in mitochondria, blood vessels, and sympathetic innervation. Brown fat is present in the neonate, continues to develop for a few weeks after birth, and recedes following infancy. It is poorly developed in the preterm neonate and is rapidly depleted during cold stress.

Thermogenesis increases oxygen consumption significantly. Lowering environmental temperature from 34° C to 24° C increases the neonate's oxygen consumption by about 50%.[59, 61] Therefore, it is important to take active measures to conserve heat during anesthetic care. The operating room should be warmed, drafts should be eliminated, radiant heat lamps and heating blankets should be employed, and the baby should be covered with a cap, blanket, and surgical drapes as feasible. Heated humidifiers for inhaled gases add bulk to the anesthetic apparatus but reduce evaporative heat loss.[62] Heating devices must be used judiciously; it is easy for a small baby to become overheated, and hyperthermia also is accompanied by increased oxygen consumption. To detect undesired heat loss or gain, temperature must be monitored during the administration of every anesthetic.

Pharmacokinetics

Hepatic microsomal enzyme systems are immature at birth, and the neonate exhibits impaired metabolism of many drugs. Oxidation and reduction, important pathways of phase I biotransformation, develop quickly and attain adult function within the first week after birth. On the other hand, conjugation pathways providing for phase II biotransformation of drugs do not mature until up to 3 months of age.[63]

Glomerular function of the kidney is also immature in the neonate. Glomerular filtration rate, as indicated by the time clearance of thiosulfate, is significantly lower until the neonate is about 3 weeks of age.[63] Urinary excretion of drugs, therefore, is impaired during this developmental period.

The immaturity of these metabolic and excretory functions in the neonate results in prolonged elimination half-lives of many drugs. The cumulative effect of repeated doses can readily lead to drug toxicity or unexpected prolongation of effect if this is not kept in mind. For example, the narcotics fentanyl and morphine are metabolized in the liver. The elimination half-life of fentanyl is at least twice as long in the neonate as in the adult[64] and appears to be even longer and more variable in preterm neonates.[35] Clearance of morphine in the neonate is less than one-half that of older infants, and elimination half-life is longer.[65] In addition, the neonate's respiratory centers appear to be more sensitive to the effects of narcotics. Thus, prolonged respiratory depression following narcotic administration is not uncommon. The elimination half-life of sufentanil (and presumably fentanyl) improves markedly by 4 weeks of age.[66]

Local anesthetics can also present such problems in neonates. The elimination half-life of lidocaine is significantly longer in the neonate than in the older child or adult (Fig. 10–6).[67, 68] Furthermore, serum concentrations of alpha-1 acid glycoprotein, the plasma protein that binds local anesthetics, are significantly lower in neonates than in older patients.[69] Thus, the unbound fraction of lidocaine is increased in

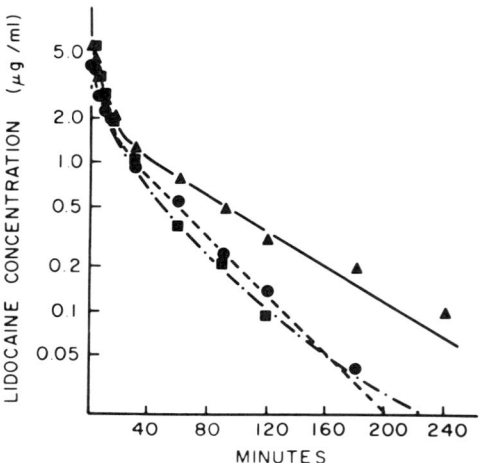

FIGURE 10–6. Like many other drugs, lidocaine has a prolonged elimination half-life in the neonate. ▲ = neonate; ● = adult; ■ = fetus. (From Morishima HO, Finster M, Pedersen H, et al.: Pharmacokinetics of lidocaine in fetal and neonatal lambs and adult sheep. Anesthesiology 50:431–436, 1979. Reprinted with permission.)

neonates, perhaps increasing the risk of toxicity. This potential risk may be partially offset by the larger volume of distribution of drugs in the neonate due to the relatively larger extracellular fluid volume.

As reviewed by Cook,[63] most sedatives and hypnotics, including barbiturates and benzodiazepines, have both prolonged elimination half-lives and increased toxicity in neonates.

BLOOD AND PARENTERAL FLUIDS

Intravenous Fluid Requirements

Maintenance intravenous fluid infusions must meet several needs of the neonate. Insensible and sensible water losses require replacement of about 100 ml per kg body weight of water each day. During the first postnatal day, the neonate shifts a large amount of intracellular water (5% to 8% of body weight) to the extracellular space, thus reducing the initial exogenous water requirement. Sodium, potassium, and chloride requirements range from 1 to 2 mEq/kg/day after the first postnatal day. Caloric requirement to meet resting metabolic needs, excluding growth, is about 50 kcal/kg/day.[70] These basic needs of the neonate can be approximately met for the short term by infusing a solution of 12.5% dextrose, to which has been added 2 mEq/100 ml each of sodium, potassium, and chloride, at a rate of 100 ml/kg/24 hours.

It must be remembered that this is a guideline and that individual requirements may vary considerably. Environmental temperature and humidity, activity level, and minute ventilation are among the factors that influence water requirements. Activity, cold stress, and growth may increase caloric requirements to 130 kcal/kg/day.[70] Abnormal losses of gastrointestinal fluids or transudates associated with disease states or surgical trauma can markedly increase fluid requirements.[71] Various parameters should be regularly monitored to assess adequacy of fluid therapy. Urine output should be 1 to 3 ml/kg/hour, with a specific gravity of 1.005 to 1.011. Serum electrolytes and blood glucose should remain within normal limits. The composition and infusion rate of intravenous fluid should be determined individually as therapy progresses.

The anesthesiologist must review the neonate's preoperative fluid management. If the maintenance fluid therapy has been satisfactory, it makes sense to continue that therapy. By continuing to administer the preoperative fluid via its infusion pump at its preoperative infusion rate, maintenance requirements for glucose, water, and electrolytes will be met. Extra fluids (usually glucose-free lactated Ringer's solution or normal saline), which are required to compensate for fluid translocation and loss during major surgical procedures, can be administered by syringe, as can colloid and blood products (see Fig. 11–3). It is our experience that discontinuing the preoperative fluid and infusion pump and replacing them with 5% dextrose in lactated Ringer's solution and a manually controlled administration set often results in unintended fluid and sugar overload. The ensuing hyperglycemia can be striking and may place the neonate at risk for complications of osmolar imbalance.

Fasting Time

Many neonates requiring anesthesia will already be fasting and receiving intravenous fluids as part of their preoperative treatment and preparation. Occasionally, however, this is not the case, and the anesthesiologist will need to designate a preanesthetic fasting period. A fasting period is necessary to minimize the risk of pulmonary aspiration of gastric contents during anesthesia. On the other hand, a prolonged fasting period can lead to dehydration, hypovolemia, and hypotension during anesthesia.

Studies of gastric emptying have been performed and their results can assist in the determination of an appropriate preanesthetic fasting time. In the nondistressed neonate, gastric emptying is nearly complete by 2 hours following a clear liquid feeding,[72] by 3 hours following a human milk feeding,[73, 74] and by 4 hours following a cow's milk formula feeding.[73] Gastric emptying is slower during the first postnatal day (this is even more pronounced in the preterm neonate)[75] and is delayed by stress and various disease states. A urine specific gravity of less than 1.012 indicates a satisfactory state of hydration during fasting.

Blood Volume

The initial blood volume of the neonate can vary, depending on parturitional losses, but is typically high, as is hematocrit. Blood volume is usually calculated to be at least 90 ml/kg body weight. During the first few months of life, red blood cells containing fetal hemoglobin succumb to age faster than new ones containing adult hemoglobin are made, leading to the "physiologic anemia" of infancy. Although this anemia is a normal occurrence, it should not be regarded lightly; oxygen-carrying capacity is impaired in proportion to the decrease in hemoglobin.

The neonate should be transfused with red blood cells intraoperatively when blood loss exceeds 10% to 15% of blood volume, or about 10 ml/kg. Factors that can alter this guideline include the preoperative hematocrit, preoperative blood balance, hemodynamic stability, and anticipated further losses.

Fetal Hemoglobin

Fetal hemoglobin (HbF) is present from early gestation; erythropoiesis takes place primarily in the reticuloendothelial system in the liver and spleen. At about 20 weeks of gestation, adult hemoglobin (HbA) production begins in the bone marrow. At birth, the hemoglobin of the preterm neonate is 90% to 95% HbF while that of the term neonate is 65% to 85% HbF. The life span of red blood cells containing HbF is less than that of cells containing HbA (110 days and 120 days, respectively). HbF production declines while HbA production continues after birth, so that by 6 months of age, the HbF level is less than 10%.[76]

Structurally, HbF contains two alpha- and two gamma-globin chains, whereas HbA has two alpha- and two beta-globin chains. Amino acid composition and sequence determine the differences between gamma and beta chains.

Functionally, HbF has greater affinity for oxygen, thus facilitating transfer of oxygen from mother to fetus in the placenta. The oxyhemoglobin dissociation curve of HbF is shifted to the left of that of HbA: the P_{50} of HbF is 19 mmHg whereas the P_{50} of HbA is 28 mmHg (see Fig. 11–1). Increasing levels of 2,3-diphosphoglycerate (2,3-DPG) in the erythrocyte during the first week after birth and continuing production of HbA cause a shift of the oxyhemoglobin dissociation curve to the right, with a P_{50} similar to that of the normal adult being attained by 4 to 6 months of age (see Fig. 11–1).[76] This facilitates release of oxygen from the blood to the tissues, an appropriate change during this period of growth and increasing activity. Transfusion of HbA red blood cells to a hypoxic neonate increases P_{50} and enhances unloading of oxygen to the tissues.[77]

CONCLUSIONS

Perianesthetic risk to the neonate is high. By combining an understanding of neonatal physiology with meticulous attention to detail and constant vigilance, the anesthesiologist can provide better care to these challenging patients.

References

1. Rackow H, Salanitre E, Green LT: Frequency of cardiac arrest associated with anesthesia in infants and children. Pediatrics 28:697–704, 1961
2. Smith RM: The pediatric anesthetist, 1950–1975. Anesthesiology 43:144–155, 1975
3. Graff TD, Phillips OC, Benson DW, et al.: Baltimore anesthesia study committee: Factors in pediatric anesthesia mortality. Anesth Analg 43:407–414, 1964
3a. Cohen MM, Cameron CB, Duncan PG: Pediatric anesthesia morbidity and mortality in the perioperative period. Anesth Analg 70:160–167, 1990
4. Avery ME, Fletcher BD, Williams RG: Lung development. In: The Lung and Its Disorders in the Newborn Infant. Philadelphia: WB Saunders, 1981, pp 3–22
5. Avery ME, Fletcher BD, Williams RG: Aeration of the lung at birth. In: The Lung

and Its Disorders in the Newborn Infant. Philadelphia: WB Saunders, 1981, pp 29–36

6. Mansell A, Bryan C, Levison H: Airway closure in children. J Appl Physiol 33:711–714, 1972
7. Nelson NM: Respiration and circulation after birth. In: Smith CA, Nelson NM (eds): The Physiology of the Newborn Infant, 4th ed. Springfield: Charles C Thomas, 1976, p 207
8. Muller NL, Bryan AC: Chest wall mechanics and respiratory muscles in infants. Pediatr Clin North Am 26:503–516, 1979
9. Keens TG, Bryan AC, Levison H, et al.: Developmental pattern of muscle fiber types in human ventilatory muscles. J Appl Physiol 44:909–913, 1978
10. Tusiewicz K, Bryan AC, Froese AB: Contributions of changing rib cage-diaphragm interactions to the ventilatory depression of halothane anesthesia. Anesthesiology 47:327–337, 1977
11. Salem MR, Bennett EJ, Schweiss JF, et al.: Cardiac arrest related to anesthesia: Contributing factors in infants and children. JAMA 233:238–241, 1975
12. Cote CJ, Liu LMP, Szyfelbein SK, et al.: Intraoperative events diagnosed by expired carbon dioxide monitoring in children. Can Anaesth Soc J 33:315–320, 1986
13. Badgwell JM, McLeod ME, Lerman J, et al.: End-tidal PCO_2 measurements sampled at the distal and proximal ends of the endotracheal tube in infants and children. Anesth Analg 66:959–964, 1987
14. Behrman RE, Kliegman RM: Noninfectious disorders of the newborn. In: Behrman RE, Vaughan VC III (eds): Nelson Textbook of Pediatrics, 12th ed. Philadelphia: WB Saunders, 1983, p 366
15. Avery ME, Fletcher BD, Williams RG: Bronchopulmonary dysplasia and other persistent pulmonary dysfunctions. In: The Lung and Its Disorders in the Newborn Infant. Philadelphia: WB Saunders, 1981, pp 263–270
16. Bryan MH, Hardie MJ, Reilly BJ, et al.: Pulmonary function studies during the first year of life in infants recovering from the respiratory distress syndrome. Pediatrics 52:169–178, 1973
17. Hickey PR: Intraoperative tension pneumopericardium with tamponade after ligation of patent ductus arteriosus in a premature neonate. Anesthesiology 64:641–643, 1986
18. Liu LMP, Cote CJ, Goudsouzian NG, et al.: Life-threatening apnea in infants recovering from anesthesia. Anesthesiology 59:506–510, 1983
19. Gregory GA, Steward DJ: Life-threatening perioperative apnea in the ex-"premie." Anesthesiology 59:495–498, 1983
20. Kurth CD, Spitzer AR, Broennle AM, et al.: Postoperative apnea in preterm infants. Anesthesiology 66:483–488, 1987
21. Avery ME, Fletcher BD, Williams RG: The perinatal circulation. In: The Lung and Its Disorders in the Newborn Infant. Philadelphia: WB Saunders, 1981, pp 37–47
22. Friedman WF, Pool PE, Jacobowitz D, et al.: Sympathetic innervation of the developing rabbit heart: Biochemical and histochemical comparisons of fetal, neonatal, and adult myocardium. Circ Res 23:25–32, 1968
23. Friedman WF: The intrinsic physiologic properties of the developing heart. Prog Cardiovasc Dis 15:87–111, 1972
24. Rao CC, Boyer MS, Krishna G, et al.: Increased sensitivity of the isometric contraction of the neonatal isolated rat atria to halothane, isoflurane, and enflurane. Anesthesiology 64:13–18, 1986
25. Cook DR, Brandom BW, Shiu G, et al.: The inspired median effective dose, brain concentration at anesthesia, and cardiovascular index for halothane in young rats. Anesth Analg 60:182–185, 1981
26. Wear R, Robinson S, Gregory GA: The effect of halothane on the baroresponse of adult and baby rabbits. Anesthesiology 56:188–191, 1982
26a. Krane EJ, Su JY: Comparison of the effects of halothane on newborn and adult rabbit myocardium. Anesth Analg 66:1240–1244, 1987
27. Diaz JH, Lockhart CH: Is halothane really safe in infancy? Anesthesiology 51:S313, 1979
28. Gregory GA: The baroresponses of preterm infants during halothane anaesthesia. Can Anaesth Soc J 29:105–107, 1982
29. Friesen RH, Henry DB: Cardiovascular changes in preterm neonates receiving isoflurane, halothane, fentanyl, and ketamine. Anesthesiology 64:238–242, 1986

30. Friesen RH, Lichtor JL: Cardiovascular depression during halothane anesthesia in infants: A study of three induction techniques. Anesth Analg 61:42–45, 1982
31. Friesen RH, Lichtor JL: Cardiovascular effects of inhalation induction with isoflurane in infants. Anesth Analg 62:411–414, 1983
32. Barash PG, Glanz S, Katz JD, et al.: Ventricular function in children during halothane anesthesia: An echocardiographic evaluation. Anesthesiology 49:79–85, 1978
33. Miller BR, Friesen RH: Oral atropine premedication in infants attenuates cardiovascular depression during halothane anesthesia. Anesth Analg 67:180–185, 1988
34. Robinson S, Gregory GA: Fentanyl-air-oxygen anesthesia for ligation of patent ductus arteriosus in preterm infants. Anesth Analg 60:331–334, 1981
35. Collins C, Koren G, Crean P, et al.: Fentanyl pharmacokinetics and hemodynamic effects in preterm infants during ligation of patent ductus arteriosus. Anesth Analg 64:1078–1080, 1985
36. Dargassies SS: Neurological Development in the Full-term and Premature Neonate. Amsterdam: Excerpta Medica, 1977, pp 248–256
37. Anand KJS, Hickey PR: Pain and its effects in the human neonate and fetus. N Engl J Med 317:1321–1329, 1987
38. Anand KJS, Sippell WG, Aynsley-Green A: Randomised trial of fentanyl anaesthesia in preterm babies undergoing surgery: Effects on the stress response. Lancet 1:243–248, 1987
39. Williamson PS, Williamson ML: Physiologic stress reduction by a local anesthetic during newborn circumcision. Pediatrics 71:36–40, 1983
40. Yaster M: The dose response of fentanyl in neonatal anesthesia. Anesthesiology 66:433–435, 1987
41. Lerman J, Robinson S, Willis MM, et al.: Anesthetic requirements for halothane in young children 0–1 month and 1–6 months of age. Anesthesiology 59:421–424, 1983
42. Cameron CB, Robinson S, Gregory GA: The minimum anesthetic concentration of isoflurane in children. Anesth Analg 63:418–420, 1984
43. LeDez KM, Lerman J: The minimum alveolar concentration (MAC) of isoflurane in preterm neonates. Anesthesiology 67:301–307, 1987
44. Levene MI, Fawer CL, Lamont RF: Risk factors in the development of intraventricular haemorrhage in the preterm neonate. Arch Dis Child 57:410–417, 1982
45. Ment LR, Duncan CC, Ehrenkranz RA, et al.: Intraventricular hemorrhage in the preterm neonate: Timing and cerebral blood flow changes. J Pediatr 104:419–425, 1984
46. Lou HC, Lassen NA, Friis-Hansen B: Impaired autoregulation of cerebral blood flow in the distressed newborn infant. J Pediatr 94:118–121, 1979
47. Strange MJ, Myers G, Kirklin JK, et al.: Surgical closure of patent ductus arteriosus does not increase the risk of intraventricular hemorrhage in the preterm infant. J Pediatr 107:602–604, 1985
48. Friesen RH, Honda AT, Thieme RE: Perianesthetic intracranial hemorrhage in preterm neonates. Anesthesiology 67:814–816, 1987
49. Friesen RH, Thieme RE, Honda AT, et al.: Changes in anterior fontanel pressure in preterm neonates receiving isoflurane, halothane, fentanyl, or ketamine. Anesth Analg 66:431–434, 1987
50. Friesen RH, Honda AT, Thieme RE: Changes in anterior fontanel pressure in preterm neonates during tracheal intubation. Anesth Analg 66:874–878, 1987
51. Perlman JM, Goodman S, Kreusser KL, et al.: Reduction in intraventricular hemorrhage by elimination of fluctuating cerebral blood-flow velocity in preterm infants with respiratory distress syndrome. N Engl J Med 312:1353–1357, 1985
52. Goudsouzian NG: Maturation of neuromuscular transmission in the infant. Br J Anaesth 52:205–213, 1980
53. Fisher DM, O'Keeffe C, Stanski DR, et al.: Pharmacokinetics and pharmacodynamics of d-tubocurarine in infants, children, and adults. Anesthesiology 57:203–208, 1982
54. Mason LJ, Betts EK: Leg lift and maximum inspiratory force, clinical signs of neuromuscular blockade reversal in neonates and infants. Anesthesiology 52:441–442, 1980
55. Lucey JF, Dangman B: A reexamination of the role of oxygen in retrolental fibroplasia. Pediatrics 73:82–96, 1984
56. Behrman RE, Vaughan VC III: Nelson Textbook of Pediatrics, 12th ed. Philadelphia: WB Saunders, 1983, p 346

57. Martyn LJ: Pediatric ophthalmology. In: Behrman RE, Vaughan VC III (eds): Nelson Textbook of Pediatrics, 12th ed. Philadelphia: WB Saunders, 1983, pp 1761–1762
58. Sinclair JC: Thermal control in premature infants. Annu Rev Med 23:129–148, 1972
59. Adamsons K Jr, Gandy GM, James LS: The influence of thermal factors upon oxygen consumption of the newborn human infant. J Pediatr 66:495–508, 1965
60. Britt BA: Temperature regulation. In: Gregory GA (ed): Pediatric Anesthesia. New York: Churchill Livingstone, 1983, pp 253–314
61. Stern L, Lees MH, Leduc J: Environmental temperature, oxygen consumption, and catecholamine excretion in newborn infants. Pediatrics 36:367–373, 1965
62. Fonkalsrud EW, Calmes S, Barcliff LT, et al.: Reduction of operative heat loss and pulmonary secretions in neonates by use of heated and humidified anesthetic gases. J Thorac Cardiovasc Surg 80:718–723, 1980
63. Cook DR: Paediatric anaesthesia: Pharmacological considerations. Drugs 12:212–221, 1976
64. Koehntop DE, Rodman JH, Brundage DM, et al.: Pharmacokinetics of fentanyl in neonates. Anesth Analg 65:227–232, 1986
65. Lynn AM, Slattery JT: Morphine pharmacokinetics in early infancy. Anesthesiology 66:136–139, 1987
66. Greeley WJ, de Bruijn NP: Changes in sufentanil pharmacokinetics within the neonatal period. Anesth Analg 67:86–90, 1988
67. Morishima HO, Finster M, Pedersen H, et al.: Pharmacokinetics of lidocaine in fetal and neonatal lambs and adult sheep. Anesthesiology 50:431–436, 1979
68. LeDez KM, Strong A, Reider M, et al.: Effect of age on the pharmacokinetics of intravenous lidocaine in pediatrics. Anesthesiology 67:A500, 1987
69. LeDez KM, Swartz J, Strong A, et al.: The effect of age on the serum concentration of alpha-1 acid glycoprotein in newborns, infants and children. Anesthesiology 65:A421, 1986
70. Sinclair JC, Driscoll JM, Heird WC, et al.: Supportive management of the sick neonate: Parenteral calories, water, and electrolytes. Pediatr Clin North Am 17:863–893, 1970
71. Shires T, Williams J, Brown F: Acute change in extracellular fluids associated with major surgical procedures. Ann Surg 154:803–810, 1961
72. Blumenthal I, Ebel A, Pildes RS: Effect of posture on the pattern of stomach emptying in the newborn. Pediatrics 63:532–536, 1979
73. Cavell B: Gastric emptying in infants fed human milk or infant formula. Acta Paediatr Scand 70:639–641, 1981
74. Tomomasa T, Hyman PE, Itoh K, et al.: Gastroduodenal motility in neonates: Response to human milk compared with cow's milk. Pediatrics 80:434–438, 1987
75. Gupta M, Brans YW: Gastric retention in neonates. Pediatrics 62:26–29, 1978
76. Delivoria-Papadopoulos M, Roncevic NP, Oski FA: Postnatal changes in oxygen transport of term, premature, and sick infants: The role of red cell 2,3-diphosphoglycerate and adult hemoglobin. Pediatr Res 5:235–245, 1971
77. Oski FA: Clinical implications of the oxyhemoglobin dissociation curve in the neonatal period. Crit Care Med 7:412–418, 1979

11. Anesthetic Management of Premature Neonates, Term Neonates, and Infants

James H. Diaz, M.D.

Portions of this chapter were adapted with permission from Diaz JH, Marino RJ: Intraoperative management. In: Goldsmith JP, Karotkin EH (eds): Assisted Ventilation of the Neonate, 2nd ed. Philadelphia: W.B. Saunders, 1988, pp 357–375.

281

INTRODUCTION

Anesthetic risks continue to be greater for neonates and infants than for older children despite significant improvements in intraoperative monitoring, anesthetic agents, and techniques of anesthetic management.[1–3] This chapter provides an update on the unique physiology, anatomy, and pathology of the premature and term neonate (first 4 weeks of life) and older infant (4 weeks to 1 year of age) requiring surgery. Anesthetic techniques, pharmacologic agents for perioperative use, and potential intraoperative management difficulties are also presented and discussed.

Anesthesiologists continue to identify causes of increased anesthetic risks in neonates and seek new ways to reduce these risks and provide safer anesthetics. In the past 35 years, anesthesiologists have made such significant contributions to neonatal medicine as an evaluation of the newborn's need for resuscitation (the Apgar score),[4] continuous distending pressure for respiratory distress syndrome (RDS),[5] the first neonatal ventilator providing intermittent mandatory ventilation (IMV),[6] systems for accurate noninvasive determination of blood pressure in neonates,[7] and safer transport systems for neonates.[8] As these contributions and other advances decreased intraoperative morbidity and mortality, a new infant group at even higher risk was recognized—premature infants with resolving lung disease and apnea.[9–11]

ANESTHETIC RISKS IN NEONATES AND INFANTS

Unlike term newborns, premature neonates cannot adapt quickly to extrauterine life. When stressed by anesthesia and surgery, premature neonates may reestablish a fetal circulatory pattern and develop altered central control of ventilation.[9] Rapid consumption of energy substrates with hypoglycemia, decreased glomerular filtration with oliguria, and thermal deregulation with nonshivering thermogenesis may also occur as a result of perioperative stress in premature neonates.[2] The most significant anesthetic risks in premature as well as term infants include increased sensitivity to the cardiodepressant effects of anesthetics, airway management difficulties, ventilatory depression, thermal instability, rapid dehydration, and nutritional imbalance.[2, 3, 12] Episodic apnea and retinopathy of prematurity, unusual in term infants, also pose significant perianesthetic risks in preterm infants. In this chapter, the unique features of preterm infants that increase intraoperative risks will be contrasted with similar features shared by term infants.

Increased Anesthetic Sensitivity

Neonatal sensitivity to the cardiodepressant effects of anesthetics is based on a number of physiologic observations made in term newborns, including poor sympathetic tone, sluggish baroreceptor responses, high resting heart rate and parasympathetic tone, and cardiac output determined more by heart rate than by stroke volume.[2, 9] Recent fetal echocardiographic studies, however, question the preeminent role of heart rate on cardiac output by demonstrating that sound-induced increases in fetal heart rates actually decreased biventricular stroke volumes but left both ejection fractions unchanged.[13] Nonetheless, all volatile anesthetics are extremely vagotonic and easily potentiate the infant's high resting vagal tone to quickly reduce heart rate and cardiac output.[1–3, 12, 14, 15]

Clinical experience has shown that term infants are extremely sensitive to the myocardial depressant effects of anesthetics.[1–3] Compared with adult populations, term infants who inhale halothane while undergoing routine surgery experience more significant cardiovascular depression and greater susceptibility to cardiac arrest.[3, 12] In 1978, significant myocardial depression and its reversal with intravenous atropine were first demonstrated by echocardiographic studies in older infants and children anesthetized with halothane.[14] Later investigations of the newer inhalational agents, enflurane and isoflurane, in term and premature neonates suggested similar cardiovascular depression was minimized but not prevented by atropine.[15, 16]

Recent investigations in infants of various ages have now documented significantly lower minimum alveolar concentrations (MAC) for halothane in term neonates[17] and isoflurane in preterm neonates[18] compared with older infants receiving the same anesthetics. Despite reduced anesthetic requirements for halothane and isoflurane in term and preterm neonates, respectively, cardiovascular depression as reflected by significant changes in heart rate and arterial blood pressure occurred with similar incidences among all infant age groups studied.[17, 18]

Airway Management Difficulties

Upper airway obstruction poses significant intraoperative risk to premature infants. Salem and others[12] actually found airway obstruction, accidental or premature tracheal extubation, and esophageal intubation to be responsible for one-half of the cardiac arrests in their study of 73 intraoperative cardiac arrests in older infants and children. Unique anatomic features predispose all neonates to airway management difficulties during anesthesia and surgery.[2] These features include a large head, a short neck with limited range of motion, a wide and flat face with small mouth and large tongue, a large and floppy epiglottis, an anterior and more cephalad glottic orifice, and a narrow cricoid ring with short trachea.[2] The more premature the neonate is, the more accentuated these features become.[2] Therefore, endotracheal intubation is frequently required for intraoperative airway control in all prematurely born infants under 6 months of postnatal age and 60 weeks of postconceptual age. These infants do not appear to be at significant risk of postextubation laryngeal edema, as are older infants and toddlers, and the risks of airway obstruction, alone or in combination with anesthetic-induced circulatory depression, far outweigh the risks of endotracheal intubation.[12, 19, 20] The longer the trachea remains intubated, however, the greater the risk of tracheal damage becomes.[21] Subglottic stenosis is a common sequel to prolonged tracheal intubation for mechanical ventilation of premature infants with bronchopulmonary dysplasia.[21] The number of atraumatic tracheal intubations, however, has little influence on the subsequent development of subglottic stenosis in premature neonates compared with tracheostomy or months of mechanical ventilation.[21]

Ventilatory Depression

Intraoperative ventilatory depression is common in neonates, especially premature infants, whose awake carbon dioxide response curves are shifted further to the right than adult response curves.[22] For this reason, narcotics, barbiturates, and volatile anesthetics cause more alveolar hypoventilation in neonates than in older infants and adults, even with the stimulation of skin incision and operation.[23]

In addition to a sluggish ventilatory response to respiratory depressants, a variety of other physiologic and anatomic factors may also predispose preterm infants to intraoperative ventilatory depression, hypoxemia, and apnea. Such factors include reduced lung volumes and capacities, high minute volumes of ventilation and oxygen consumption, and poorly developed primary and accessory muscles of ventilation.[24-28]

Although tidal volume and dead space are nearly equal on a volume per weight basis in infants and adults, newborn vital capacity is one-half that of the adult, and respiratory rate is twice that of the adult.[24] Minute volume of ventilation and minute consumption of oxygen per body weight are also two to three times greater in newborns than in adults.[24] Correspondingly smaller lung volumes and capacities can be expected for premature babies and even term babies who are small for gestational age. Narcotics, barbiturates, and volatile anesthetics have a more pronounced effect on ventilatory rate than volume of gas moved and may cause more respiratory depression in premature infants whose minute ventilation is more dependent on rate than on volume.[24] As noted in the previous chapter, all inhaled anesthetics, particularly halothane, may also impair intercostal muscle function promoting hypoventilation, further reduction in functional residual capacity (FRC), and closure of small airways, especially in preterm neonates.[25] For these reasons, controlled ventilation of anesthetized, paralyzed infants provides better alveolar ventilation with less mismatching of ventilation and lung perfusion than spontaneous ventilation. Muscle relaxants may, therefore, provide better operating conditions in preterm infants and permit reduced dosages of intravenous or inhaled anesthetics with less cardiovascular depression during surgery and less respiratory depression after surgery.[20]

Several anatomic factors described in Chapter 10 combine with the physiologic factors noted to predispose premature infants to ventilatory depression during anesthesia and surgery. Acting together, the premature infant's elastic chest wall, bulging abdomen, and weak thoracoabdominal musculature generate less negative intrathoracic pressure than in an older child or adult, shrinking FRC and promoting early airway closure, often during tidal breathing and especially during hypoventilation.[26-28]

Thermal Instability

Intraoperative hypothermia is quite common in premature infants and imposes such severe stresses that cardiovascular depression and hypoperfusion acidosis may result. Reasons for infant temperature instability, which are now well recognized, include poor central thermoregulation, thin insulating fat, high minute volume of ventilation, reduced muscle mass with poor shivering capacity, and, most importantly, an exaggerated body surface area to mass ratio that is 2.7 times that of an adult.[29-32] The more premature the neonate, the more exaggerated this critical ratio becomes, with the smallest premature infants having body surface area to mass ratios of up to 3.5 times that of an adult.[31, 32]

Like the term neonate, the premature neonate responds to cold stress by trying to limit heat loss through cutaneous vasoconstriction and by increasing intrinsic heat production through nonshivering thermogenesis.[30] Although designed to compensate for heat loss, these mechanisms, described in Chapter 10, are all ineffective in preterm infants.[30] Cutaneous vasoconstriction is limited by poor sympathetic tone and by thin layers of skin, subcutaneous tissues, and insulating fat.[30] Shivering, a heat-producing mechanism for the larger preterm and term neonate, is limited in its ability to produce heat by underdeveloped muscle tone and small muscle mass.[30, 33] Like shivering, nonshivering thermogenesis rapidly consumes tissue oxygen stores and is ineffective at maintaining body temperature in cold-stressed preterm infants.[34] Nonshivering thermogenesis occurs in specialized brown fat that is poorly developed in preterm infants and accounts for only 2% or less of body weight.[32, 34] Even the fuel substrates for nonshivering thermogenesis, primarily glucose and free fatty acids, are limited in preterm infants.[34, 35]

Physicians now recognize the need for warmed ambient temperatures, no drafts, warming mattresses between the patient and the cold operating table, heated humidification of inspired gases, and warmed skin-cleansing solutions during all neonatal procedures and especially during surgery in premature infants.[36] A warmed operating room without cold drafts provides more thermal stability with greater safety in term newborns than do heating lamps, warming mattresses, radiant warmers, warmed inspired gases, or warm antiseptic solutions.[36, 37] A variety of infant radiant warmers now permit surgical exposure and access, a warm patient environment with little discomfort to medical attendants, and continuous servocontrolled thermoregulation in preterm neonates during most operative procedures. However, as noted in the previous chapter, heating devices can easily overheat small preterm infants and should be used cautiously in servocontrolled modes with continuous monitoring of the device's heat output and the patient's body temperature to prevent hyperthermia with increased oxygen consumption and tachyarrhythmias.

Rapid Dehydration

Like hypothermia, rapid intraoperative dehydration may cause neonatal circulatory collapse by depleting circulating fluid volume, reducing stroke volume, and promoting hypoperfusion acidosis. The premature infant's large extracellular fluid volume (40% or more of body weight) is rapidly reduced by fasting, insensible and operative fluid losses, and gastrointestinal and respiratory fluid losses. Renal maturation is only 80% complete by age 4 weeks in term neonates and cannot provide for large urine volumes during fluid overload, concentrated urine during hypovolemic dehydration, or easy reabsorption of bicarbonate during hypoperfusion acidosis.[38–40] Thus, neonates, especially premature neonates, are brought to surgery unable to handle fluid overloads or deficits, and with strong tendencies toward rapid salt and water losses promoting early dehydration with hypovolemia and acidosis with cardiovascular depression.[40] In premature infants, these physiologic disadvantages are even more pronounced with decreasing gestational age. Adequate fluid hydration with water and electrolytes should be provided during all infant operations. Adequacy of intraoperative fluid therapy can be closely monitored by accurate determinations of heart rate and blood pressure, effect of positive pressure ventilation on blood pressure, and urine output.

Nutritional Imbalance

A final physiologic risk factor common to all neonates intraoperatively is a tendency toward nutritional imbalance, hypoglycemia, and starvation ketosis due to low hepatic glycogen stores and stress-increased metabolic workloads. In addition to water and electrolytes, intravenous dextrose should be administered perioperatively to maintain nutritional balance and provide energy substrates for metabolism during fasting and surgery. An intraoperative glucose infusion providing 4 to 7 mg/kg/min and not exceeding 10 mg/kg/min should maintain normoglycemia.[41] However, attempts to completely replace large intraoperative fluid losses in preterm neonates solely with glucose infusions may produce hyperglycemia with ketoacidosis, fluid overload with cardiovascular instability, and neurologic depression from cerebral edema, intracranial hemorrhage, or hyponatremia.[41]

ANESTHETIC IMPLICATIONS OF PREMATURE INFANT PATHOPHYSIOLOGY

Premature infants are more predisposed than term infants to a variety of unique pathophysiologic conditions with significant anesthetic implications, including infant RDS, anemia, patent ductus arteriosus, intracranial hemorrhage, episodic apnea, and retinopathy of prematurity (ROP). Infant RDS, anemia, intracranial hemorrhage, and ROP were described in Chapter 10 and will only be treated here as they apply to preterm neonates.

Respiratory Distress Syndrome

Lung development is incomplete at birth, especially in preterm infants, and continues until adolescence.[42] At about 24 weeks' gestation, terminal sacs resembling fluid-filled alveoli form in the fetal lung.[42] At the time, specialized cells lining these sacs, known as type II alveolar epithelial cells, begin to produce the chemical detergent, surfactant, that will coat the inside of the alveolus, reduce surface tension, and keep the alveolus open when first expanded by air at birth.[42, 43] Extracellular surfactant deficiency promotes alveolar collapse and causes idiopathic RDS of the newborn. The younger the infant is, the greater the surfactant deficiency, and the greater the likelihood of severe RDS.[42-44] Unless the fetus is 24 weeks' gestation or older, there is little likelihood that a premature infant will survive.[42-44] After 24 weeks, alveolar and pulmonary capillary development continues, alveolar pressure–volume stability improves, and type II cells increase in size and number.[42-44] By 26 to 28 weeks, effective gas exchange can occur at preterm birth.[42-44] Despite accelerated surfactant production by stress-released glucocorticoids, RDS occurs in up to 60% of preterm neonates.[42-44] Of those who survive RDS, 20% will develop bronchopulmonary dysplasia (BPD) with severe pulmonary dysfunction lasting throughout infancy and into early childhood.[42-45] BPD is characterized pathologically by interstitial pulmonary fibrosis and numerous small cysts alternating with areas of collapsed lung.[44, 45] Pathophysiologically, BPD is characterized by gross impairment of ventilatory mechanics and respiratory gas exchanges and occurs most commonly in preterm infants mechanically ventilated for prolonged periods with inspired oxygen concentrations over 70%.[44, 45]

With rapid improvements in neonatal nutritional support and long-term assisted ventilation, more premature infants now survive RDS and require such surgical procedures as ligation of a patent ductus arteriosus (PDA), ventriculoperitoneal shunting, bowel resection for necrotizing enterocolitis, inguinal hernia repair, or central venous cannulation early in life, often during the course of treatment for RDS.[20] The special problems preterm infants with RDS bring to the operating room may include hypoxemia, hypercapnia, reduced pulmonary compliance, and anemia.[20] Other acquired problems may include subglottic stenosis, pulmonary barotrauma, pulmonary oxygen toxicity, pulmonary interstitial emphysema, and bronchopulmonary dysplasia.[46]

Anemia

Despite high initial blood volumes and hematocrits, preterm infants are susceptible to anemias caused by combinations of decreased erythropoiesis, hemolysis of vitamin E deficiency, short erythrocyte life span, bouts of sepsis, and frequent blood sampling for laboratory investigations.[47]

At birth, expanded blood volumes of 90 to 105 ml/kg may result from uteroplacental transfusion and delayed cord clamping.[47, 48] High hematocrits and hemoglobin levels (16.0 to 17.0 g/dl) result from hemoconcentration within hours of birth and from fetal hemoglobin (HbF) produced in the fetal liver and spleen.[48, 49] Adult hemoglobin (HbA) is also present in the fetus and neonate, but its production, which commences in fetal bone marrow at 20 weeks, lags behind that of HbF.[48, 49] At birth, the preterm infant's hemoglobin is 90% to 95% HbF, compared with 65% to 85% HbF in the term infant.[48–50] The differences in HbF contribution to total hemoglobin at birth are important in determining red cell longevity, oxygen-carrying capacity, and tissue oxygenation.[49, 50]

As noted in the previous chapter, the hemoglobins differ in structure, function, and life span.[49] HbF has greater affinity for oxygen than HbA, limited ability to bind with 2,3-diphosphoglycerate (2,3-DPG), and impaired oxygen-releasing capabilities (Fig. 11–1).[49, 50] These physiologic characteristics of HbF are beneficial to the fetus competing with the mother for oxygen but detrimental to the preterm neonate whose tissues may be starving for oxygen by the stresses of RDS or surgery (see Fig. 11–1; Table 11–1).[49, 51]

Recent clinical investigations have demonstrated that an increase in HbA concentration by blood transfusion in preterm neonates with PDA may enhance ductal closure and alleviate congestive heart failure.[52, 53] Possible mechanisms for transfusion-mediated ductal closure include reversal of the HbF:HbA ratio, improved blood oxygen content, better

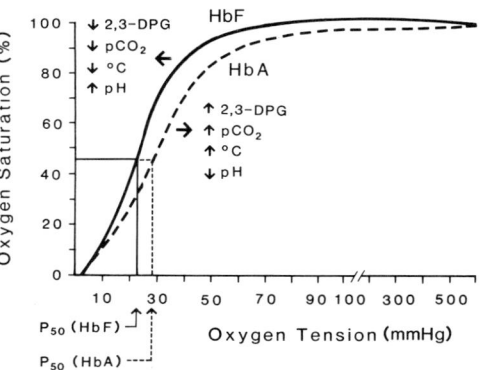

FIGURE 11–1. Oxyhemoglobin dissociation curves for fetal and adult hemoglobin. Factors that shift the oxyhemoglobin dissociation curves of the hemoglobins include temperature (°C), hydrogen ion concentration (pH), partial pressure of CO_2 in the blood (PCO_2), and red cell 2,3-diphosphoglycerate (2,3-DPG). HbF is shifted to the left of HbA. P_{50} is the partial pressure of O_2 at which each hemoglobin is 50% saturated. P_{50} (HbF) = 18 to 24 mmHg. P_{50} (HbA) = 25 to 29 mmHg. (Data from Delivoria-Papadopoulos M, Roncevic NP, Oski FA: Postnatal changes in oxygen transport of term, premature, and sick infants: The role of red cell 2,3-diphosphoglycerate and adult hemoglobin. Pediatr Res 5:235, 1971; and Oski FA: Clinical implications of the oxyhemoglobin dissociation curve in the neonatal period. Crit Care Med 7:412, 1979.)

Table 11–1. Mean Hemoglobin Changes in Preterm and Term Neonates
During First Year of Life

Value	Gestational Age			Chronologic Age				
	28 Weeks	34 Weeks	Term	Day 1	Day 7	Day 14	6 Months	1 Year
Hemoglobin (g/dl)	14.5	15.0	16.8	18.4	17.0	16.8	10–15	14–18
Hematocrit (%)	45	47	53	58	54	52	30–40	31–43

Data from Glader BE: Erythrocyte disorders in infancy. In: Avery ME, Taeusch HW (eds): Schaffer's Diseases of the Newborn, 5th ed. Philadelphia: W.B. Saunders, 1984, pp 581–615; and from Goldsmith JP, Karotkin MD: Appendix 26. In: Goldsmith JP, Karotkin EH (eds.): Assisted Ventilation of the Neonate, 2nd ed. Philadelphia: W.B. Saunders, 1988, p 452.

tissue oxygenation, and oxygen-induced ductal smooth muscle constriction.[52, 53]

In term infants, the hemoglobin concentration falls rapidly and reaches a nadir of 9.0 to 11.0 g/dl (hematocrit 30% to 33%) by 9 to 12 weeks.[54] In preterm infants, this fall is greater and faster, reaching its nadir of 7.0 to 8.0 g/dl (hematocrit 28% to 30%) by 4 to 8 weeks.[54, 55] Preterm infant anemia is thus greater than term infant anemia, and its severity is directly related to the degree of prematurity.[54, 55] Despite rapid falls in hemoglobin levels, tissue oxygenation continues as HbA levels rise, 2,3-DPA levels increase, and the oxyhemoglobin dissociation curve moves to the right (see Fig. 11–1).[49, 50] By the third or fourth month, hemoglobin levels stabilize at 11.0 to 12.0 g/dl in term infants and slightly lower in preterm infants.[54, 55] By 1 year, hemoglobin levels of term and preterm infants are comparable (see Table 11–1).[51, 54, 56] Hemoglobin changes during the first year of life in term and premature infants are indicated in Table 11–1.[51, 54, 56]

Patent Ductus Arteriosus

Patency of the ductus arteriosus in utero appears to be related to circulating prostaglandins, particularly PGE_1 and PGE_2, and closure at birth is probably mediated by falling prostaglandin levels and oxygen-directed constriction of ductal smooth muscle.[57] Persistent PDA after birth may occur in three different groups of neonates: full-term infants otherwise normal, premature infants, and infants with congenital heart disease.[58] Premature infants have the highest incidence of PDA and are the most difficult to manage because of accompanying lung disease.[58, 59]

The incidence of PDA in preterm infants can be correlated with age and birth weight. Hemodynamically significant PDA occurs with an incidence of 1 per 10,000 live births in term infants and 1 per 7000 live births in preterm infants less than 36 weeks' gestation.[58, 59] In the National Collaborative Study on PDA in Premature Infants,[59] hemodynamically significant PDA occurred in 42% of premature infants with birth weights less than 100 g and in only 7% of infants weighing 1500 to 1750 g at birth. The hemodynamic significance of the PDA in this study was determined by clinical, radiographic, and echocardiographic criteria, and resulted in life-threatening circulatory volume overload.[59]

The degree of left-to-right shunting through a PDA is determined by the size of the shunt, myocardial performance, and systemic and pulmonary vascular resistances. Underlying lung disease often modifies these determinants of shunting by increasing pulmonary vascular resistance.[59, 60] In premature infants with PDA and RDS, pulmonary vascular resistance remains high after birth and can reduce or even reverse left-to-right shunting through the PDA. As RDS improves, the left-to-right shunt returns to cause fluid overload and heart failure.[58, 59] Premature infants with RDS and PDA often remain ventilator-dependent and, if weaned, tire quickly and again need ventilator support.[58, 59] In premature infants without lung disease, impaired myocardial capability, inability to handle volume overload, and/or rapidly falling pulmonary vascular resistance after birth will increase the magnitude of the left-to-right shunt through a PDA and precipitate heart failure by the first 1 or 2 weeks of life.[58, 59]

The clinical manifestations of PDA in premature infants are also modified by lung disease. In the absence of RDS, heart failure with tachycardia, feeding difficulty, poor weight gain, and hepatomegaly occur within weeks.[58, 59] The heart is hyperactive, producing palpable thrills and loud continuous murmurs often with diastolic rumbles and multiple clicks.[58, 59] Peripheral pulses are bounding and cyanosis is absent.[58] In a preterm infant recovering from RDS, the clinical manifestations of PDA are not as clear-cut and may require further diagnostic investigation to differentiate them from the overlapping manifestations of lung disease.[58, 59] In 10% of preterm infants with PDA and RDS, heart murmurs are absent.[58, 59] When present, murmurs are systolic rather than continuous and have no associated sounds.[58] The chest x-ray film in preterm infants with both PDA and heart failure shows cardiomegaly, pulmonary vascular engorgement, and pulmonary edema.[58–60]

The echocardiographic relationship of left atrial (LA) diameter to aortic (AO) diameter can provide a valuable ratio (LA:AO) that, if large (>1.3) or increasing over time (>0.3 from previous study), confirms the presence of a hemodynamically significant PDA in infants with few clinical manifestations.[58, 59] Cardiac catheterization may rarely be necessary to differentiate PDA from aortopulmonary window or large ventricular septal defect.[58] In most cases, the ductus permits angiographic catheter access to the descending aorta through the right ventricle and provides a large step-up in oxygen saturation between the right ventricle and pulmonary artery.[58]

The treatment of PDA in preterm infants with or without RDS is controversial and may include red cell transfusion for anemia, fluid restriction without diuretics, intravenous indomethacin administration, or surgical ligation.[53, 60–62] Postulated mechanisms for transfusion-directed ductal closure with reversal of the HbF:HbA ratio have been presented.[53] Diuretic therapy with furosemide has actually been shown to increase the incidence of PDA in premature infants with RDS by stimulating increased renal synthesis of PGE_2.[60] On the other hand, simple limitation of fluid intake to amounts estimated to meet requirements for excretion, insensible loss, and growth will reduce the risks of PDA and heart failure in premature infants.[61, 62]

By inhibiting synthesis of PGE_2, indomethacin therapy can constrict and close the PDA in up to 71% of preterm infants with hemodynamically significant PDA.[62, 63] However, a 35% incidence of spontaneous closure of the ductus has also been reported in preterm infants managed with fluid restriction and an indomethacin placebo.[61–63] The complications of indomethacin therapy in PDA appear to be minimal, and, in the absence of contraindications, three doses of intravenous indomethacin (0.2 to 0.3 mg/kg) administered 8 to 12 hours apart are recommended in preterm infants with PDA.[61–63] Contraindications to indomethacin therapy include renal dysfunction, platelet count below 50,000, evidence of intracranial or other bleeding, and necrotizing enterocolitis (NEC).[61–63] If indomethacin is contraindicated or fails to close the ductus, surgical ligation of the ductus is indicated and is associated with little surgical risk, quick ventilator weaning, and good long-term survival.[62, 63]

For the preterm infant with PDA, other problems evident before or after ductal closure will determine outcome and have been correlated with a 16% hospital mortality.[58, 59] Such problems have included bronchopulmonary dysplasia, intracranial hemorrhage, necrotizing enterocolitis, sepsis, and renal dysfunction and are equally distributed in premature infants receiving indomethacin or having surgical closure of a PDA.[58, 59, 62, 63] The development of indomethacin therapy for PDA has improved the understanding of ductal patency and closure and has spawned the development of intravenous PGE_1 therapy (0.1 to 1.0 μg/kg/min) for maintaining ductal patency in such ductal-dependent heart defects as pulmonary and aortic outflow tract obstructions.[59, 62, 63]

Intracranial Hemorrhage

Infants with birth weights less than 700 g exhibit a higher incidence of intracranial hemorrhage (62% versus 25%) than premature infants with birth weights of 701 to 1500 g.[64] Intracranial hemorrhage (ICH) in the smallest preterm infants is more severe, occurs earlier, and is more often associated with a fatal outcome than in preterm infants weighing more than 700 g.[64–67] ICH in preterm infants is most commonly periventricular-intraventricular, but it may also be subdural, subarachnoid, or intra-cerebellar.[66–68]

Periventricular-intraventricular hemorrhage originates in the capillaries of the subependymal germinal matrix that are poorly supported by connecting tissue.[64] Initial hemorrhagic lesions usually occur near the caudate nucleus in premature infants less than 28 weeks' gestation and at the choroid plexus in older preterm infants.[64–66] Approximately 80% of cases of periventricular hemorrhage rupture through the ependyma to fill the ventricular system with blood that often pools in the posterior fossa, causing obliterative arachnoiditis and subsequent hydrocepha-lus.[65–68]

The pathogenesis of ICH in preterm infants appears to be related to several etiologies that may be divided into endothelial, vascular, and extravascular factors.[64] The endothelial factors include immaturity and fragility of the periventricular capillary bed. Endothelial factors cannot be modified in the perioperative period as can vascular and extravascular factors.[64, 65, 69] Vascular causes of ICH include impaired cerebral autoregulation,[69] a disproportionate amount of total cerebral blood flow entering the periventricular circulation,[69, 70] fluctuating arterial hypertension,[69, 70] and anatomic susceptibility to venous engorgement in the periventricular capillary bed.[64, 68–70] Extravascular factors in ICH may include increased fibrinolytic activity in the periventricular region,[70] congenital or acquired hypocoagulability,[70–72] heparin administration,[73] and the rapid intravenous administration of colloids,[74] saline,[75] or sodium bicarbonate.[75] Such etiologic factors may combine in a premature infant, particularly one subjected to a perinatal asphyxial insult, to produce periventricular-intraventricular hemorrhage.[64, 65, 68]

A number of commonly performed procedures have been associated with significant intracranial hypertension in preterm infants, including intratracheal suctioning,[76] awake tracheal intubation,[77] and asynchronous mechanical ventilation during spontaneous breathing.[78, 79] Such procedures may predispose the preterm infant to a greater risk of ICH.[76–79] On the other hand, surgical closure of PDA has not been shown to increase the risk of ICH in preterm infants.[80]

As noted in Chapter 10, eliminating fluctuations in blood pressure and cerebral blood flow by confining tracheal intubation, suctioning, and mechanical ventilation to anesthetized, paralyzed preterm infants has been shown to reduce intracranial pressure and possibly the risk of ICH (see Fig. 10–5).[76–78, 81] Even barbiturate sedation of preterm infants recovering from RDS has reduced the incidence of ICH in a susceptible population by eliminating stress-induced increases in arterial pressure during prolonged neonatal intensive care unit stays.[81]

Since the administration of halothane, isoflurane, fentanyl, or ketamine does not increase intracranial pressure in preterm neonates as it does in adults, premature neonates should receive an appropriate amount of anesthesia in surgery to eliminate fluctuations in intracranial pressure and reduce the perianesthetic risks of ICH.[79, 82, 83] An adequate plane of general anesthesia with inhaled and/or intravenous anesthetics and muscle relaxants can be maintained in most preterm infants needing surgery, reserving light anesthetics with muscle paralysis for infants who are moribund or in shock.[79, 82, 83]

Episodic Apnea

Episodic apnea occurs frequently in premature infants, usually worsens when oxygen and ventilatory therapy ceases, and can often be induced by feeding or upper airway suctioning.[84] Episodic apnea can be a brief respiratory pause of less than 15 seconds (periodic breathing) or a prolonged apneic pause of greater than 15 seconds.[84, 85] Apnea lasting longer than 15 seconds is often accompanied by heart rates of less than 100 beats/min for at least 5 seconds.[84, 85] In most cases, the incidence of perioperative apnea may be inversely correlated with gestational age and weight.[84–87] Despite significant advances in the perioperative management of premature infants, apnea and/or bradycardia still pose one of the greatest risks following anesthesia and surgery in these patients.[84, 87]

In a retrospective review of infants undergoing herniorrhaphy in the first months of life, Steward[9] was among the first to report that preterm infants were more likely to develop postoperative apnea than were full-term infants. Later, Liu and associates[10] reported a significant incidence of prolonged apnea in premature neonates younger than 41 weeks' postconceptual age compared with infants older than 46 weeks' postconceptual age. Recently, Kurth and associates[11] reported a 37% incidence of postoperative prolonged apnea in infants 32 to 55 weeks' postconceptual age and recommended postoperative apnea monitoring for up to 60 weeks' postconceptual age in preterm infants. This study also documented initial episodes of prolonged apnea occurring as late as 12 hours following anesthesia.[11]

The methylxanthines theophylline and caffeine are often administered orally or intravenously as respiratory stimulants in the management of apnea of prematurity.[85, 88–91] Recently, Welborn and associates[85] recommended intravenous caffeine therapy (5 to 10 mg/kg after induction) for preterm infants with episodic apnea as being more effective and less arrhythmogenic than theophylline. The pharmacologic basis for methylxanthine therapy in episodic apnea of prematurity appears to be related more to central stimulation of medullary breathing centers than to pulmonary bronchodilation and augmented diaphragmatic function.[89, 90] Methylxanthine therapy should be continued perioperatively in preterm infants with episodic apnea, and long-acting anesthetic adjuvants, especially ketamine, barbiturates, narcotics, and tranquilizers, should probably be avoided.[85–88, 91]

The risk of sudden infant death syndrome (SIDS) is significantly increased in premature infants who have episodic apnea, and SIDS is a potential postoperative consequence.[92] All prematurely born infants up to 60 weeks' postconceptual age, survivors of SIDS and their siblings, and infants with episodic apnea may be at greater risk of sudden postoperative death than term infants and should be carefully monitored for apnea both in the immediate postanesthetic period and for at least 12 to 24 hours postoperatively.[9–11, 87, 92] Postoperative pain in premature infants with episodic apnea is better managed with non-narcotic analgesics or regional nerve blocks that are less likely to cause ventilatory depression than narcotics and tranquilizers (see Regional Anesthesia).

Retinopathy of Prematurity

Retrolental fibroplasia or, more appropriately, retinopathy of prematurity (ROP) is a poorly understood disorder causing intense vasoconstriction of immature retinal vessels with retinal edema on exposure to high inspired oxygen concentrations with development of high PaO_2 in retinal vessels.[93–95] Retinal hemorrhage, neovascularization, fibroproliferation, and retinal detachment and scarring may follow and result in blindness in severe cases or myopia in milder cases.[93–95] Prenatal factors predisposing infants to ROP are prematurity, low birth weight, and immaturity of the retinal vessels.[94] Postnatal factors predisposing infants to ROP include prolonged O_2 therapy, long-term mechanical ventilation, high inspired O_2 concentrations, and high PaO_2 (greater than 70 to 90 mmHg) and SaO_2 (greater than 92% to 95%) in the retinal vessels.[94–99] Although ROP usually afflicts the sickest and smallest infants, it has occurred infrequently in room air in term infants up to 44 weeks' postconceptual age,[94, 95] in cyanotic infants,[95] and even after short-term administration of intraoperative O_2 to term infants.[96, 97]

To avoid ROP, infants at greatest risk must be identified and examined by indirect ophthalmoscopy preoperatively for evidence of ROP. As emphasized in Chapter 10, intraoperative inspired O_2 fractions (FiO_2) should provide a measured preductal PaO_2 between 50 and 80 torr in the right radial artery,[96–101] a transcutaneous PO_2 between 45 and 70 torr,[96–101] or a transcutaneous O_2 saturation between 88% and 92%.[96–101] Short-term (1 to 3 minutes) administration of high concentrations of O_2 before a hypoxic challenge such as tracheal intubation, extubation, or prolonged suctioning is considered acceptable and desirable and should not be avoided for fear of ROP.[101]

PREOPERATIVE EVALUATION

Meticulous preoperative evaluation of neonates and infants, particularly those requiring mechanical ventilation, should assess activity, size, and skin color and carefully examine the upper airway, cardiopulmonary system, and volume status. Prior anesthetic history, drug allergy or therapy, ventilatory management, and family history should also be noted. An organized plan for intraoperative management including premedication, if any, fasting status, and need for postoperative ventilation should be documented in a preanesthetic note.

Physical Examination

Physical examination may begin with evaluation of the head, neck, and upper airway for nasal patency, craniofacial deformity, and cervical range of motion, so as to predict quality of mask fit and ease of tracheal intubation. Existing uncuffed endotracheal tubes should be checked for appropriate size,[102] for positioning by auscultation and chest x-ray film, and, most importantly, for tracheal air leak at 20 to 25 cm H_2O positive peak airway pressure.[19] Baseline vital signs[103] should be determined (Table 11–2) and mechanical ventilator settings noted, especially FiO_2, rates of mechanical and spontaneous ventilation, use of continuous positive airway pressure (CPAP) or positive end-expiratory pressure (PEEP), peak airway pressures and flows, and inspiratory-to-expiratory time ratios. Uninterrupted oxygen and ventilatory therapy for RDS with either an anesthesia bag or a pressure-limited, timed-cycle ventilator should be maintained during transport to the operating room and during the operative procedure. Baseline arterial blood or capillary gases will confirm adequacy of oxygenation and ventilation (Table 11–3).[104] Transcutaneous oxygen tension ($PTCO_2$) or saturation ($STCO_2$) probes provide good trend indicators of oxygenation and tissue perfusion and may prove helpful during transport of ventilated neonates. Since even a short trip

Table 11–2. Normal Mean Blood Pressures and Heart Rates in Preterm and Term Neonates

Age	Systolic Blood Pressure (torr)	Diastolic Blood Pressure (torr)	Heart Rate (bpm)
0–12 hours (preterm)	49	26	160
0–12 hours (term)	70	44	120
4 days	75	50	135
6 weeks	95	55	160
1 year	95	60	140

Data from Goldsmith JP, Karotkin EH: Appendices 23, 24, and 31. In: Goldsmith JP, Karotkin EH (eds): Assisted Ventilation of the Neonate, 2nd ed. Philadelphia: W.B. Saunders, 1988, pp 448, 449, 455.

Table 11–3. *Normal Mean (± SD) Arterial Blood Gases in Preterm and Term Neonates**

	Preterm (<34.5 Weeks)			Term		
	Birth (3–5 Hours)	24 Hours	1 Week	Birth (5 hours)	24 Hours	1 Week
pH	7.32 (0.038)	7.46 (0.0)	7.37 (0.043)	7.33 (0.028)	7.36 (0.032)	7.37 (0.026)
$Paco_2$ (mmHg)	47 (8.5)	28 (8.4)	36 (4.2)	36 (3.6)	33 (3.1)	35 (3.1)
Pao_2 (mmHg)	59 (7.7)	69 (15.2)	80 (12.0)	63 (12.0)	72 (9.5)	73 (9.7)
BE (mEq/L)	−3.7 (1.5)	−4.7 (3.3)	−2.9 (2.3)	−6.3 (1.2)	−5.2 (1.3)	−3.2 (1.3)

*BE = base excess; SD = standard deviation.
Data from Goldsmith JP, Karotkin EH: Appendix 5. In: Goldsmith JP, Karotkin EH (eds): Assisted Ventilation of the Neonate, 2nd ed. Philadelphia: W.B. Saunders, 1988, p 434.

to the operating room can compromise a stable neonate, transport incubators or radiant warmers with compressed gases are necessary to maintain thermal stability and permit continuous ventilatory therapy. Some neonatal intensive care units have the capabilities, extra space, and personnel to permit certain surgical procedures (e.g., ligation of PDA; gastrostomy) on site to avoid the potential dangers of transport.

Roentgenographic Evaluation

In infants requiring assisted ventilation, a preoperative chest x-ray film will confirm endotracheal tube position, evaluate heart size, and rule out extra-alveolar air accumulations in pneumothorax, lobar emphysema, pulmonary interstitial emphysema, pneumomediastinum, or pneumoperitoneum, which can all be expanded by intraoperative administration of nitrous oxide (N_2O).[46, 105] Congestive heart failure, usually secondary to a PDA, requires preoperative evaluation (often by echocardiography) and appropriate management before elective surgery. Wet lung syndrome (transient tachypnea of the newborn) in the larger preterm infant will also require roentgenographic evaluation preoperatively and appropriate management before elective surgery.

Ophthalmologic Evaluation

Preoperative indirect ophthalmoscopy by an experienced ophthalmologist will confirm the degree of retinal maturity or severity of ROP in infants requiring long-term oxygen and ventilatory therapy for RDS.[98–101] It is necessary to ascertain the degree of retinal maturity or extent of existing damage before the administration of anesthetics and O_2.[96–99]

Laboratory Evaluation

In addition to hemoglobin and hematocrit, preoperative laboratory studies in premature infants should include serum glucose, electrolytes, and urinalysis (Table 11–4).[106] Hypoglycemia should be corrected. Parenteral hyperalimentation should be continued intraoperatively to avoid rebound hypoglycemia. Normovolemia is indicated by a urinary output of 0.5 to 1.0 ml/kg/hour or greater, a urine specific gravity of 1.010 to 1.015, serum sodium of 140 to 145 mEq/L, and serum potassium of 4.0 to 5.5 mEq/L (see Table 11–4).[106]

Physical findings of severe dehydration such as weight loss, dry mucous membranes, poor skin turgor, sunken fontanelles, sunken eyes, and hypotension should be sought, confirmed by laboratory studies, and corrected preoperatively. Respiratory distress, short-term oxygen dependency, or both are also contraindications to semielective surgery (e.g., non–life-threatening bowel obstruction) in preterm neonates with RDS and in term infants with transient tachypnea. These patients should be managed with nasogastric suction and intravenous nutrition until the respiratory problems have resolved to avoid intraoperative exacerbations of respiratory failure with pulmonary hypertension and, possibly, a return to the fetal circulatory pattern. All anesthetics unmask preoperative hypovolemia quickly and, in addition to their anticipated vagal effects on heart rate, can significantly reduce cardiac output, causing electromechanical dissociation or cardiac arrest without warning.[1, 3, 12]

Fasting Status

Fasting status in premature infants being fed orally or by gavage should be limited to 2 hours for clear liquids and 4 hours for formula. All infants, particularly premature infants with such neurologic disorders

Table 11–4. *Normal Mean with Range Laboratory Values in Preterm and Term Neonates*

	Preterm (1500–1750 g)			Term		
	1 Week	1 Month	2 Months	Birth	1 Day	3 Days
Na (mEq/L)	139	136	137	143	145	149
	(133–146)	(133–148)	(133–142)	(124–156)	(132–159)	(139–162)
K (mEq/L)	5.6	5.5	5.7	6.4	6.3	5.9
	(4.6–6.7)	(4.5–6.6)	(4.6–7.1)	(5.3–7.3)	(5.3–8.9)	(5.0–7.7)
Cl (mEq/L)	108	107	107	100	103	103
	(100–117)	(100–115)	(101–115)	(90–111)	(87–114)	(93–112)
Ca (mg/dl)	9.2	9.4	9.5	8.4	7.8	7.9
	(6.1–11.6)	(8.6–10.5)	(8.6–10.8)	(7.3–9.2)	(6.9–9.4)	(5.9–9.7)
Glu (mg/dl)	—	—	—	63	63	59
				(40–97)	(42–104)	(40–90)

Glu = serum glucose; — = no data available prior to milk feedings.
Data from Goldsmith JP, Karotkin EH: Appendix 25. In: Goldsmith JP, Karotkin EH (eds): Assisted Ventilation of the Neonate, 2nd ed. Philadelphia: W.B. Saunders, 1988, pp 450, 451.

as hydrocephalus, hypoxic encephalopathy, or intracranial hemorrhage, have poor upper airway protective reflexes and reduced gastroesophageal sphincter tone. Delayed gastric emptying occurs in premature infants with RDS, neurologically depressed infants, and infants with gastrointestinal reflux, and it may cause feedings to remain in the stomach for prolonged periods. Regurgitation and aspiration of gastric contents are common regardless of fasting status and underscore the need for swift orogastric decompression, when indicated, and for early establishment of a tracheal airway to protect the lungs and ensure ventilation. When fasting begins in any compromised neonate, an intravenous infusion of glucose should be started to prevent hypoglycemia and dehydration.

Premedication

Oral premedication in neonates is contraindicated due to poor airway-protective reflexes, reduced gastroesophageal sphincter tone, and undetermined gastric absorption. Parenteral premedication with such cardiorespiratory depressants as barbiturates, narcotics, and tranquilizers can worsen common preexisting conditions like apnea, hypoventilation, hypoxemia, and hypotension. Preoperative anticholinergics like atropine or glycopyrrolate reduce high vagal tone and dry oral secretions. Anticholinergics, especially atropine, also reduce the incidence and severity of intraoperative bradycardia and hypotension from vagal stimulation (nasogastric suctioning, endotracheal intubation) and anesthetic agents, like halothane[14] and isoflurane.[16] Premedication with anticholinergics may be given in two doses. First, a subcutaneous dose may be administered 30 minutes prior to induction of anesthesia to control secretions. Then an intravenous dose may be administered immediately prior to or during induction, and before endotracheal intubation, to maintain heart rate and cardiac output. Atropine is more vagolytic than scopolamine and glycopyrrolate.[107] The drying effects of anticholinergics or secretions must be remembered when premedicating intubated infants so that steps may be taken to prevent plugging of the endotracheal tube with inspissated bronchial secretions.

ANESTHETIC PHARMACOLOGY

Although immature neurophysiologically, premature neonates perceive pain at 28 weeks' postconceptual age or even earlier and react to pain with a stress response that includes tachycardia, hypertension, sweating, and release of catechols and corticosteroids.[108] The preterm infant's physiologic stress response to surgical pain may be so massive as to promote hyperglycemia, protein catabolism, cardiovascular instability, or arterial hypertension associated with increased intracranial pressure and intracranial hemorrhage.[79, 108] With appropriate perioperative monitoring, an adequate plane of general anesthesia with inhaled and/or intravenous anesthetics and muscle relaxants can and should be provided to even the sickest preterm infants.

For satisfactory surgical anesthesia, infants require higher delivered concentrations of halothane, enflurane, and isoflurane than older children and adults (Table 11–5).[17, 18, 109–111] Uptake and excretion of inhaled anesthetics also occur more rapidly in neonates than in older children and adults.[109–112] Rapid uptake and distribution of inhaled anesthetics in neonates and older infants appear to be related to several factors, especially higher cardiac output, greater alveolar ventilation, and smaller FRC than in older children and adults.[109–112]

Increased inhaled anesthetic requirements in infants have been quantitated as effective doses (ED_{50})[113] and minimum alveolar concentrations (MAC)[109–111] in comparison with anesthetic requirements in older children and adults (see Table 11–5).[17, 18, 109–111] Increased dose requirements may result from rapid anesthetic uptake, quick alveolar saturation, rapid vascular distribution, hyperdynamic cardiovascular tone and metabolism, and immaturity of the central nervous system, kidneys, and liver.[109–112] Though higher than adult requirements, anesthetic requirements in preterm and term neonates appear to be significantly lower than in older infants and children.[17, 18] Presently, combinations of N_2O, volatile anesthetic agents, muscle relaxants, narcotics, and barbiturates are the most widely employed anesthetic techniques in neonates and older infants.[114] Among inhaled anesthetics, halothane and N_2O have been studied more extensively in infants than the newer agents enflurane and isoflurane.

Despite increased anesthetic requirements in comparison with adults, term neonates have significantly lower MAC values for halothane than do older infants.[17] Induction and recovery of inhalation anesthesia were significantly shorter with enflurane than with equipotent halothane

Table 11–5. Mean Minimum Alveolar Concentration in Preterm and Term Neonates and Adults

Inhaled Anesthetics	MAC (%)		
	Preterm	*Term*	*Adult*
Halothane	—	0.87	0.76
Enflurane	—	—	1.7
Isoflurane	1.28 (<32 weeks)	1.6	1.15
	1.41 (32–37 weeks)		

MAC = minimum alveolar concentration; − = no data available.
Data from Lerman J, Robinson S, Willis MM, et al.: Anesthesiology 59:421, 1983; Le Dez KM, Lerman J: Anesth Analg 56:501, 1977; Govaerts MJM, Sanders M: Br J Anaesth 47:877, 1975; Cameron CB, Robinson S, Gregory GA: Anesth Analg 63:418, 1984; and Diaz JH, Marino RJ: Intraoperative management. In: Goldsmith JP, Karotkin EH (eds): Assisted Ventilation of the Neonate, 2nd ed. Philadelphia: W.B. Saunders, 1988, pp 357–375.

concentrations in infants and children.[110] Enflurane requirements, however, have not been determined in term and preterm neonates.[110]

Interestingly, recent clinical investigations have shown that term newborns require less inspired isoflurane than anticipated, compared with equipotent halothane doses.[111] These findings suggest that in newborns, even smaller inhaled dosages of isoflurane provide satisfactory surgical anesthesia with faster emergence than with halothane.[111] Preterm neonates require significantly less inspired isoflurane for anesthesia than do term neonates.[18] The MAC of isoflurane in preterm neonates of less than 32 weeks' gestation is significantly less than that in preterm neonates of 32 to 37 weeks' gestation (see Table 11–5).[17, 18, 109–111] Both preterm age groups, however, show a similar drop in systolic arterial pressure at equi-MAC concentrations of isoflurane.[18]

The more potent volatile agents, halothane, enflurane, and isoflurane, produce more cardiovascular depression than combinations of N_2O and muscle relaxants.[114] Due to minimal hemodynamic compromise, the popularity of N_2O and muscle relaxant anesthesia with reversal of muscle relaxation at the end of the operative procedure has increased.[114] During N_2O–muscle relaxant anesthesia, additional analgesia with narcotics is often needed.[114] Intravenous narcotics or barbiturates added to N_2O inhalation in adults promote more cardiovascular instability than N_2O in O_2 alone.[114, 115] Narcotics or barbiturates should be carefully titrated intravenously in infants to avoid untoward intraoperative effects (e.g., hypotension, hypoventilation) and postoperative effects (e.g., delayed emergence, respiratory depression).[112]

N_2O is no longer considered an innocuous inhaled anesthetic, especially in premature neonates.[112] N_2O dilutes inspired oxygen concentrations, becomes a potent cardiovascular depressant when combined with narcotics,[115] and rapidly expands extra-alveolar air-containing cavities that are not being adequately decompressed, such as pneumothoraces, congenital lung cysts, lobar and interstitial emphysema, or obstructed stomach or bowel.[46, 105, 112] Compressed air or helium may also serve as O_2-diluting carrier gases in premature infants in whom N_2O is contraindicated.[112]

Muscle Relaxants

Shortly after the introduction of succinylcholine as a muscle relaxant in the 1950s, Stead[116] suggested that when equipotent doses of succinylcholine were administered in infants and adults, less profound neuromuscular relaxation occurred in infants. In 1966, Nightingale and associates[117] reported that infants were more resistant to the muscle-relaxant properties of succinylcholine than were adults and recommended a greater dose per unit of body weight. Cook and associates[118] later confirmed that infants have greater requirements for succinylcholine than do older children or adults because of greater distribution of the drug in a larger volume of extracellular fluid. In infants, non-neuromuscular effects of succinylcholine may include dysrhythmias, particularly sinus bradycardia, hyperkalemia, myoglobinemia, and increased intraocular pressure.[118, 119] Succinylcholine has been associated with malignant hyperthermia in older children and adolescents.[120] Distribution and elimination of succinylcholine are rapid, with intravascular hydrolysis by plasma pseudocholinesterases beginning on injection and providing short-lived muscular relaxation, even in premature infants.[118, 119, 121]

In contrast to succinylcholine requirements, earlier studies suggested that newborns were more sensitive than older children and adults to the nondepolarizing muscle relaxants curare and pancuronium. Goudsouzian[121] and Cook[119] have now demonstrated that neonates have no increased sensitivity to these agents but do vary widely in twitch response, such that some newborns are quite sensitive and others relatively resistant to muscular relaxation. The nondepolarizing agents curare, metocurine, pancuronium, gallamine, atracurium, and vecuronium should be titrated to effect with small initial doses and reduced maintenance doses and should be monitored by twitch response and adequately antagonized at the conclusion of surgery with combinations of anticholinesterases (neostigmine, pyridostigmine) and anticholinergics (atropine, glycopyrrolate).[112, 119, 121] Recovery times, often not applicable to premature and critically ill infants, range from 10 to 15 minutes for atracurium and vecuronium to 20 to 50 minutes for pancuronium, curare, and metocurine.[112, 119, 121] Non-neuromuscular effects of nondepolarizing relaxants in infants range from histamine-mediated hypotension with curare, metocurine, and large doses of atracurium to vagolytic tachycardia with gallamine and pancuronium.[112, 119, 121] Variable neuromuscular response and resistance to antagonism are quite common in infants and could indicate the need for postoperative mechanical ventilation.[112, 119, 121] Hypothermia, hypocalcemia, and concomitant aminoglycoside antibiotic therapy often potentiate nondepolarizing neuromuscular relaxants and interfere with adequate reversal.[112, 119, 121]

Intravenous Anesthetics

Despite their increasing popularity and use in adult anesthesia, most intravenous agents have not been well studied in infants, particularly in premature neonates. Most available information on narcotics and barbiturates in immature subjects is derived from animal models.[122, 123] Narcotics and barbiturates produce more cardiorespiratory depression in newborns than in adults.[122, 123] Meperidine may cause less respiratory depression and more cardiovascular depression than morphine.[124] Morphine clearance and elimination half-life are significantly prolonged in term neonates compared with older infants receiving equivalent intravenous doses of morphine.[125] Compared with adults, newborns given morphine anesthesia display prolonged postoperative cardiorespiratory depression due to higher initial plasma concentrations, slower clearance rates, and delayed hepatorenal elimination.[125] New, ultrapotent narcotics like fentanyl, sufentanil, and alfentanil maintain better perioperative hemodynamic stability than morphine and can be administered as single large intravenous boluses or by continuous infusion.[126–129] Fentanyl, ten times more potent than morphine, has a significantly longer elimination half-life in both term and preterm infants than in older infants receiving equivalent intravenous doses of fentanyl.[126, 127] Postoperative rebounds in plasma fentanyl levels have now been observed after fentanyl anesthesia in term newborns and may promote prolonged hypoventilation.[126, 127] Such rebounds in narcotic levels are felt to result from surgically induced hepatic hypoperfusion; increased intra-abdominal pressure with reduced cardiac output, delayed drug distribution, biotransformation, and clearance; and hepatic sequestration of unbound drug.[126, 127] Ventilatory support is often required in neonates receiving more than 10 μg/kg of fentanyl for general anesthesia.[126, 127] Sufentanil, ten times more potent than fentanyl (100 times more potent than morphine), also results in higher initial plasma levels, slower clearance rates, and longer elimination half-lives in term neonates than in older infants and adults receiving equivalent intravenous doses.[128, 129] The pharmacokinetics of sufentanil have not been studied in premature infants, and alfentanil, less potent and shorter acting than fentanyl, has not been studied in neonates or older infants.

Intravenous barbiturates, specifically thiopental, appear to be more dangerous in newborn than in adult rats and guinea pigs.[123] Rectal barbiturates, though effective in older infants and children, have not been studied extensively in newborns, have variable effects on cardiorespiratory status depending on uptake, and should be avoided in neonates. Though cardiorespiratory-depressant effects of narcotics and barbiturates may be difficult to interpret from animal studies, these effects in infants may be due to combinations of increased cardiovascular sensitivity, altered central control of ventilation, limited protein binding, and prolonged excretion from delayed hepatic biotransformation and reduced renal excretion.[112] Premature infants with episodic apnea, neurologic disorders, or pulmonary diseases that produce alveolar hypoventilation should not receive narcotics, barbiturates, or tranquilizers intraoperatively unless prolonged postoperative mechanical ventilation is planned.[112]

Ketamine, a phencyclidine derivative initially developed for veterinary use, is a newer intravenous anesthetic adjuvant that produces potent musculoskeletal analgesia and sedation.[130] Shortly after its introduction, ketamine was recommended for pediatric anesthesia because of greater cardiovascular stability, less respiratory depression, and better maintenance of airway protective reflexes.[130] Ketamine does provide greater cardiovascular stability in infants compromised by shock and heart failure, but it also causes prolonged sedation, increased oropharyngeal secretions, and more respiratory depression and upper airway compromise than initially imagined.[112, 130] Ketamine has proved most useful as an intravenous anesthetic in the sickest infants with cyanotic congenital heart disease who require prolonged postoperative ventilation.[112, 130] Ketamine is not a good anesthetic choice for premature neonates with episodic apnea or for preterm infants who will be weaned from mechanical ventilation immediately following surgery.[112] When indicated, intravenous ketamine titrated to effect produces significantly shorter recovery times in older children and adults than when given as large intramuscular boluses.[112]

In summary, all intravenous anesthetics can produce unpredictable effects in neonates and premature infants and should be carefully titrated in reduced dosages at induction of anesthesia to avoid significant postoperative apnea and sedation. The reversible intravenous agents, such as short-acting narcotics and muscle relaxants, may offer more versatility and less risk of postoperative apnea than inhalation anesthetics and the longer-acting irreversible intravenous agents, such as barbiturates, tranquilizers, and ketamine.

INTRAOPERATIVE ANESTHETIC MANAGEMENT

Intraoperative anesthetic management of infants should provide a closely monitored continuum of analgesia, amnesia, and surgical relaxation with complete upper airway control, ventilatory support, and maintenance of circulatory and homeostatic stability. Such a perfect anesthetic state cannot always be achieved, especially in the high-risk premature infant. Frequent adjustments may be necessary in levels of anesthesia and surgical muscle relaxation. Compared with the nursery course, the intraoperative course of most neonates is one of fluctuating cardiopulmonary and volume status, temperature instability, neuromuscular irritability, and loss of muscle tone.

Monitoring

Intra-anesthetic monitoring of neonates and infants must be at least as extensive as that employed preoperatively in specialized care units and perhaps more so, depending on the experience of the anesthesiologist and the surgical procedure. Minimum intra-anesthetic monitoring of all neonates should include use of a precordial or esophageal stethoscope, temperature probe, and blood pressure cuff of appropriate size; an accurate, noninvasive method for determining blood pressure; continuous electrocardiogram; and pulse oximetry. Critically ill neonates may require more invasive monitoring, such as direct blood pressure monitoring by radial artery cannula or umbilical artery catheter. Central venous pressure catheters to assist fluid therapy are sometimes indicated in preterm neonates who are in cardiorespiratory failure or undergoing cardiac surgery, but they can often offer more risk than benefit even in the sickest infants.[131] Pulmonary artery catheters have seldom been used in neonates and infants, and at present no reliable data exist on their use, indications, contraindications, or complications.

Intraoperative Airway Management

For the physiologic reasons discussed, endotracheal intubation is recommended for intraoperative upper airway management and inhalation anesthesia in all premature neonates, term neonates, and older preterm infants to at least 6 months of postnatal age and 60 weeks or more of postconceptual age. Some additional practical points of airway management in premature infants include quality of mask fit, selection of laryngoscope blade, selection of endotracheal tube, awake versus anesthetized tracheal intubation, and nasotracheal versus orotracheal intubation.

A better mask fit for preoxygenation or bag–mask ventilation can often be achieved by a clear plastic, contoured Rendell-Baker-Soucek mask (size 0–1), which permits observation of oral secretions and color and provides a minimal dead space of 4 ml or less.[132] A straight, not curved, laryngoscope blade (Miller 0–1) affords better glottic visibility, occupies less space in a small mouth, and can be modified to provide continuous oxygen or anesthetic insufflation.[133] The appropriate sterile endotracheal tube is nontapered, made of implantation-tested polyvinylchloride, fits the glottis easily (external diameter 2.5 to 3.0 cm), and provides an audible tracheal air leak at 20 to 25 cm H_2O peak airway pressure.[19, 102]

Premature infants with hemodynamic instability, gastric or intestinal obstruction, or airway anomalies should undergo preoxygenation and awake tracheal intubation to prevent pulmonary aspiration and airway obstruction, which commonly complicate intravenous and mask inductions in such patients. Inhalation or intravenous induction of general anesthesia with muscular paralysis can follow establishment of a secure upper airway and auscultation of bilaterally equal breath sounds in such compromised infants. Stable preterm neonates, however, may undergo tracheal intubation following induction of intravenous or inhalation anesthesia and muscle paralysis. A nasotracheal tube offers more stability than an orotracheal tube in neonates requiring prolonged postoperative ventilation, but it is more difficult to place, often requires Magill forceps to insert, and can cause epistaxis. Also, in at least one study, nasotracheal intubation was associated with a higher evidence of postextubation atelectasis than the orotracheal approach, particularly in preterm infants with birth weights less than 1500 g.[134]

Intraoperative Ventilatory Management

Intraoperative ventilatory management of premature infants should provide for inhalation of anesthetic gases, appropriate oxygenation, and adequately assisted or controlled ventilation. As noted, spontaneous ventilation is not recommended during anesthesia in neonates and infants because of anesthetic-induced depression of alveolar ventilation and widening of the alveolar to arterial oxygen gradient (A-aDo$_2$). Neonates in respiratory failure preoperatively need similar oxygen and ventilatory management intraoperatively, with careful titration of inspired oxygen, monitored peak inspiratory pressures, and positive end-expiratory pressure, when indicated (Fig. 11–2).[46] The adequacy of oxygenation and ventilation should be continuously assessed by evaluation of color, breath sounds, chest excursion, transcutaneous oxygen tension or saturation, and arterial blood gases. Transcutaneous oximetry provides more reliable noninvasive monitoring of oxygenation than does transcutaneous oxygen tension because of frequent anesthetic-induced alterations in skin perfusion and fluctuating skin temperature.[135] Recommended inspired oxygen fractions and safe limits for arterial and tissue oxygenation in neonates have been presented in Chapter 10.

Apparatus for administering gas anesthesia and ventilating the neonate and infant during surgery should have minimal dead space and little resistance to breathing, should eliminate carbon dioxide adequately, and should provide for assisted or controlled ventilation. Anesthesia breathing circuits should be compact, lightweight, and easy to clean, and should permit heated humidification of inspired gases. To meet these needs, various non-rebreathing modifications of Ayre's T-piece system[136] have been developed, including the Jackson-Rees[137] modification, the Mapleson D system,[138] and the Bain[139] modification of the Mapleson D system (see Fig. 11–2).[46] These breathing systems require a fresh gas flow of at least twice minute ventilation to prevent rebreathing and carbon dioxide retention.[137–139] Hand ventilation with these breathing circuits may afford better appreciation of subtle changes in lung compliance and lower airway resistance than mechanical ventilation. The use of mechanical ventilation with a non-rebreathing circuit or an infant circle system and soda-lime carbon dioxide absorption is advocated for surgical procedures

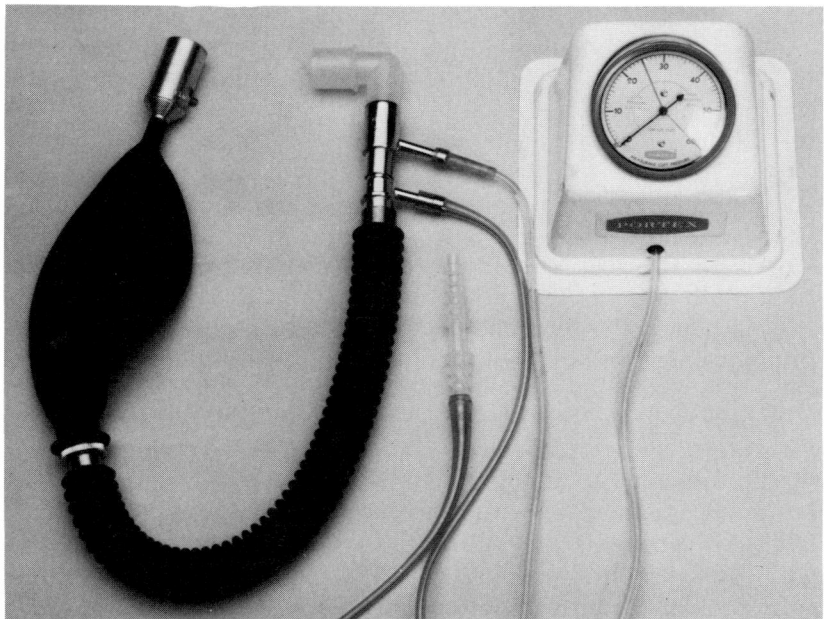

FIGURE 11–2. Simple system for continuous manometric monitoring of delivered airway pressures in an infant non-rebreathing anesthesia circuit, such as a Jackson-Rees (as shown), Mapleson D, or Bain circuit. (Reprinted with permission from the International Anesthesia Research Society from Tension pneumoperitoneum-pneumothorax during repair of congenital diaphragmatic hernia, by JH Diaz. Anesth Analg 66:577, 1987.)

lasting more than 1 or 2 hours and for cardiothoracic surgery. The intraoperative use of adult circle systems and adult ventilators for infants can be accomplished with careful attention to airway pressures, but this is not recommended, especially in premature infants.

With appropriate monitors and alarms, mechanical ventilation is safe in neonates. Inspiratory and expiratory pressures should be carefully monitored and documented during intraoperative mechanical ventilation. Mechanical ventilators for intraoperative use in infants should be equipped with high-pressure and low-pressure alarms that will clearly signal unsafe peak pressures, hypoventilation, or ventilator disconnect. During thoracic surgery, especially for ligation of a PDA, preexisting ventilator settings often will be inadequate during periods of lung compression in the lateral decubitus position. The use of the intraoperative monitoring systems described will allow moment-to-moment adjustment of ventilator settings throughout the surgical procedure. We have found that measurement of mean airway pressure ($P_{\overline{aw}}$) is particularly useful in monitoring mechanical ventilation during thoracic surgery. For PDA ligation in an infant with very low birth weight (<1500 g), an increase of $P_{\overline{aw}}$ of approximately 30% will be needed during lung compression to maintain the infant's respiratory status at acceptable blood gas ranges. The use of muscle relaxants to eliminate diaphragmatic excursion and improve surgical access during the PDA ligation will also require increased mechanical ventilator support intraoperatively.

Pulse oximetry will provide accurate and inexpensive continuous monitoring of effective oxygenation during mechanical ventilation in infants and can be correlated with capillary or arterial blood gases when suspicious readings occur after technical difficulties are eliminated.[135, 140, 141] In mechanically ventilated infants, intraoperative end-tidal capnometry by infrared analysis correlates closely with arterial carbon dioxide tension, provided distal endotracheal tube air is sampled and severe cardiopulmonary disease is excluded.[142] Unfortunately, these limitations make end-tidal capnometry a less reliable monitor of alveolar ventilation than arterial carbon dioxide in the smallest premature infants with cardiopulmonary disorders.[142–144] However, prolonged transcutaneous carbon dioxide monitoring in mechanically ventilated premature infants has been well correlated with arterial carbon dioxide tensions and has detected hypocapnea ($PaCO_2$ < 35 torr) and hypercapnea ($PaCO_2$ > 45 torr) in 74% of a preterm neonatal intensive care unit population during a recent analysis of 586 paired values.[144] Transcutaneous carbon dioxide monitoring in infants is, however, limited by frequent calibration drifts in monitor electrodes, the necessity of repositioning sensors to minimize the risk of burns, and loss of signal when blood pressure is low.[144]

Intraoperative Fluid Therapy

Unlike fluids required daily, intraoperative fluid therapy for all neonates and infants undergoing surgery should restore preoperative fluid deficits, continue maintenance fluids, replace surgical fluid losses through hemorrhage and third-space extravasation, and replace respiratory losses, especially during inhalation of dry anesthetic gases. Administration of crystalloid solutions, colloids, and blood products should be regulated by calibrated infusion pumps or given intermittently by manual syringe injection of specific volumes (Fig. 11–3). Acute blood loss of up to 10% of estimated blood volume can be replaced with crystalloid solutions, provided the preoperative hematocrit is 40% or higher in the term newborn or premature infant and 30% or higher in older infants.[145, 146] Blood losses greater than 10% of estimated blood volume should be replaced with warmed infusions of salt-poor albumin, fresh-frozen plasma, or, preferably, packed erythrocytes, as indicated by serial hematocrits, measured bleeding, and cardiovascular and clotting status.[145, 146]

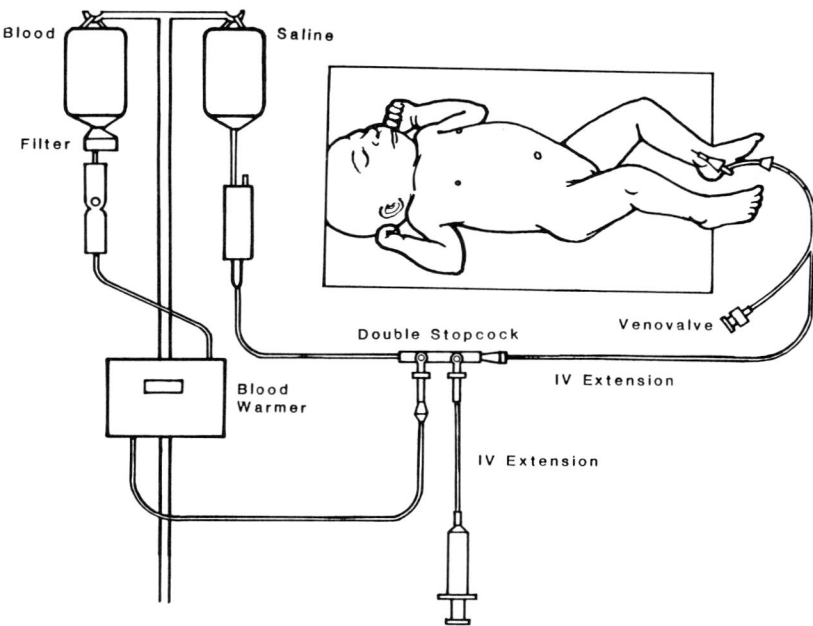

FIGURE 11–3. Simple system for intravenous administration of warmed blood products by manual syringe injection of specific volumes.

Estimated blood volumes for neonates range from 80 to 90 ml/kg for term infants to 90 to 105 ml/kg for premature infants.[145, 146] Maintenance fluids for preterm infants should be supplied as 5% to 12.5% dextrose with normal electrolytes (2 mEq/100 ml each of sodium, potassium, and chloride), with fluid requirements ranging from 2 to 4 ml/kg/hour depending on dietary, cardiopulmonary, and renal status.[145, 146] Preoperative fluid deficits are calculated by multiplying hours of fasting by maintenance fluid requirements.[145, 146] Infants receiving intravenous fluid therapy preoperatively should have no fluid deficits at surgery.[145, 146] Intraoperative urinary output, if measured, should be at least 0.5 to 3.0 ml/kg/hour, with a specific gravity between 1.005 and 1.015.[145, 146] Maximum urine concentration in a premature infant is indicated by a specific gravity of 1.018 (or 800 mOsm/L) but may be as high as 1.025 (1000 mOsm/L) in term infants.[145, 146] Specific gravity of preterm neonatal urine may be spuriously elevated by solutes of high molecular weight, such as sugars or proteins. Under normal circumstances, urine volume is a more useful parameter of hydration in premature neonates than specific gravity. Replacement fluid requirements depend on the surgical procedure, ranging from 1 to 2 ml/kg/hour for minor procedures to 5 to 10 ml/kg/hour for major procedures, and should be administered as normal saline or dextrose-free lactated Ringer's solution, provided that maintenance glucose needs have been met.[41, 145, 146] No more than 7 to 8 mg/kg/min of glucose should be administered while replacing intraoperative losses to avoid hyperglycemia and the risks of osmolar imbalance.[41, 145, 146] Frequently infants transported to surgery with hyperalimentation solutions infusing get boluses of these fluids that exceed their glucose capacity, resulting in hyperglycemia. Exposure of bowel and body cavities to high-intensity surgical lights causes fluid evaporation that should be replaced at 2 ml/kg/hour, and exposure of lung requires 4 ml/kg/hour of extra intravenous fluids.[145, 146] Very premature neonates may have tremendous fluid requirements, up to 10 ml/kg/hour or greater.[145, 146] Care must be taken not to exceed the infant's cardiovascular and renal capacity when high volumes of fluid are needed for replacement.

Regional Anesthesia

Caudal anesthesia with lidocaine, mepivacaine, and bupivacaine has been used successfully to provide anesthesia for term newborns and older infants undergoing lower abdominal and lower extremity surgery, but dosages have been difficult to determine.[147, 148] Recently, spinal anesthesia with tetracaine has been recommended as an alternative to general anesthesia in premature neonates and "ex-premature" infants undergoing minor surgical procedures.[149, 150] Dosages for spinal anesthesia range from 0.25 to 0.5 mg/kg for injected volumes of 0.2 to 0.4 ml, depending on the addition of hyperbaric diluent or epinephrine.[149, 150] Regional nerve blocks may be especially useful in managing postoperative pain in preterm infants with episodic apnea without the respiratory depression commonly caused by narcotic analgesics or tranquilizers.[112]

Local anesthetics may present unique problems in preterm infants with limited plasma protein binding capabilities and immature hepatic biotransformation systems. The elimination half-life of lidocaine is significantly prolonged in fetal and neonatal lambs as compared with adult sheep[151] and in human neonates as compared with older infants.[152] Recently, LeDez and associates[153] noted significantly lower serum concentrations of alpha-1 acid glycoprotein, the plasma protein that binds local anesthetics, in neonates than in older infants and children. Limited plasma protein binding of local anesthetics in preterm infants can provide for larger unbound active fractions of local anesthetics, increasing risks of neurologic and cardiovascular toxicity.[153] Local anesthetic toxicity, even at therapeutic doses, occurs frequently in acidotic patients, who can trap basic local anesthetics in their stomachs normally and in their hearts and brains when hypoxic.[153]

Successful regional anesthesia in preterm infants does not ensure cardiopulmonary stability or airway patency and is not recommended as the sole anesthetic for unstable infants who may require assisted ventilation. Regional anesthesia may be combined with general anesthesia in neonates and infants to reduce inspired anesthetic fractions and provide better postoperative analgesia, especially after perineal or lower extremity surgery.[112]

Termination of Anesthesia

At completion of surgery, several decisions must be made, including whether to reverse neuromuscular blockade, when to extubate the trachea, and what the course of postoperative pulmonary management is to be. Massive blood loss, systemic hypotension, hypothermia, or hypocalcemia contraindicates reversal of nondepolarizing muscle relaxants. Only when the infant is conscious and vigorous may the endotracheal tube be removed. Before tracheal extubation, a critically ill premature neonate may need a short trial of spontaneous breathing with supplemental oxygen via endotracheal tube with continuous positive airway pressure (CPAP). Premature neonates should not be connected to a "T" piece or have an endotracheal tube simply left in place to "protect the airway" without CPAP or mechanical ventilation.[112] CPAP or intermittent mandatory ventilation (IMV) should always be continued until extubation to prevent atelectasis and avoid the added work of breathing imposed by the high resistance of small-caliber endotracheal tubes.[112]

Reassessment of adequacy of oxygenation and ventilation will then determine the proper timing of tracheal extubation. Endotracheal tubes that will remain in place postoperatively must be reevaluated for proper placement and patency and may have to be carefully repositioned or changed at the completion of surgery. Infants who have manipulation of the airway during surgery (i.e., repair of tracheoesophageal fistula) are especially prone to blood clots plugging the endotracheal tube postoperatively.

POSTANESTHETIC MANAGEMENT

Postoperatively, all neonates and infants should be swiftly transported in warmed isolettes to postanesthetic recovery areas (recovery rooms, term nurseries, or pediatric or neonatal intensive care units). Careful monitoring for apnea, hypotension, hypothermia, and prolonged sedation should continue for a period before discharge to nonintensive care areas. Several scoring systems are available to evaluate infant cardiopulmonary and neurobehavioral well-being in postanesthetic recovery areas.[154] Premature neonates up to 60 weeks' postconceptual age, survivors of sudden infant death syndrome and their siblings, and all preterm or term infants with episodic apnea should be carefully monitored for apnea for at least 12 to 24 hours postoperatively.

Postoperative alveolar hypoventilation may be the result of inadvertent intraoperative hypocarbia, hypothermia, prolonged narcosis, inadequate reversal of neuromuscular blockade, or hypocalcemia. A timed, 30- to 60-second trial of apnea will usually allow sufficient rise in $PaCO_2$ to initiate spontaneous ventilation in hypocarbic neonates accustomed to retention of carbon dioxide from RDS or bronchopulmonary dysplasia. Prolonged narcosis may require a diagnostic dose (0.005 mg/kg) of naloxone, which will result in dramatic recovery in cases in which narcotics have caused postoperative apnea. The likelihood of rebound narcosis after naloxone antagonism wears off is great, necessitating prolonged observation after naloxone therapy, especially in preterm infants. Inadequate reversal of nondepolarizing muscle relaxants can be easily excluded as a cause of postoperative hypoventilation by evaluating twitch and post-tetanic response to electrical stimulation of a peripheral motor nerve. If hypothermia, hypocalcemia, and concomitant aminoglycoside antibiotic therapy can be excluded, a second dose of atropine and neostigmine can be administered to antagonize residual neuromuscular block.

Postoperative cardiovascular monitoring with electrocardiography, pulse oximetry, and accurate blood pressure determinations by Doppler, Dinamap, or arterial line should continue throughout the nursery course. Thermal and fluid balance should be maintained.

COMPLICATIONS OF ANESTHESIA IN PREMATURE NEONATES AND INFANTS

Recognition of anesthetic risks and careful attention to the details of airway management, ventilatory control, and vigilant monitoring will prevent the most common intraoperative problems in neonates and infants, such as cardiovascular and respiratory accidents. Several less serious intraoperative complications in neonates and infants include corneal abrasions, lip lacerations, intravenous line infiltrations, electrocautery or heating lamp burns, endobronchial intubation, and postextubation laryngeal edema. These complications may be prevented by careful attention to such details as taping the eyelids, performing gentle laryngoscopy, covering intravenous sites with transparent dressings that allow frequent inspection, grounding the electrocautery, keeping radiant heaters at least 2 feet away from the patient, and auscultating often for bilateral, equal breath sounds. A high index of suspicion for both endobronchial intubation and accidental tracheal extubation proves most valuable in the smallest premature infants intubated for prolonged periods and moved frequently for nursing care and respiratory therapy.

Sounds of air movement in the esophagus may be mistaken for breath sounds in the trachea and lung. Movement of the apices of the chest wall is a better indicator of endotracheal intubation than the auscultation of breath sounds.

Postextubation laryngeal edema manifesting as inspiratory stridor is unusual in premature infants and most common between the ages of 2 and 5 years.[19] Initial management should be conservative, with humidification, steroids, and nebulized racemic epinephrine. No improvement or worsening of stridor may require endoscopic evaluation to rule out congenital anomalies, acquired subglottic stenosis, or laryngeal damage. Premature neonates who have required prolonged endotracheal intubation and assisted ventilation for respiratory failure are at higher risk for acquired subglottic stenosis and postextubation stridor.[21]

INTRAOPERATIVE MANAGEMENT OF SURGICAL EMERGENCIES IN PREMATURE NEONATES AND INFANTS

A variety of congenital anomalies require early surgical correction in the premature or term newborn. Such disorders include tracheoesophageal fistula, diaphragmatic hernia, omphalocele, gastroschisis, intestinal obstruction, pyloric stenosis, patent ductus arteriosus, myelomeningocele, and necrotizing enterocolitis. Some disorders, like diaphragmatic hernia and gastroschisis, require more immediate surgical correction than others. Prematurity and RDS often coexist with various congenital deformities and complicate management. When feasible, delay of semi-elective surgery (e.g., bowel obstruction) until the resolution of the respiratory illness should make anesthetic management safer and improve outcome. Suggestions for anesthetic management of common newborn and infant surgical emergencies are presented in Table 11–6.[112]

CONCLUSIONS

Successful intraoperative management of neonates and infants requires timing, teamwork, an appreciation of the risks involved, and a firm understanding of infant physiology. The pediatric anesthesiologist does not regard the preterm infant as a small term infant and has developed the skills and equipment needed to provide optimum intraoperative care to the high-risk premature infant. The pediatrician should not regard the preterm infant's intraoperative course as an extension of a stable nursery course. Surgical environments are constantly changing and are radically different from nursery environments that emphasize growth and nutrition. New problems are frequently encountered in the operating room on a moment-to-moment basis, and dedicated clinical efforts by

Table 11–6. *Perioperative Management of Neonatal Emergencies*

Surgical Diagnosis	Preoperative Considerations	Special Monitoring	Suggested Inhalation Anesthetic	Suggested Intravenous Adjuvants	Postoperative Considerations
Diaphragmatic hernia	Hypoplastic lungs Asphyxia, shock Gastric distention Pneumothorax Cardiac defects	Nasogastric tube Airway manometer Right radial arterial line Controlled low-pressure ventilation	Low-dose halothane or isoflurane with O_2 only	Low-dose fentanyl or morphine Muscular relaxation with pancuronium	Controlled ventilation Muscular relaxation Pulmonary artery vasodilators Extracorporeal membrane oxygenation
Gastroschisis	Hypovolemia Asphyxia, shock Hypothermia Gastric distention Sepsis	Nasogastric tube Airway manometer Radial arterial line	Halothane or isoflurane in air/O_2 N_2O can further distend bowel	Muscle relaxants may permit inappropriate primary closure and should be used judiciously	Hypovolemia Tight closure with hypoventilation and caval compression Prolonged ileus Controlled ventilation
Intestinal obstruction	Hypovolemia, shock Regurgitation Aspiration Cystic fibrosis Down's syndrome	Nasogastric tube for gastrointestinal drainage Large-bore IV	Halothane or isoflurane in air/O_2 N_2O can further distend bowel	Muscle relaxants often indicated to permit reduced doses of inhaled anesthetics in unstable infants	Hypovolemia Regurgitation with aspiration risk continues Prolonged IV or gastrostomy feeding
Myelomeningocele	Hypothermia Sepsis Increased intracranial pressure	Careful positioning with foam padding Large-bore IV Esophageal stethoscope	Halothane or isoflurane in N_2O/O_2	Muscle relaxants may interfere with identification of nerve roots by electrical nerve stimulator	Hypovolemia Hypothermia Raised intracranial pressure Future ventriculoperitoneal shunt may be necessary Avoid prolonged sedation and hypoventilation from narcotics

Condition	Problems/Concerns	Monitoring	Anesthetic Agents	Muscle Relaxants	Complications
Omphalocele	Hypovolemia Hypotension Hypothermia Gastric distention Cardiac defects	Airway manometer	Halothane or isoflurane in air/O_2 N_2O may further distend bowel	Muscle relaxants may permit primary closure and should be used judiciously	Hypovolemia Tight closure with hypoventilation and caval compression Prolonged ileus
Patent ductus arteriosus	Heart failure Extreme prematurity RDS Cardiac defects	Airway manometer Arterial line helpful Large-bore IV	Halothane or isoflurane in N_2O/O_2 Consider narcotics with air/O_2 in smallest premature infants with congestive heart failure	Short-acting muscle relaxants (e.g., atracurium or vecuronium)	Mechanical ventilation for RDS Cyanosis suggests ductal-dependent cardiac lesion Recurrent laryngeal nerve injury
Pyloric stenosis	Vomiting, aspiration Gastric distention Hypokalemia Hypochloremia Metabolic alkalosis, then hypoperfusion acidosis	Nasogastric tube	Halothane or isoflurane in air/O_2 N_2O may further distend stomach	Rapid-sequence intravenous induction with pentothal and succinylcholine during cricoid pressure; nondepolarizing muscle relaxants usually not required	Respiratory depression Hypoglycemia
Tracheoesophageal fistula	Oral secretions Aspiration Gastric distention Cardiac defects	Nasogastric tube Gastrostomy tube Endotracheal tube below fistula Arterial line helpful	Halothane or isoflurane in air/O_2 N_2O may distend stomach prior to gastrostomy	Muscle relaxants often indicated	Tracheomalacia Esophageal reflux Chronic aspiration Aspiration pneumonitis

Data from Diaz JH, Marino RJ: Intraoperative management. In: Goldsmith JP, Karotkin EH (eds): Assisted Ventilation of the Neonate, 2nd ed. Philadelphia: W. B. Saunders, 1988, pp 357–375.

anesthesiologists are required to return all neonates to postoperative nursery environments in homeostatic balance.

References

1. Rackow H, Salinitre E, Green LT: Frequency of cardiac arrest associated with anesthesia in infants and children: Report of 66 original cases. Pediatrics 28:697, 1961
2. Smith RM: The pediatric anesthetist, 1950–1975. Anesthesiology 43:144, 1975
3. Keenan RL, Boyan CP: Cardiac arrest due to anesthesia. A study of incidence and causes. JAMA 253:2373, 1985
4. Apgar V: A proposal for evaluation of the newborn infant. Anesth Analg 32:260, 1953
5. Gregory GA, Kitterman JA, Phibbs RH, et al.: Treatment of the idiopathic respiratory distress syndrome with continuous positive airway pressure. N Engl J Med 284:1333, 1971
6. Kirby RR, Robison EJ, Schulz J, et al.: Continuous-flow ventilation as an alternative to assisted or controlled ventilation in infants. Anesth Analg 51:871, 1972
7. Janis KM, Kemmerer WT, Kirby RR: Intraoperative Doppler blood pressure measurements in infants. Anesthesiology 33:361, 1970
8. Hackel A: A medical transport system for the neonate. Anesthesiology 43:258, 1975
9. Steward DJ: Premature infants are more prone to complications following minor surgery than are term infants. Anesthesiology 56:304, 1982
10. Liu LMP, Cote CJ, Goudsouzian NG: Life-threatening apnea in infants recovering from anesthesia. Anesthesiology 59:506, 1983
11. Kurth CD, Spitzer AR, Broennle AM, et al.: Postoperative apnea in preterm infants. Anesthesiology 66:483, 1987
12. Salem MR, Bennett EJ, Schweiss JF, et al.: Cardiac arrest related to anesthesia: Contributing factors in infants and children. JAMA 233:238, 1975
13. Kenny J, Plappert T, Doubilet P, et al.: Effects of heart rate on ventricular size, stroke volume, and output in the normal human fetus: A prospective Doppler echocardiographic study. Circulation 76:52, 1987
14. Barash PG, Glanz S, Katz JD, et al.: Ventricular function in children during halothane anesthesia: An echocardiographic evaluation. Anesthesiology 49:79, 1978
15. Barash PG, Katz JD, Firestone S, et al.: Cardiovascular performance in children during induction: An echocardiographic comparison of enflurane and halothane. Anesthesiology 51:S531, 1979
16. Friesen RH, Lichtor JL: Cardiovascular effects of inhalation induction with isoflurane in infants. Anesth Analg 62:411, 1983
17. Lerman J, Robinson S, Willis MM, et al.: Anesthetic requirements for halothane in young children 0–1 month and 1–6 months of age. Anesthesiology 59:421, 1983
18. LeDez KM, Lerman J: The minimum alveolar concentration (MAC) of isoflurane in preterm neonates. Anesthesiology 67:301, 1987
19. Koka BV, Jeon IS, Andre JM, et al.: Postintubation croup in children. Anesth Analg 56:501, 1977
20. Diaz JH: Halothane anesthesia in infancy: Identification and correlation of preoperative risk factors with intraoperative arterial hypotension and postoperative recovery. J Pediatr Surg 20:502, 1985
21. Jones R, Bodnar A, Roan Y, et al.: Subglottic stenosis in newborn intensive care graduates. Am J Dis Child 135:367, 1981
22. Brooks JG: Apnea of infancy and sudden infant death syndrome. Am J Dis Child 136:1012, 1982
23. Olsson AK, Lindahl SGE: Ventilation, dynamic compliance and ventilatory response to CO_2: Effects of age and body weight in infants and children. Anaesthesia 40:229, 1985
24. Hatch DJ, Sumner E: Neonatal Anaesthesia and Perioperative Care. London: Edward Arnold, 1986
25. Tusiewicz K, Bryan AC, Froese AB: Contributions of changing rib cage-diaphragm interactions to the ventilatory depression of halothane anesthesia. Anesthesiology 47:327, 1977

26. Muller NL, Bryan AC: Chest wall mechanics and respiratory muscles in infants. Pediatr Clin North Am 26:503, 1979
27. Keens TG, Bryan AC, Levison H, et al.: Developmental pattern of ventilatory muscles. J Appl Physiol 44:909, 1978
28. Mansell A, Bryan AC, Levison H: Airway closure in children. J Appl Physiol 33:711, 1972
29. Motil KJ, Blackburn MG: Temperature regulation in the newborn infant. Clin Pediatr 12:634, 1973
30. Sinclair JC: Thermal control in premature infants. Annu Rev Med 23:129, 1972
31. Bruck K: Temperature regulation in the newborn. Biol Neonat 3:65, 1961
32. Klaus M, Fanaroff A, Martin RJ: The physical environment. In: Klaus MH, Fanaroff AA (eds): Care of the High-Risk Neonate, 2nd ed. Philadelphia: W.B. Saunders, 1979, pp 94–104
33. Adamsons K, Gandy GM, James LS: The influence of thermal factors upon oxygen consumption of the newborn human infant. J Pediatr 66:495, 1965
34. Britt BA: Temperature regulation. In: Gregory GA (ed): Pediatric Anesthesia. New York: Churchill Livingstone, 1983, pp 253–314
35. Stern L, Lees NH, Leduc J: Environmental temperature, oxygen consumption, and catecholamine excretion in newborn infants. Pediatrics 36:367, 1965
36. Hey E: The care of babies in incubators. In: Gairdner D, Hull D (eds): Recent Advances in Pediatrics. London: Churchill Livingstone, 1971, pp 171–209
37. Heiser MS, Downes JJ: Temperature regulation in the pediatric patient. Semin Anesth 3:37, 1984
38. Dierdorf SF, Krishna G: Anesthetic management of neonatal surgical emergencies. Anesth Analg 60:204, 1981
39. Arant BS: Developmental patterns of renal function maturation compared to the human neonate. J Pediatr 92:705, 1978
40. Edelmann CM, Soriano JR, Boichis H, et al.: Renal bicarbonate reabsorption and hydrogen ion excretion in normal infants. J Clin Invest 46:1309, 1967
41. Lowk C, Mitchell AA, Epstein MF, et al.: Risk factors for neonatal hyperglycemia associated with 10% dextrose infusion. Am J Dis Child 139:783, 1985
42. Avery ME, Fletcher BD, Williams RG: Aeration of the lung at birth. In: Avery ME, Fletcher BD, Williams RG: The Lung and Its Disorders in the Newborn Infant. Philadelphia: W.B. Saunders, 1981, pp 29–36
43. Avery ME, Fletcher BD, Williams RG: Bronchopulmonary dysplasia and other persistent pulmonary dysfunctions. In: Avery ME, Fletcher BD, Williams RG: The Lung and Its Disorders in the Newborn Infant. Philadelphia: W.B. Saunders, 1981, pp 263–270
44. Bryan MH, Hardie MJ, Reilly BJ, et al.: Pulmonary function studies during the first year of life in infants recovering from the respiratory distress syndrome. Pediatrics 52:169, 1973
45. Northway WH Jr, Rosan RC, Porter DY: Pulmonary disease following respiratory therapy of hyaline membrane disease: Bronchopulmonary dysplasia. N Engl J Med 276:357, 1967
46. Diaz JH: Tension pneumoperitoneum-pneumothorax during repair of congenital diaphragmatic hernia. Anesth Analg 66:577, 1987
47. Todres ID: Growth and development. In: Ryan JF, Todres ID, Cote CJ, et al. (eds): A Practice of Anesthesia for Infants and Children. Orlando: Grune & Stratton, 1986, pp 5–17
48. Usher R, Lind J: Blood volume of the newborn premature infant. Acta Paediatr Scand 54:419, 1965
49. Delivoria-Papadopoulos M, Roncevic NP, Oski FA: Postnatal changes in oxygen transport of term, premature, and sick infants: The role of red cell 2,3,-diphosphoglycerate and adult hemoglobin. Pediatr Res 5:235, 1971
50. Oski FA: Clinical implications of the oxyhemoglobin dissociation curve in the neonatal period. Crit Care Med 7:412, 1979
51. Goldsmith JP, Karotkin EH: Appendix 10. In: Goldsmith JP, Karotkin EH (eds): Assisted Ventilation of the Neonate, 2nd ed. Philadelphia: W.B. Saunders, 1988, p 437
52. Rosenthal A: Hemodynamics in physiologic anemia of infancy. N Engl J Med 306:538, 1982
53. Lister G, Hellenbrand WE, Kleinman CS, et al.: Physiologic effects of increasing

hemoglobin concentration in left-to-right shunting in infants with ventricular septal defects. N Engl J Med 306:502, 1982

54. Glader BE: Erythrocyte disorders in infancy. In: Avery ME, Taeusch HW (eds): Schaffer's Diseases of the Newborn, 5th ed. Philadelphia: W.B. Saunders, 1984, pp 581–615

55. O'Brien RT, Pearson HA: Physiologic anemia of the newborn infant. J Pediatr 79:132, 1971

56. Goldsmith JP, Karotkin EH: Appendix 26. In: Goldsmith JP, Karotkin EH (eds): Assisted Ventilation of the Neonate, 2nd ed. Philadelphia: W.B. Saunders, 1988, p 452

57. Coceani P, Olley PM: The response of the ductus arteriosus to prostaglandins. Can J Physiol Pharmacol 51:220, 1973

58. Freed MD: Congenital cardiac malformations. In: Avery ME, Taeusch HW (eds): Schaffer's Diseases of the Newborn, 5th ed. Philadelphia: W.B. Saunders, 1984, pp 278–281

59. Ellison RC, Peckham GJ, Lang P, et al.: Evaluation of the preterm infant for patent ductus arteriosus. Pediatrics 71:364, 1983

60. Green TP, Thompson TR, Johson DE, et al.: Furosemide promotes patent ductus arteriosus in premature infants with the respiratory distress syndrome. N Engl J Med 308:743, 1983

61. Bell EF, Warburton D, Stonestreet BS, et al.: Effect of fluid administration on the development of symptomatic patent ductus arteriosus and congestive heart failure in premature infants. N Engl J Med 302:598, 1980

62. Mikhail M, Lee W, Toews W, et al.: Surgical and medical experience with 734 premature infants with patent ductus arteriosus. J Thorac Cardiovasc Surg 83:349, 1982

63. Olley P, Coceani F: Use of prostaglandins in cardiopulmonary diseases of the newborn. Semin Perinatol 4:135, 1980

64. Levene ME, Fawer CL, Lamont RF: Risk factors in the development of intraventricular haemorrhage in the preterm neonate. Arch Dis Child 57:410, 1982

65. Ment LR, Duncan CC, Ehrenkranz RA, et al.: Intraventricular hemorrhage in the preterm neonate: Timing and cerebral blood flow changes. J Pediatr 104:419, 1984

66. Perlman JM, Volpe JJ: Intraventricular hemorrhage in extremely small premature infants. Am J Dis Child 140:1122, 1986

67. Volpe JJ: Current concepts in neonatal medicine: Neonatal intraventricular hemorrhage. N Engl J Med 304:886, 1981

68. Pape KE, Wigglesworth JS: Haemorrhage, Ischemia and the Perinatal Brain. Philadelphia: J.B. Lippincott, 1979

69. Lou HC, Lassen NA, Friis-Hansen B: Impaired autoregulation of cerebral blood flow in the distressed newborn infant. J Pediatr 94:118, 1979

70. Fujimura M, Salisbury DM, Robinson RO, et al.: Clinical events relating to intraventricular haemorrhage in the newborn. Arch Dis Child 54:409, 1979

71. Gilles FH, Price RA, Kerry SV, et al.: Fibrinolytic activity in the ganglionic eminence of the premature human brain. Biol Neonate 18:426, 1971

72. McDonald MM, Johnson ML, Rumack CM, et al.: Role of coagulopathy in newborn intracranial hemorrhage. Pediatrics 74:26, 1984

73. Lesko SM, Mitchell AA, Epstein MF, et al.: Heparin use as a risk factor for intraventricular hemorrhage in low-birth-weight infants. N Engl J Med 314:1156, 1986

74. McDonald MM, Koops BL, Johnson ML, et al.: Timing and antecedents of intracranial hemorrhage in the newborn. Pediatrics 74:32, 1984

75. Wheeler AS, Sadri S, Gutsche BB, et al.: Intracranial hemorrhage following intravenous administration of sodium bicarbonate or saline solution in the newborn lamb asphyxiated in utero. Anesthesiology 51:517, 1979

76. Fanconi S, Duc G: Intratracheal suctioning in sick preterm infants: Prevention of intracranial hypertension and cerebral hypoperfusion by muscle paralysis. Pediatrics 79:538, 1987

77. Friesen RH, Honda AT, Thieme RE: Changes in anterior fontanel pressure in preterm infants during tracheal intubation. Anesth Analg 66:874, 1987

78. Perlman JM, Goodman S, Kreusser KL, et al.: Reduction in intraventricular hemorrhage by elimination of fluctuating cerebral blood flow velocity in preterm infants with respiratory distress syndrome. N Engl J Med 312:1353, 1985

79. Freisen RH, Honda AT, Thieme RE: Perianesthetic intracranial hemorrhage in preterm neonates. Anesthesiology 67:814, 1987
80. Strange MJ, Myers G, Kirklin JK, et al.: Surgical closure of the patent ductus arteriosus does not increase the risk of intraventricular haemorrhage in the preterm infant. J Pediatr 107:602, 1985
81. Donn SM, Roloff DW, Goldstein GW: Prevention of intraventricular haemorrhage in preterm infants by phenobarbitone. Lancet 2:215, 1981
82. Friesen RH, Thieme RE, Honda AT, et al.: Changes in anterior fontanel pressure in preterm neonates receiving isoflurane, halothane, fentanyl, or ketamine. Anesth Analg 66:431, 1987
83. Berry FA, Gregory GA: Do premature infants require anesthesia for surgery? Anesthesiology 67:291, 1987
84. Kattwinkel J: Apnea in the neonatal period. Pediatr Rev 2:115, 1980
85. Welborn LG, DeSoto H, Hannallah RS, et al.: The use of caffeine in the control of postanesthetic apnea in former premature infants. Anesthesiology 68:796, 1988
86. Welborn LG, Ramirez N, Oh TH, et al.: Postanesthetic apnea and periodic breathing in infants. Anesthesiology 65:658, 1986
87. Gregory GA, Steward DJ: Life-threatening perioperative apnea in the ex-"premie." Anesthesiology 59:495, 1983
88. Aranda JV, Gorman WB, Bergsteinsson H, et al.: Efficacy of caffeine in the treatment of apnea in the low-birthweight infant. J Pediatr 90:467, 1977
89. Aranda JV, Gorman W, Outerbridge EW: Pharmacokinetic disposition of caffeine in premature neonates with apnea (abstract). Pediatr Res 11:414, 1977
90. Aranda JV, Trumen T: Methylaxanthines in apnea of prematurity. Clin Perinatol 6:87, 1979
91. Durand DJ, Goodman A, Ray P, et al.: Theophylline treatment in the extubation of infants weighing less than 1250 grams: A controlled trial. Pediatrics 80:684, 1987
92. Brooks JG: Apnea of infancy and sudden infant death syndrome. Am J Dis Child 136:1012, 1982
93. Kinsey VE, Arnold HJ, Kalina RE, et al.: PaO_2 levels and retrolental fibroplasia: A report of the cooperative study. Pediatrics 60:655, 1977
94. Shohat M, Reisner SH, Krikler R, et al.: Retinopathy of prematurity: Incidence and risk factors. Pediatrics 72:159, 1983
95. Weiter JJ: Retrolental fibroplasia: An unsolved problem. N Engl J Med 305:1404, 1981
96. Betts EK, Downes JJ, Schaffer DB, et al.: Retrolental fibroplasia and oxygen administration during general anesthesia. Anesthesiology 47:518, 1977
97. Phibbs RH: Oxygen therapy: A continuing hazard to the premature infant. Anesthesiology 147:486, 1977
98. Lucey JF, Dangman B: A reexamination of the role of oxygen in retrolental fibroplasia. Pediatrics 73:82, 1984
99. Behrman RE, Vaughan VC III (eds): Nelson Textbook of Pediatrics, 12th ed. Philadelphia: W.B. Saunders, 1983
100. Martyn LT: Pediatric ophthalmology. In: Behrman RE, Vaughan VC III (eds): Nelson Textbook of Pediatrics, 12th ed. Philadelphia: W.B. Saunders, 1983, pp 1761–1762
101. Tsai B: Anesthetic considerations in the premature infant. Clinical Proceedings, Children's Hospital National Medical Center, Washington, D.C. 35:279, 1979
102. Smith RM: Anesthesia for Infants and Children, 4th ed. St. Louis: C.V. Mosby, 1980, p 175
103. Goldsmith JP, Karotkin EH: Appendices 23, 24, and 31. In: Goldsmith JP, Karotkin EH (eds): Assisted Ventilation of the Neonate, 2nd ed. Philadelphia: W.B. Saunders, 1988, pp 448, 449, 455
104. Goldsmith JP, Karotkin EH: Appendix 5. In: Goldsmith JP, Karotkin EH (eds): Assisted Ventilation of the Neonate, 2nd ed. Philadelphia: W.B. Saunders, 1988, p 434
105. Eger EI, Saidman LJ: Hazards of nitrous oxide anesthesia in bowel obstruction and pneumothorax. Anesthesiology 26:61, 1965
106. Goldsmith JP, Karotkin EH: Appendix 25. In: Goldsmith JP, Karotkin EH (eds): Assisted Ventilation of the Neonate, 2nd ed. Philadelphia: W.B. Saunders, 1988, pp 450, 451
107. Eger EI: Atropine, scopolamine and related compounds. Anesthesiology 23:365, 1965
108. Anand KJS, Sippell WG, Aynsley-Green A: Randomised trial of fentanyl anaesthesia

in preterm babies undergoing surgery: Effects of the stress response. Lancet 1:243, 1987

109. Gregory GA, Eger EI, Munson ES: The relationship between age and halothane requirement in man. Anesthesiology 30:488, 1969
110. Govaerts MJM, Sanders M: Induction and recovery with enflurane and halothane in paediatric anaesthesia. Br J Anaesth 47:877, 1975
111. Cameron CB, Robinson S, Gregory GA: The minimum anesthetic concentration of isoflurane in children. Anesth Analg 63:418, 1984
112. Diaz JH, Marino RJ: Intraoperative management. In: Goldsmith JP, Karotkin EH (eds): Assisted Ventilation of the Neonate, 2nd ed. Philadelphia: W.B. Saunders, 1988, pp 357–375
113. Nicodemus HF, Nassiri-Rahimi C, Bachman L, et al.: Median effective doses (ED 50) of halothane in infants and children. Anesthesiology 31:344, 1969
114. Vivori E: Induction and maintenance of anaesthesia. In: Rees GT, Gray TC (eds): Paediatric Anaesthesia: Trends in Current Practice. London: Butterworths, 1981, pp 101–114
115. McDermott RW, Stanley TH: The cardiovascular effects of low concentrations of nitrous oxide during morphine anesthesia. Anesthesiology 41:89, 1974
116. Stead AL: The response of the newborn infant to muscle relaxants. Br J Anaesth 27:124, 1955
117. Nightingale DA, Glass AG, Bachman L: Neuromuscular blockade by succinylcholine in children. Anesthesiology 27:736, 1966
118. Cook DR, Wingard LB, Taylor FH: Pharmacokinetics of succinylcholine in infants, children, and adults. Clin Pharmacol Ther 20:493, 1976
119. Cook DR: Muscle relaxants in infants and children. Anesth Analg 60:335, 1981
120. Nelson TE, Flewellen EJ: Current concepts: The malignant hyperthermia syndrome. N Engl J Med 309:416, 1983
121. Goudsouzian NG: Maturation of neuromuscular transmission in the infant. Br J Anaesth 52:205, 1980
122. Kupferberg HJ, Way EL: Pharmacologic basis for the increased sensitivity of the newborn rat to morphine. J Pharmacol Exp Ther 141:105, 1963
123. Carmichael EB: The median lethal dose (LD_{50}) of pentothal sodium for both young and old guinea pigs and rats. Anesthesiology 8:589, 1947
124. Way WL, Costley EC, Way EL: Respiratory sensitivity of the newborn infant to meperidine and morphine. Clin Pharmacol Ther 6:454, 1965
125. Lynn AM, Slattery JT: Morphine pharmacokinetics in early infancy. Anesthesiology 66:136, 1987
126. Koehntop DE, Rodman JH, Brundage DM, et al.: Pharmacokinetics of fentanyl in neonates. Anesth Analg 65:227, 1986
127. Collins C, Koren G, Crean P, et al.: Fentanyl pharmacokinetics and hemodynamic effects in preterm infants during ligation of patent ductus arteriosus. Anesth Analg 64:1078, 1985
128. Davis PJ, Cook DR, Stiller RL, et al.: Pharmacodynamics and pharmacokinetics of high-dose sufentanil in infants and children undergoing cardiac surgery. Anesth Analg 66:203, 1987
129. Greeley WJ, deBruijin NP, Davis DP: Sufentanil pharmacokinetics in pediatric cardiovascular patients. Anesth Analg 66:1067, 1987
130. White PF, Way WL, Trevor AJ: Ketamine—Its pharmacology and therapeutic uses. Anesthesiology 56:119, 1982
131. Morgan BC: Complications from intravascular catheters. Am J Dis Child 138:425, 1984
132. Rendell-Baker L, Soucek DH: New paediatric face masks and anaesthetic equipment. Br Med J 1:1690, 1962
133. Diaz JH: Further modifications of the Miller blade for difficult pediatric laryngoscopy. Anesthesiology 60:612, 1984
134. Spitzer AR, Fox WW: The use of oral versus nasal endotracheal tubes in newborn infants. J Calif Perinat Assoc 4:32, 1984
135. Swedlow DB, Stern S: Continuous noninvasive oxygen saturation monitoring in children with a new pulse-oximeter. Crit Care Med 11:228, 1983
136. Ayre P: Anaesthesia for intracranial operation. Lancet 1:561–563, 1937
137. Rees GJ: Anaesthesia in the newborn. Br Med J 2:1419, 1950

138. Mapleson WW: The elimination of rebreathing in various semi-closed anaesthetic systems. Br J Anaesth 26:323–332, 1954
139. Bain JA, Spoerel WE: Flow requirements for a modified Mapleson D system during controlled ventilation. Can Anaesth Soc J 20:629–636, 1973
140. Peevy KJ, Hall MW: Transcutaneous oxygen monitoring: Economic impact on neonatal care. Pediatrics 75:1065–1067, 1985
141. Rooth G, Huch A, Huch R: Transcutaneous oxygen monitors are reliable indicators of arterial oxygen tension (if used correctly). Pediatrics 79:283, 1987
142. Badgwell JM, McLeod ME, Lerman J, et al.: End-tidal P_{CO_2} measurements sampled at the distal and proximal ends of the endotracheal tube in infants and children. Anesth Analg 66:959, 1987
143. Lindahl SGE, Yates AP, Hatch DJ: Relationship between invasive and noninvasive measurements of gas exchange in anesthetized infants and children. Anesthesiology 66:168, 1987
144. Bucher HU, Fanconi S, Fallenstein F, et al.: Transcutaneous carbon dioxide tension in newborn infants: Reliability and safety of continuous 24-hour measurements at 42°C. Pediatrics 78:631, 1986
145. Furman EB, Roman GD, Lemmer LAS, et al.: Specific therapy in water, electrolyte, and blood-volume replacement during pediatric surgery. Anesthesiology 42:187, 1975
146. Furman EB: Blood and fluid replacement for paediatric patients. In: Steward DJ (ed): Some Aspects of Paediatric Anaesthesia. Amsterdam: Excerpta Medica, 1982, pp 79–100
147. Hassan SZ: Caudal anesthesia in infants. Anesth Analg 56:686, 1977
148. Takasaki M, Dohi S, Kawabata Y, et al.: Dosage of lidocaine for caudal anesthesia in infants and children. Anesthesiology 47:527, 1977
149. Abajian JC, Mellish RWP, Browne AF, et al.: Spinal anesthesia for surgery in the high-risk infant. Anesth Analg 63:359, 1984
150. Blaise G, Roy WL: Spinal anesthesia in children. Anesth Analg 63:1140, 1984
151. Morishima HO, Finster M, Pedersen H, et al.: Pharmacokinetics of lidocaine in fetal and neonatal lambs and adult sheep. Anesthesiology 50:431, 1979
152. LeDez KM, Strong A, Reider M, et al.: Effect of age on the pharmacokinetics of intravenous lidocaine in pediatrics. Anesthesiology 67:A500, 1987
153. LeDez KM, Swartz J, Strong A, et al.: The effect of age on the serum concentration of alpha-1 acid glycoprotein in newborns, infants, and children. Anesthesiology 65:A421, 1986
154. Aldrete JA, Kroulik D: A postanesthetic recovery score. Anesth Analg 49:924, 1974

12. Perioperative Management of Neonatal Emergencies

Robert M. Arensman, M.D.

INTRODUCTION

In the field of pediatric surgery, neonates are the patients furthest removed from the realm of general surgery, having a series of unique surgical problems that are encountered only in the neonatal period and never again (see Table 11–6). In addition, physiologic and surgical responses are different for this group of patients. Neonatal surgery is often performed in the first week of life in unstable infants compromised by patent ductus arteriosus, pulmonary hypertension, electrolyte imbalance, and metabolic stress.

As a child matures, surgical illnesses and their pathophysiologic manifestations will more closely resemble those encountered in adults.

322

As this happens, pediatric perioperative care begins to resemble adult perioperative care. During the neonatal period, however, only special attention to unique surgical diagnoses and pathophysiologic reactions will improve chances of successful surgical outcome and long-term survival. A discussion of perioperative management of neonatal emergencies follows and focuses on preparation and diagnostic evaluation of neonates with surgical diseases. Postoperative and postsurgical management techniques are presented and discussed in Chapter 14.

PREOPERATIVE STABILIZATION AND MANAGEMENT OF SURGICAL ILLNESSES IN NEONATES

Before making specific surgical diagnoses and planning their operative management, the pediatric surgeon's attention is directed to the preoperative stabilization and management of surgical illnesses in neonates. Such attention includes the selection and establishment of intravenous access; intravenous fluid and electrolyte therapy; parenteral antibiotic therapy; intravascular monitoring; gastric decompression; and the insertion of chest tubes, urinary catheters, and endotracheal tubes when indicated.

Intravenous Access

Intravenous infusions should be established preoperatively in neonates with major thoracoabdominal illnesses needing surgical therapy. In the term neonate, intravenous line placement is not usually a major problem. Subcutaneous veins are often easily seen, lie close to the skin's surface, and are not obscured by the layer of subcutaneous fat that becomes so prominent in children between 6 months and 2 years of age. Veins on the dorsum of the hands, scalp, and dorsal and lateral surfaces of the feet and especially the greater saphenous veins at the ankles are often easily identified and can be cannulated with 22- to 24-gauge intravenous catheters. In larger babies, 20-gauge intravenous catheters can often be inserted percutaneously into greater saphenous veins without the need for cutdowns. Nontapered, silastic intravenous catheter-over-the-needle units are preferred to butterfly needles or tapered catheters.

Intravenous Fluid and Electrolyte Therapy

Electrolyte abnormalities are rare within hours of birth unless the neonate has been vomiting since delivery. However, hypoglycemia is not unusual within hours of birth because of stress-increased consumption of limited hepatic glycogen and is best prevented by administering intravenous glucose solutions during careful monitoring of serum glucose concentrations. Surgical illnesses contraindicate fluid restriction during the first 24 to 48 hours of newborn life, and increased intravenous hydration is often required to maintain adequate organ and tissue perfusion and restore circulatory volume. In older neonates with acute surgical illnesses, especially gastric outlet obstructions (e.g., pyloric stenosis, duodenal atresia, annular pancreas), hypoglycemia is less of a problem than major electrolyte and acid–base disturbances, particularly hypochloremic, hypokalemic metabolic alkalosis. Suspected derangements in serum electrolytes and acid–base status should be confirmed by laboratory determinations and corrected preoperatively by accurate replacement of calculated deficits in serum electrolytes and circulating fluid volume.

Hyperalimentation is rarely indicated in the perioperative management of neonates except in babies with intractable gastroesophageal reflux or prolonged vomiting from pyloric stenosis. Significant malnutrition in such cases could make immediate operative correction hazardous and, perhaps, inadvisable. In cases in which surgery can be safely deferred, preoperative intravenous alimentation to restore nutrition and nitrogen balance may reduce postoperative wound complications, intestinal malabsorption, and adynamic ileus. Such markers of adequate nutrition as serum albumin, serum prealbumin, and total lymphocyte count can be monitored to determine adequate protein repletion prior to operation and permit better timing of elective surgery.

Intravascular Monitoring

Invasive vascular monitors, like central venous and intra-arterial catheters for pressure monitoring and blood gas determinations, have been used less frequently in neonates than in older children and adults with comparable surgical illnesses. In the past, limited availability of small-bore catheters made invasive monitoring in neonates technically difficult and unfeasible. Several companies now supply small-bore central monitoring cannulas that can be inserted percutaneously into the subclavian or jugular (external or internal) veins over previously inserted guide wires. Our experience indicates that central venous catheters can be reliably inserted in neonates weighing as little as 500 g. Intra-arterial catheters are also easily placed percutaneously in larger children or by cutdown in smaller infants and premature neonates. Vascular catheters currently available for intravenous insertion are also appropriate for use as arterial lines, usually in gauges 20 to 24. Commonly used safe sites for arterial cannulation include the radial, dorsalis pedis, and posterior tibial arteries. More rarely, the ulnar artery is cannulated. The superficial temporal arteries are easily located just anterior to the ear, but their cannulation carries an increased risk of ischemic injury to the external ears, may be associated with intracranial bleeding, and is no longer recommended for intra-arterial monitoring in neonates. A reliable Allen's test is difficult to conduct in neonates prior to radial artery cannulation because a neonate cannot maintain a clenched fist for long or on command. Nevertheless, both distal end arteries should be identified by palpation or by Doppler ultrasound before intra-arterial catheters are inserted at the wrist or at the ankle. In a modified Allen's test, the artery to be cannulated can be compressed and, with distal flow occluded, skin color in an area of collateral circulation can be noted to ensure long-term distal perfusion to the hand or foot demonstrating adequacy of collateral perfusion. Despite adequate collateral circulation in an ipsilateral extremity, reinstitution of intra-arterial monitoring should be in the contralateral extremity. Femoral and brachial arterial pressure monitoring has been associated with ischemic complications distally and loss of digits, arms, and legs. Recently, transcutaneous oxygen saturation monitors have offered an alternative to invasive arterial monitoring, especially in neonates showing steady improvement with diminishing oxygen requirements or with poor peripheral circulation.

Gastric Decompression

Gastric decompression is easily achieved in neonates but often delayed or forgotten in seriously ill neonates, with deleterious results. Continuous sump tubes, sizes 8 to 10 French, may be inserted into the stomach through the nose or mouth in premature infants to produce greater efficiency in removing intragastric gas and fluid than single-lumen Levine or feeding tubes. Although sumps can be connected to intermittent suction, they are designed for continuous low-pressure or Venturi suction with little risk of occlusion or mucosal irritation. Migration of gastric tubes due to continuous manipulation by the infant's tongue is reduced when the tube is placed through the nose. Neonates breathing spontaneously, however, may be better suited for orogastric decompression, reserving both nares for nasal breathing.

In the past, tube gastrostomy inserted under local anesthesia was a reliable method of gastric decompression.[1] Fewer open gastrostomies are now performed in neonates because of improvements in transnasal or transoral gastric decompression. Nevertheless, surgical gastrostomy continues to play a role in gastric decompression, providing a larger lumen for gastric decompression, a more secure method of tube fixation, and easy access to the distal gastrointestinal tract for long-term enteral alimentation.

Chest Tubes

Tube thoracostomy is a simple but highly effective minor surgical technique that can prove lifesaving when fluid or air is accumulating under tension in the thoracic cavity. Midline mediastinal structures are highly mobile in neonates and can shift easily into the contralateral hemithorax during tension pneumothorax, occluding venous return to the heart, reducing cardiac output, and often precipitating cardiac arrest. In acute tension pneumothorax, thoracostomy with large-bore catheter-over-the-needle devices (gauges 14 to 18) will decompress the hemithorax quickly and restore cardiac output. In elective thoracostomy, a standard chest tube (sizes 8 to 16 French) may be inserted. Most chest tubes have end and side ports for efficient gas or fluid removal, radiopaque markers for radiographic confirmation of intrathoracic placement, and grooves or flanges to assist their external fixation at the chest wall.

Although the general principles of chest tube placement (high in the chest for air drainage and low in the chest for fluid drainage) are sound, previous recommendations that chest tubes for air egress should be inserted in the midclavicular line through the pectoralis major muscle are no longer recommended for the following reasons. First, larger neonates have substantial pectoralis muscle masses, which can make correct identification of intercostal spaces difficult. Second, tube thoracostomy on the anterior chest wall may result in insertion through the breast bud or the axillary tail of Spence, causing subsequent breast disfigurement or scarring, abscess formation, or traumatic fat necrosis. Chest tube placement at the lateral edge of the pectoralis major muscle allows insertion in a thinner area of the chest wall that contains only skin, subcutaneous tissue, and intercostal muscle. This site of insertion allows the resulting scar to be hidden beneath the arm.

Once a thoracostomy tube is placed, its end should be sealed immediately by placing it beneath a water seal. A pneumothorax may persist during drainage without suction, but tension pneumothorax and mediastinal shift will not occur. Most infants and children can easily survive a pneumothorax without tension until suction is placed on the chest tube. Chest tube suction for air and fluid is usually achieved by using one of the commercially available chest tube suction chambers that incorporate a water seal, a suction chamber, and a collection chamber all in one. When connected to continuous suction, modern chest drain devices will maintain slightly negative intrathoracic pressure, clear fluid and gas from the pleural space, measure chest tube drainage, and maintain suction force at a safely preset level.

Urinary Catheter

Most neonates, including the smallest premature infants, may now have their urinary bladders catheterized with appropriately gauged Foley catheters (sizes 3 to 6 French). The risks of urosepsis and urethral stricture, especially in males, makes long-term bladder catheterization hazardous, but short-term perioperative catheterization is often indicated during rapid fluid loss and replacement therapy.

Endotracheal Intubation

Securing the upper airway by endotracheal intubation permits effective ventilation and ensures tissue oxygenation. For brief periods, it often is sufficient to maintain gas exchange by bag-and-mask ventilation. A mask of proper size and fit encompassing the nose and mouth is required, along with a rebreathing bag and oxygen source. Although ventilatory stabilization of neonates with acute surgical illnesses may be achieved in this manner, conversion to endotracheal tube and bag ventilation or mechanical ventilation may be required. In most cases, orotracheal intubation is quicker and easier than nasotracheal intubation. Bilateral breath sounds and equal chest excursions are good indicators of correct endotracheal tube placement, but radiographic confirmation is also recommended, especially if the neonate will require long-term mechanical ventilation.

In rare cases of intubation failure or airway anomalies in neonates, cricothyroid puncture or tracheostomy may be indicated in apneic neonates. A catheter-over-the-needle unit (gauges 18 to 22) may be inserted through the cricothyroid membrane and its central needle removed, leaving its outer catheter in place for connection to a 5.0-mm endotracheal tube adapter for oxygen insufflation. Cricothyroid puncture does not provide effective ventilation, only a temporary source of oxygen until a more reliable access for carbon dioxide removal can be established, usually an endotracheal tube or tracheostomy.[2-4]

The ease and success of endotracheal intubation have virtually eliminated the need for emergency tracheostomy in neonates. A controlled tracheostomy over a previously inserted endotracheal tube is preferred to a blind stab wound in the neck of an apneic neonate. Recent experience suggests that neonates may remain intubated endotracheally for several months without major damage to the trachea or need for tracheostomy. If there is concern about potential tracheal damage during prolonged intubation, periodic bronchoscopy will permit complete evaluation of the vocal cords, tracheal mucosa, and tracheal cartilages. If progressive damage is noted, upper airway access may be converted from an endotracheal tube to a tracheostomy, again with an endotracheal tube in place to guide the surgeon and provide full perioperative control of the upper airway.

CLASSIFICATION OF NEONATAL SURGICAL EMERGENCIES

In general, neonatal surgical emergencies may be classified into two major groups by anatomy and clinical presentation. Thoracic emergencies begin with respiratory distress and hypoxemia; abdominal emergencies begin with abdominal distention and bilious vomiting. Thoracic lesions are frequently more emergent than abdominal disorders because of acute respiratory failure. Thoracic emergencies to be considered include diaphragmatic hernia, tracheoesophageal fistula, congenital lobar emphysema, cystic adenomatoid malformation, intrathoracic masses (pulmonary sequestration and bronchogenic cysts), and patent ductus arteriosus. Abdominal emergencies to be considered include anterior abdominal wall defects (gastroschisis/omphalocele), small bowel obstruction (duodenal stenosis/atresia, jejunoileal atresia, malrotation, or meconium ileus), and colonic obstructions (Hirschsprung's disease, meconium plug syndrome, and hypoplastic left colon syndrome).

Thoracic Surgical Emergencies in Neonates

Congenital Diaphragmatic Hernia. Congenital diaphragmatic hernia (CDH) with onset of respiratory failure at birth has one of the most dramatic presentations of all thoracic surgical emergencies in neonates.[5-8] Neonates in gravest danger are deeply cyanotic and make no respiratory effort. Neonates in less severe respiratory failure manifest varying degrees of tachypnea and cyanosis. Rarely, a neonate with CDH shows no symptoms during the first few hours or even days of life. These children with late onset of respiratory symptoms generally have small diaphragmatic defects. This group may also have defects on the right side where the liver blocks significant herniation of abdominal contents into the right hemithorax. In general, neonates who develop diaphragmatic hernia after the first day of life recover quickly after surgical repairs without pulmonary hypertension or prolonged respiratory failure.

Infants in acute respiratory distress from CDH at birth require prompt surgical evaluation and management. Before the hernia can be reduced and the hemidiaphragm repaired, the immediate management of acute respiratory failure includes tracheal intubation for mechanical ventilation with rapid ventilatory rates and low peak inspired pressures. Ventilator-induced respiratory alkalosis with hyperoxygenation has now been shown to improve the systemic acidosis, hypoxemia, and pulmonary hypertension that characterize large diaphragmatic defects. The goal of preoperative mechanical hyperventilation in CDH is to achieve the highest possible PaO_2, lower the $PaCO_2$ gradually to 25 to 35 mmHg, and maintain serum pH above 7.45 by a combination of hyperventilation and intravenous sodium bicarbonate therapy. In other words, the goal is to control persistent pulmonary hypertension.[9]

With respiratory failure stabilized, insertion of reliable intravenous and arterial lines may follow. Pulmonary hypertension with CDH causes massive right-to-left shunting of unoxygenated blood across the patent ductus arteriosus, away from the lungs, and into the aorta and systemic circulation. Consequently, only the right radial artery will consistently provide preductal arterial blood for gas analysis, while the umbilical artery provides postductal arterial blood for analysis. Many studies, however, have reported survival results and treatment protocols in CDH based on postductal arterial gas determinations from the umbilical artery or lower extremities.[10] Preductal and postductal arterial monitoring sites may be desirable for differential arterial blood gas comparisons to detect and quantitate pulmonary shunting after CDH repair. A combination of a preductal arterial line and a postductal transcutaneous oximeter will provide a less invasive but equally reliable shunt study.

Tension pneumothorax frequently complicates ventilatory management in CDH because of the high inspired pressures required to inflate the lungs, both of which are compressed by bowel contents (ipsilateral lung) or mediastinal structures (contralateral lung) and are often severely hypoplastic. Tension pneumothorax may occur in either side of the chest in CDH, causing loss of breath sounds on the affected side, mediastinal shifting into the opposite hemithorax, and cardiovascular collapse from insufficient venous return. A chest x-ray film will confirm tension pneumothorax, determine its site of origin, and direct immediate treatment. A catheter-over-the-needle unit (gauge 18 to 22) should be inserted quickly above one of the ribs high on the breathless hemithorax and its central needle removed to decompress the lung, release trapped air, and confirm the diagnosis of tension pneumothorax. Placement of the proper sized thoracostomy tube follows when the neonate is stabilized. Prophylactic insertion of a chest tube in the contralateral hemithorax is often recommended before air evacuation of neonates with CDH to regional neonatal centers or after vigorous cardiopulmonary resuscitation with prolonged delivery of high inspired pressures by rebreathing bags or mechanical ventilators.

Following surgical reduction of the thoracic hernia and primary or patch repair of the hemidiaphragm, a chest tube is often placed on the affected side to allow fluid drainage and maintain a centrally located mediastinum. Postoperatively, the mediastinum often shifts to occupy the void created by a hemithorax emptied of its abdominal contents and minimally occupied by a hypoplastic lung. Air added to or withdrawn from the chest tube will keep the heart and mediastinum in a central position, promoting adequate venous return and maximizing cardiac output.

A gastric tube should be inserted as soon as possible in all neonates with CDH to decompress the stomach, which is often distended by positive-pressure ventilation, and to reduce the air and fluid contents of the viscera in the thoracic hernia (Fig. 12–1). In the past, a gastric tube inserted preoperatively in neonates with CDH would have been replaced

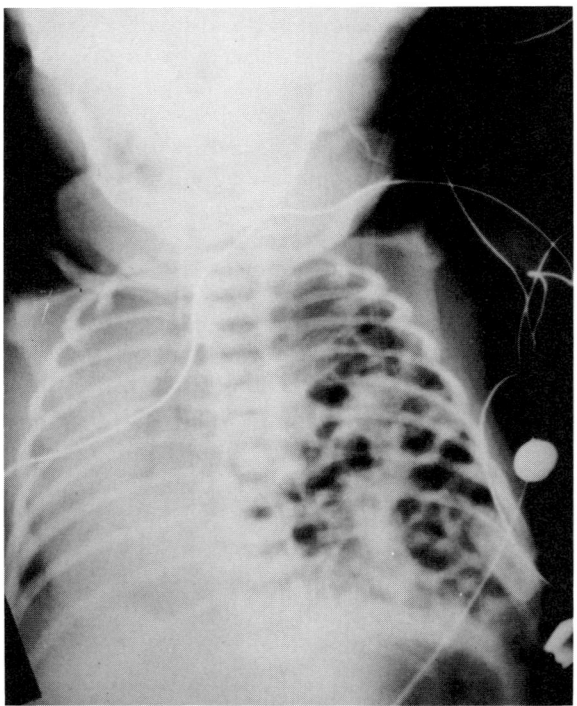

FIGURE 12–1. Chest radiograph showing common left-sided congenital diaphragmatic hernia with distended gastric shadow and multiple air-filled loops of small bowel in the left hemithorax.

with a gastrostomy in the postoperative period. However, with the recent introduction of postoperative anticoagulation for extracorporeal membrane oxygenation (ECMO), incidental operations like gastrostomy and appendectomy are often eliminated after CDH repair to lessen the likelihood of hemorrhage should anticoagulation for ECMO become necessary. Postoperative gastrostomy following CDH repair should be reserved for neonates with specific indications for gastrostomy, such as coexisting gastrointestinal anomalies.

Bladder drainage by Foley catheter is not routinely required in children with CDH because most neonates are able to void into an external collection bag for monitoring of urinary output. Of course, bladder catheterization must be individualized in every case depending on hemodynamic status.

Tracheoesophageal Fistula. Tracheoesophageal fistula (TEF) may present as one of four common varieties, all characterized by varying degrees of esophageal atresia and/or fistula connections between a trachea and esophagus.[11, 12] Neonates with TEF may have minimal symptoms or profound respiratory embarrassment. In the common forms of TEF, respiratory distress begins when orogastric secretions spill into the tracheobronchial tree, causing aspiration pneumonitis and bronchospasm.

Once the diagnosis of TEF in a neonate is entertained, an oral sump tube placed in the proximal esophagus will prevent spillage of saliva from the obstructed esophagus into the trachea (Fig. 12–2). Esophageal obstruction in TEF may be due to a blind esophageal pouch in 87% of cases (Fig. 12–2) or to an esophageal atresia. Since the more common varieties of TEF do not have an esophagus patent to the stomach, gastric decompression usually is impossible. Should abdominal distention and restricted ventilation occur in TEF with a blind esophageal pouch, a decompressive gastrostomy for drainage of gastric contents is necessary. If esophageal suction is instituted quickly in neonates with TEF, the need for immediate gastric decompression by gastrostomy is often lessened. Historically, the repair of a TEF began with decompressive gastrostomy before right thoracotomy. Now attention to anesthetic technique with careful positioning of the endotracheal tube tip (above the carina but below the fistula) and low peak inspiratory pressures permits a safer approach to the fistula without first decompressing the stomach. Once the fistula is divided, further distention of the gastrointestinal tract from positive-pressure ventilation does not occur. A nasogastric tube may be positioned carefully across the esophageal anasto-

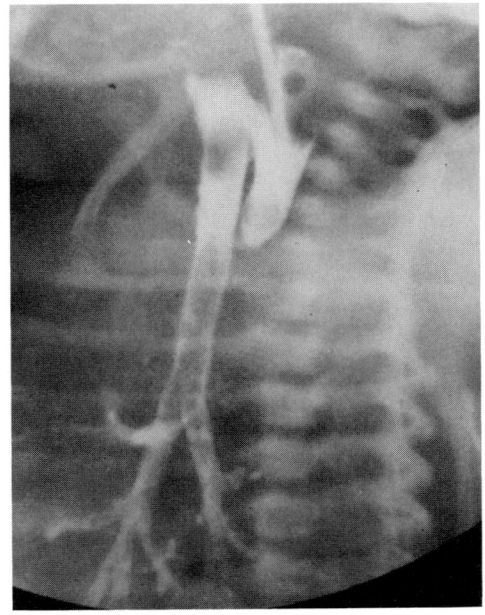

FIGURE 12–2. Most common form of tracheoesophageal fistula (C-type) with small amount of radiographic contrast material in the blind proximal esophageal pouch and tracheobronchial tree.

mosis during surgery, with its tip in the stomach for postoperative gastric drainage. If, however, the nasogastric tube is accidentally withdrawn postoperatively, great care must be taken in reinserting it because of the risk of esophageal perforation.

Immediate endotracheal intubation in neonates with TEF is often unnecessary unless the infant is very premature or has severe underlying lung disease or aspiration pneumonitis. Term neonates with excessive salivation and TEF identified shortly after birth may be easily managed preoperatively with esophageal pouch decompression and intravenous hydration. Careful attention to pouch decompression usually prevents aspiration pneumonia and allows adequate time for further diagnostic evaluation before unhurried TEF repair.

Premature neonates and infants with severe underlying lung disease or aspiration pneumonitis may often require prolonged endotracheal intubation for mechanical ventilation postoperatively. Since surgical repair of TEF leaves a fresh suture line on the posterior wall of the trachea, tracheal extubation is desirable as soon as possible postoperatively to avoid further tracheal trauma. Term neonates with stable cardiopulmonary status and no preexisting lung disease may have their tracheas extubated at the completion of uncomplicated TEF repair. Of course, if tracheal reintubation is indicated in the postoperative period, it must be performed with extreme care to prevent tracheal perforation at the suture line.

Central venous, urinary, and intra-arterial catheters are all useful adjuncts in unstable patients with TEF, but none of these monitors is used routinely in uncomplicated TEF repairs. Transcutaneous oxygen saturation monitoring is useful to confirm adequate tissue perfusion and oxygenation. Postoperative care and monitoring may be modified as necessary should the neonate develop postsurgical complications, hemodynamic instability, or respiratory compromise from unrecognized lung disease.

Congenital Lobar Emphysema and Cystic Adenomatoid Malformation. Congenital lobar emphysema (CLE) and cystic adenomatoid malformation (CAM) are two neonatal thoracic emergencies characterized by lung hyperinflation that are difficult to differentiate clinically and radiographically.[13–15] In CLE, air trapping occurs within one or more lung lobes at birth, producing obstructive emphysema (Fig. 12–3). Air trapping in CLE is usually limited to the upper lobes (see Fig. 12–3). CAM is also lobar in its distribution but is generally confined to one or more lower lobes. In CAM, cystic dilatation of the lower lobes with air and fluid produces lobar hyperexpansion. As a result of lobar hyperexpansion in both CLE and CAM, adjacent mediastinal structures such as the heart and the contralateral heart are compressed and displaced.

Tachypnea, tachycardia, and inadequate cardiac preload are the most

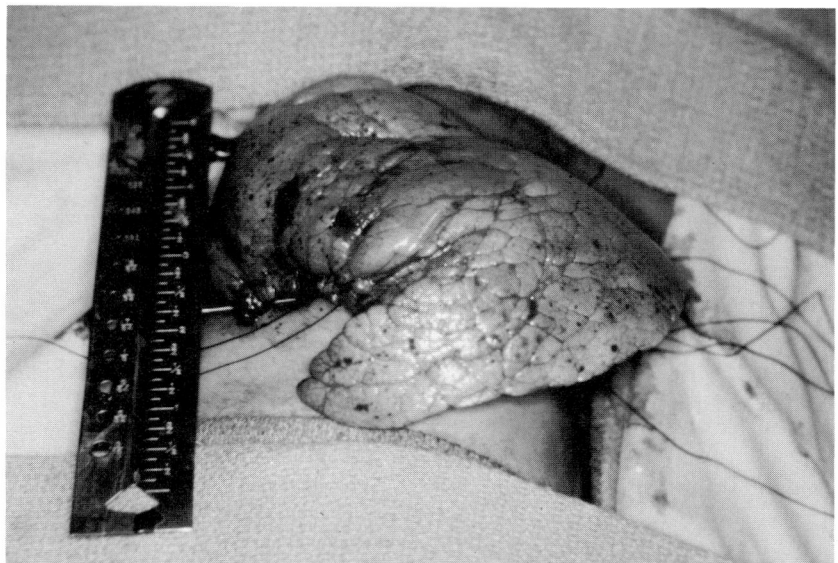

FIGURE 12–3. Overexpanded left upper lobe and lingula herniated from the left chest at thoracotomy due to congenital lobar emphysema.

common presenting features in both CLE and CAM. Tracheal intubation and mechanical ventilation are often required for immediate pulmonary stabilization in CLE and CAM. Gastric distention from air swallowing will require early nasogastric decompression. The suddenness of symptom onset in CLE or CAM is often variable. Many neonates show respiratory distress at birth; others are asymptomatic for hours, days, or, rarely, for several weeks after birth. The rapidity and severity of clinical presentation in CLE or CAM will determine the timing of surgical intervention.

Overzealous ventilation by bag and mask or mechanical ventilator may actually aggravate respiratory distress in CLE or CAM by increasing air trapping and mediastinal shifting or causing tension pneumothorax. Frequently, urgent chest decompression by large-bore needle or thoracostomy tube may be needed to drain a tension pneumothorax or overdistended lobe that causes hemodynamic compromise. Although the disruption of pulmonary parenchyma during tube decompression may be lifesaving, surgical exploration of the involved hemithorax should follow immediately for definitive therapy and to stop any pulmonary hemorrhage caused by blind needle or tube insertion through the lung.

In neonates with CLE or CAM, pulmonary resection is usually necessary. Although the pulmonary tissue to be resected contributes little to respiration, intra-arterial monitoring in radial or umbilical arteries is recommended during the perioperative period for frequent blood gas measurements. Following thoracotomy and lobectomy, one or more chest tubes are inserted to drain residual fluid and air and prevent postoperative pneumothorax. Since the condition of most neonates with CLE or CAM is improved dramatically by removal of the affected lobe, intra-arterial lines are generally needed for only a short time postoperatively.

Bronchogenic Cyst and Pulmonary Sequestration. Bronchogenic cyst (BC) and pulmonary sequestration (PS) are two of the more common intrathoracic mass lesions in neonates.[16–18] Although both lesions cause congenital chest masses, they are often asymptomatic at birth and are usually diagnosed on routine chest x-ray films during evaluation of upper respiratory infections. If the mass effect of BC or PS produces respiratory distress during the neonatal period, the mass must be of sufficient size to cause normal lung displacement and compression. A paratracheal bronchogenic cyst may compromise tracheal air flow and cause expiratory stridor. More peripherally located pulmonary sequestrations will compress branch bronchi and cause bronchomalacia, atelectasis, obstructive emphysema, and expiratory wheezing.

If BC and PS are symptomatic in the neonatal period, perioperative management follows that recommended for CLE and CAM. Immediate tracheal intubation is indicated for severe respiratory compromise at birth. This is seldom the case, however, and tracheal intubation is normally performed at the time of thoracotomy. Normal pulmonary tissue is not usually damaged during the removal of a BC or PS, allowing tracheal extubation at the conclusion of uncomplicated surgery. Intra-arterial monitoring is useful for intraoperative blood gas monitoring but can be discontinued postoperatively and replaced by transcutaneous oxygen saturation monitoring. Thoracostomy tubes are regularly placed during chest closure to drain trapped intrathoracic fluids and air. Nasogastric decompression, if indicated preoperatively for gastric distention or during mechanical ventilation, may be discontinued in the postoperative period after tracheal extubation.

Patent Ductus Arteriosus. Patent ductus arteriosus (PDA) is a common congenital defect in neonates, especially premature neonates, and rarely requires emergency left thoracotomy for repair unless excessive left-to-right shunting causes medically unmanageable cardiorespiratory failure. The size of the PDA and the direction and flow of its shunt flow can be determined precisely by ultrasonographic examination. When medical management of PDA with fluid restriction and intravenous indomethacin fail to close the ductus, elective surgical closure is indicated to manage chronic congestive heart failure. Perioperative management in PDA ligation requires insertion of an endotracheal tube, if one is not already in place for preoperative mechanical ventilation. A dependable intravenous line is indicated for fluid therapy and transfusion if necessary. On occasion, the thin posterior wall of the patent ductus leaks or ruptures during closure. Blood loss associated with such a catastrophe is sudden and heavy, making available blood products necessary prerequisites for PDA ligation. If transcutaneous monitoring of either oxygen tension or saturation is available, a urinary catheter and intra-arterial line may not be indicated to monitor end-organ perfusion during PDA ligation.

Controversy continues about the need for a thoracostomy tube on the side of operation after PDA ligation. Neonates who are receiving only minimal ventilatory support preoperatively, have no evidence of pulmonary interstitial emphysema, and show no signs of thoracic bleeding or pleural air leak at the conclusion of surgery may have the hemithorax closed without tube drainage. On the other hand, if chances of a pneumothorax or bleeding are reasonably high, a chest tube should be inserted during closure to prevent the sudden onset of hemothorax or tension pneumothorax.

Abdominal Surgical Emergencies in Neonates

Omphalocele and Gastroschisis. Omphalocele and gastroschisis, the most common congenital defects of the anterior abdominal wall, share clinical presentations at birth. Surgical repair is more urgent in gastroschisis due to greater risks of sepsis and hypovolemic shock.[19] Both defects will require similar medical care at birth. Early nasogastric decompression of the stomach and intestines will reduce emesis and risk of aspiration. Immediate nasogastric decompression is especially critical in neonates with gastroschisis, since the abdominal defect through which herniation of abdominal viscera has occurred is frequently quite small and results in partial or total obstruction of the gastrointestinal tract. Neither condition is likely to cause respiratory problems immediately at birth, so many of these neonates do not require tracheal intubation and mechanical ventilation until surgery. Maintenance and replacement fluids are administered by a dependable intravenous line along with broad-spectrum antibiotics to prevent bacterial contamination of the exposed (gastroschisis) or membrane-draped (omphalocele) bowel loops. Surgical closure of the abdominal wall defect should follow preoperative stabilization and may be complete primary closure, as in most gastroschises and small omphaloceles, or staged reduction and secondary closure with silo placement, as in large omphaloceles.[20] Since neonates with omphalocele do have complete bowel coverage by chorioamnionic membranes, they may await unhurried, elective reduction and closure of their defects unless their omphalocele ruptures (Fig. 12–4).

Neither condition routinely demands intra-arterial monitoring, urinary drainage, or prolonged postoperative tracheal intubation and mechanical

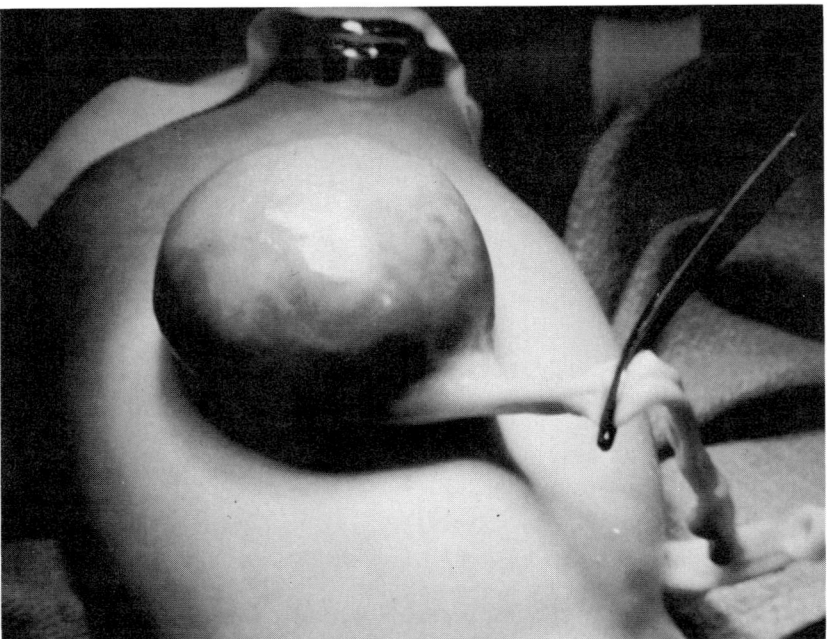

FIGURE 12-4. Preoperative photograph of moderate sized omphalocele sac containing a large portion of the liver and showing the umbilical cord attached to the lower left of the sac.

ventilation. Nasogastric decompression by nasogastric tube or, rarely, gastrostomy should be continued postoperatively until the bowel is functioning properly. Care should be taken to investigate fully for associated congenital anomalies, especially in a child with a large omphalocele, which is frequently accompanied by congenital cardiac defects.[21]

Obstructive Lesions of the Small Bowel. Obstructive lesions of the small intestines may all have a similar clinical presentation, with abdominal distention and bilious vomiting. The more common congenital causes of small bowel obstruction include duodenal obstruction (by atresia, stenosis, web, or annular pancreas),[22] midgut malrotation,[23] jejunoileal atresia[24] (Fig. 12–5), and meconium ileus.[25] Lower sites of obstruction (jejunoileal atresia and meconium ileus) have the greatest amounts of associated abdominal distention and a delayed onset of bilious vomiting. On the other hand, upper small bowel obstruction, as in duodenal atresia, usually results in vomiting with the first feeding or even sooner. In addition, the abdominal contour in duodenal obstructions may appear flat because abdominal distention is limited to the stomach, which

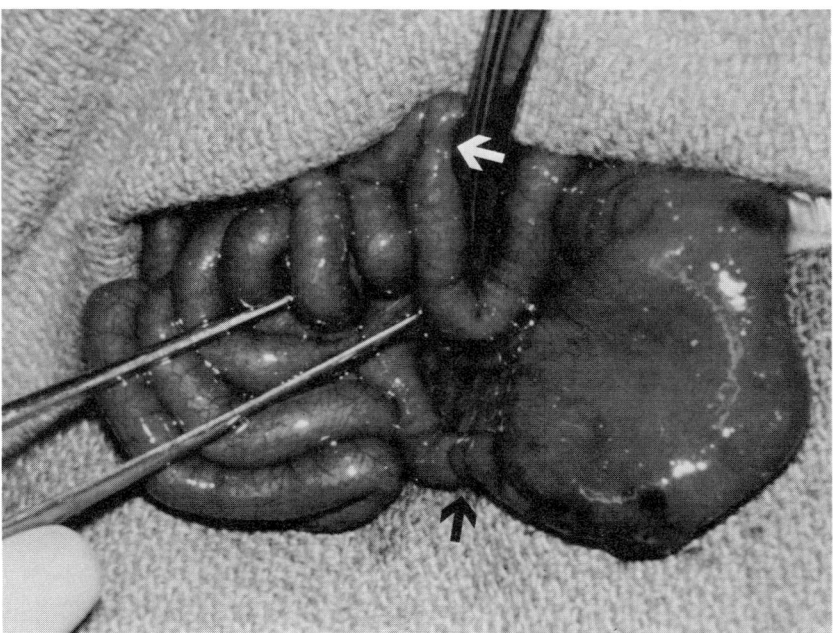

FIGURE 12–5. Intraoperative photograph of child with jejunoileal atresia (small bowel obstruction) demonstrating marked discrepancy in bowel size before and after the atretic segment *(black arrow).* Note normal peristaltic wave in distal small bowel *(white arrow).*

elevates the hemidiaphragms and not the anterior abdominal wall as it distends.

Patients with jejunoileal obstructions may feed for 1 to 3 days before emesis occurs, despite marked abdominal distention. Palpable and even visible loops of dilated bowel may be present from birth in neonates with jejunoileal small bowel obstructions (see Fig. 12–5).

Presurgical management of upper small bowel obstructions includes dependable intravenous line insertion for fluid resuscitation and early gastric decompression. Nasogastric decompression will prevent further emesis with hypovolemia and electrolyte imbalance, remove swallowed air from the distended stomach, and relieve the respiratory restrictions imposed by elevated hemidiaphragms. Further monitoring is not routinely necessary in these neonates unless sepsis or massive fluid losses have compromised hemodynamic stability.

Accurate radiographic diagnosis of the level of obstruction may follow stabilization with intravenous fluids and nasogastric decompression. Air shadows and air-fluid levels within the small bowel are often sufficient to confirm the radiographic diagnosis of small bowel obstructions. The double-bubble pattern of duodenal obstructions on plain abdominal x-ray films (Fig. 12–6) is quite characteristic and often eliminates the need for additional contrast (barium) studies. The multiple air–fluid levels of lower small bowel obstructions are not diagnostic radiographically but may be sufficient to justify laparotomy without additional contrast studies.

Malrotation of the midgut is always a neonatal surgical emergency. Blood supply to most of the small bowel is compromised by midgut malrotation. If the bowel is not untwisted quickly, total gut infarction may occur. Marked distention is apparent on physical examination, although abdominal radiographs often show little air. Malrotation creates a closed-loop obstruction as intestinal air is absorbed from the bowel lumen, which fills with lymph and edema fluid. Abdominal x-ray films of a closed-loop intestinal obstruction show a hazy or "ground glass" appearance with little intraluminal air. Historically a barium enema was performed to detect malposition of the cecum and confirm the diagnosis of midgut malrotation. Today, pediatric radiologists often perform a double-contrast diagnostic study with one contrast agent in the colon and another in the duodenum. Such a study will not only show the malrotated colon and cecum but also will detect rarer cases of midgut malrotation with malposition of the ligament of Treitz and normal colon rotation. Final confirmation of the type of midgut malrotation will occur at early laparotomy for surgical correction.

Meconium ileus often secondary to the pancreatic insufficiency of

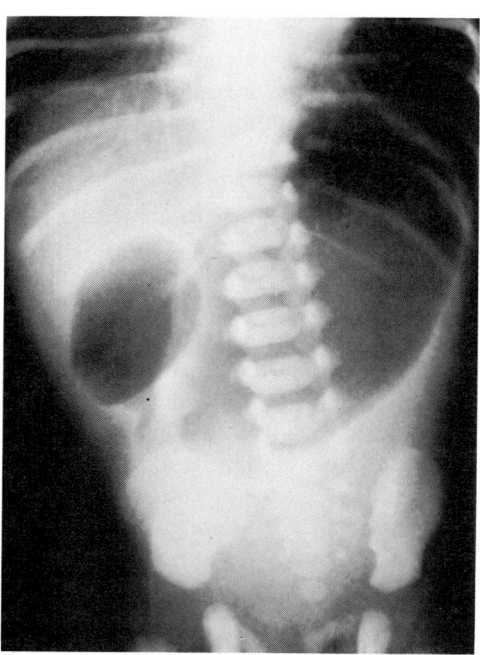

FIGURE 12–6. Abdominal film demonstrating the double-bubble sign of duodenal atresia with the air-filled fundal bubble on the left and the smaller air-filled pyloric bubble on the right.

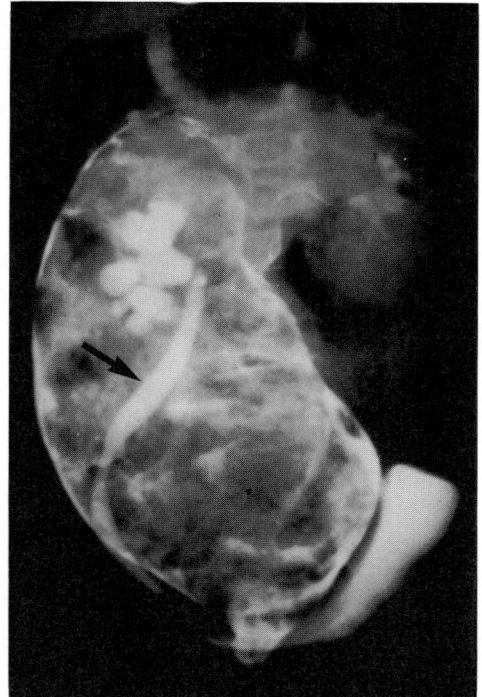

FIGURE 12-7. Colonic obstruction. Barium enema and intravenous pyelogram demonstrating massive colonic distention associated with congenital megacolon (Hirschsprung's disease) with ureteral compression at the pelvic brim and secondary hydroureter (*arrow*).

cystic fibrosis resembles jejunoileal atresia or malrotation in its clinical presentation. Abdominal distention is prominent, and onset of bilious emesis is often delayed beyond the first few feedings. A family history of cystic fibrosis suggests the diagnosis, which will require confirmation by abdominal radiography showing a flocculent intraluminal appearance to the bowel in the right lower quadrant. Gastrografin enema may be both diagnostic and therapeutic in meconium ileus by demonstrating the ileal plug, softening it, and promoting its expulsion during bowel movement after the enema.

Endotracheal intubation in neonates with upper small bowel obstructions is usually indicated only during surgical correction by bowel resection and anastomosis. Postoperative invasive monitoring or prolonged mechanical ventilation is indicated by the neonate's clinical condition or coexisting diseases, especially respiratory distress syndrome.

Colonic Obstruction. Clinical presentation of colonic obstruction in neonates may mimic symptoms of distal small bowel obstruction, with marked abdominal distention and copious bilious vomiting. Plain abdominal x-rays may suggest the distal location of the intestinal obstruction but cannot differentiate distal small bowel from colonic obstructions.

Colonic obstruction may be confirmed by barium enema, which differentiates common colonic obstructions (Hirschsprung's disease, meconium plug syndrome) from the common distal small bowel obstructions (meconium ileus, ileal atresia, and ileocecal intussusception) (Fig. 12–7).

Presurgical management of neonates with congenital colonic obstructions includes insertion of dependable intravenous lines for volume and electrolyte therapy and of nasogastric tubes for gastric decompression and aspiration prophylaxis. Further invasive monitoring depends on the severity of illness (hypovolemic shock, acidosis) or the presence of coexisting illnesses (PDA, respiratory distress syndrome). During surgery, bladder drainage is recommended to provide better surgical access below the pelvic brim if multiple colonic biopsies near the peritoneal reflection or a diverting, left lower quadrant colostomy are required.

CONCLUSIONS

In neonates, surgical abnormalities constitute a unique series of conditions seldom encountered in any other age group. Careful attention to perioperative critical care and hemodynamic stabilization allows these tiny infants to undergo major corrective surgery with reduced risk. Today, many new modalities of diagnosis and therapy are available to the neonatal caregiver to ensure good care for babies both before and during complex operative procedures.

References

1. Holder TM, Gross ER: Temporary gastrostomy in pediatric surgery. Experience with 187 cases. Pediatrics 26:36, 1960
2. Brantigan CO, Grow JB Sr: Cricothyroidotomy: Elective use in respiratory problems requiring tracheotomy. J Thorac Cardiovasc Surg 71:72, 1976
3. Levinson MM, Scuderi PE, Gibson RL, et al.: Emergency percutaneous transtracheal ventilation (PTV). J Am Coll Emerg Phys/Ann Emerg Med 8(10):396, 1979
4. Kress TD, Balasubramaniam S: Cricothyroidotomy. Ann Emerg Med 11:197, 1982
5. Bochdalek VA: Einige Betrachtungen über die Entstehung des angeborenen Zwerchfellbruches. Als Beitrag zur pathologischen Anatomie der Hernien. Vierteljahresschrift Prakt Heilkund 3:89, 1848
6. Adelman S, Benson CD: Bochdalek hernias in infants: Factors determining mortality. J Pediatr Surg 11:569, 1976
7. Boix-Ochoa J, Natal A, Canals J: The important influence of arterial blood gases on the prognosis of congenital diaphragmatic hernia. World J Surg 1:783, 1977
8. Adzick NS, Harrison MR, Glick PL, et al.: Diaphragmatic hernia in the fetus: Prenatal diagnosis and outcome in 94 cases. J Pediatr Surg 20:357, 1985
9. Fox WW, Shahaz S: Persistent pulmonary hypertension in the neonate: Diagnosis and management. J Pediatr 103:505, 1983
10. Raphaely RC, Downes JJ Jr: Congenital diaphragmatic hernia: Prediction of survival. J Pediatr Surg 8:815, 1973
11. Gross RE: Surgery of Infancy and Childhood: Its Principles and Techniques. Philadelphia: W.B. Saunders, 1953, pp 75–102
12. Kluth D: Atlas of esophageal atresias. J Pediatr Surg 11:901, 1976
13. Bolande RB, Schneider AF, Boggs JD: Infantile lobar emphysema: Etiological concept. AMA Arch Pathol 61:289, 1956
14. Cremin BJ, Movsowitz H: Lobar emphysema in infants. Br J Radiol 44:692, 1971

15. Buntain WL, Isaacs H Jr, Payne VC Jr, et al.: Lobar emphysema, cystic adenomatoid malformation, pulmonary sequestration and bronchogenic cyst in infancy and children: A clinical group. J Pediatr Surg 9:85, 1974
16. Haller JA, Golladay ES, Pickard LR, et al.: Surgical management of lung bud anomalies: Lobar emphysema, bronchogenic cysts, cystic adenomatoid malformations, and intrapulmonary sequestration. Ann Thorac Surg 28:33, 1979
17. Telander RL, Lennox C, Sieber W: Sequestration of the lung in children. Mayo Clin Proc 51:578, 1976
18. Takahashi M, Ohno M, Mihara K, et al.: Intralobar pulmonary sequestration with special emphasis on bronchial communication. Radiology 114:543, 1975
19. Schuster SR: Omphalocele, hernia of the umbilical cord and gastroschisis. In: Ravitch MM, Welch KJ, Benson CD, et al. (eds): Pediatric Surgery, 3rd ed. Chicago: Year Book Medical Publishers, 1979, pp 778–801
20. Allen RG, Wrenn EL Jr: Silon as a sac in the treatment of omphalocele and gastroschisis. J Pediatr Surg 4:3, 1969
21. Cantrell JR, Haller JA, Ravitch MM: A syndrome of congenital defects involving the abdominal wall, sternum, diaphragm, pericardium and heart. Surg Gynecol Obstet 107:602, 1958
22. Lynn HB: Duodenal obstruction: Atresia, stenosis and annular pancreas. In: Ravitch MM, Welch KJ, Benson CD, et al. (eds): Pediatric Surgery, 3rd ed. Chicago: Year Book Medical Publishers, 1979, pp 902–911
23. Andrassy RJ, Mahour GH: Malrotation of the midgut in infants and children. Arch Surg 116:158, 1981
24. Nixon HH, Tawes R: Etiology and treatment of small intestinal atresia: Analysis of a series of 127 jejeunoileal atresias and comparison with 62 duodenal atresias. Surgery 69:41, 1971
25. Kalayoglu M, Sieber WK, Rodnan JB, et al.: Meconium ileus: A critical review of treatment and eventual prognosis. J Pediatr Surg 6:290, 1971

13. Perioperative Management of Conjoined Twins Undergoing Separation Surgery

James H. Diaz, M.D.
Eric B. Furman, M.B., B.Ch., D.A., FFA(SA)

Portions of this chapter were adapted with permission from Diaz JH, Furman EB: Perioperative management of conjoined twins. Anesthesiology 66:1039–1042, 1987

HISTORY AND CLASSIFICATION

Some 600 sets of conjoined twins have now been reported worldwide.[1] Historians cite the earliest reference to conjoined twins as Janus, the mythical Roman gatekeeper god of beginnings and endings, depicted as two bearded heads back to back.[1] There have been many reports of conjoined twins throughout history.[1,2] A variety of written and oral reports of conjoined twins may have gone unnoticed, or when passed on orally, resulted in the creation of mythological idols, like Janus, or frequently told stories about two-headed monsters (Fig. 13–1).[1,2] Early written records of conjoined twins and attempts at their surgical separation were made in the tenth century.[3] In 945 A.D., male omphalopagus twins from Constantinople were described, and after the death of one, surgical separation allowed the surviving twin to live for 3 days.[4] Later, in 963 A.D., the death of xiphopagus twins at age 25 years was noted after another unsuccessful separation.[5] In 1100 A.D., a comprehensive written record of conjoined twins was made in Latin of the Biddendon girls, born in England, who were joined ventrally from shoulders to hips with only one pair of arms and legs.[6]

During the Renaissance, several detailed medical reports and illustrations of conjoined twins were published.[7] In his sixteenth century text, *Of Monsters and Prodigies*, the French surgeon Ambroise Paré accurately described conjoined twins and proposed 11 etiologic factors now

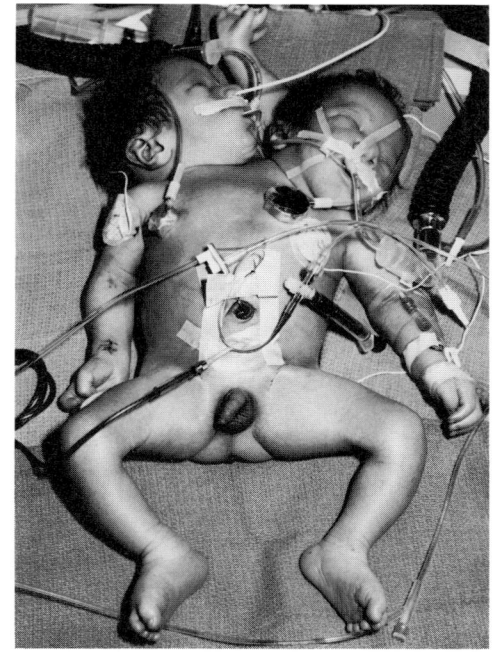

FIGURE 13–1. Thoraco-omphalo-ischiopagus twins anesthetized by the author (J.H.D.) 24 hours after birth for urgent exploratory laparotomy with diverting colostomy. They had two heads and three arms (rudimentary third arm projects cephalad between the heads), and shared a common trunk with two legs, male genitalia, and imperforate anus. The twins died 2 weeks postoperatively from cardiorespiratory arrest during upper gastrointestinal series. Surgical separation would have been difficult in this case because of the shared pulmonary circulations and would have resulted in the intentional sacrifice of one twin.

known to be invalid.[7] Today, conjoined twins are said to result from an aberrant twinning process with incomplete fission of the zygote's primitive streak during the second week of gestation or 20 days postovulation.[8] This hypothesis has been supported by observations of identical sex in almost every reported case of conjoined twins.[9] There is little scientific support for suggestions that conjoined twins may result from the fusion of two separate fertilized ova.[8]

Conjoined twins are classified by their most prominent site of connection. Such sites may include the thorax (thoracopagus), upper abdomen (xiphopagus), lower abdomen (omphalopagus), pelvis (ischiopagus), sacrum (pygopagus), or skull (craniopagus). Compound classifications may be used to describe all possibilities for joining (Fig. 13–1). For example, omphalo-ischiopagus tripus twins are fused at the lower abdomen and pelvis and have two arms and one common leg. The major types of conjoined twins, their frequency of occurrence, sites of musculoskeletal attachments, and possible organs shared are described in Table 13–1.[7]

König performed the first successful surgical separation of conjoined twins in 1689. He separated omphalopagus twins joined at the umbilicus

Table 13–1. *Classification of Conjoined Twins*

Type of Twin	Frequency (%)	Site of Joining	Possible Organs Shared					
			Heart and Great Vessels	Biliary Tract	Upper GI Tract	Lower GI Tract	GU Tract	CNS
Thoracopagus	40	Sternum, diaphragm, upper abdominal wall	Yes	Yes	Yes	No	No	No
Xiphopagus or Omphalopagus	34	Xiphoid, anterior abdominal wall, umbilicus	No	Yes	Yes	Yes	Yes	No
Pygopagus	18	Buttocks, coccyx, sacrum	No	No	No	Yes	Yes	Yes
Ischiopagus	6	Lower abdomen, pelvis, sacrum, lower extremity	No	Possible	Possible	Yes	Yes	Possible
Craniopagus	2	Cranial vault, dural venous sinuses	No	No	No	No	No	Yes

GI = gastrointestinal; GU = genitourinary; CNS = central nervous system.
Adapted with permission from Filler RM, Crocker D: Conjoined twins. In: Ravitch MM, Benson CD, Aberdeen E, et al. (eds): Pediatric Surgery, 3rd ed, vol 2. Chicago: Year Book Medical Publishers, 1979, pp 809–814.

by slowly tightening an encircling tourniquet and constricting and necrosing the connecting bridge. This technique is still in use today, particularly in the staged separation of craniopagus twins.[10] Now over 60 reports documenting successful separation of various types of conjoined twins have been published. Most surgical separations have been performed in the past 25 years.[7] Craniopagus[11] and pygopagus[12] twins were first separated in 1952 and 1953, respectively. Ischiopagus twins were first separated successfully in 1966.[13] Thoracopagus twins with joined hearts were first separated in 1979.[14] The single survivor of cardiac separation was a twin with a normal heart who shared only an interatrial vascular bridge with the nonsurviving twin, who had multiple heart defects.[14] There have been no long-term survivors of separation procedures in thoracopagus conjoined twins with a shared, common myocardium, also referred to as "cardiopagus" twins.[15]

By far the world's best known and among the longest lived conjoined twins were never separated.[16] Chang and Eng Bunker were born in Siam (now Thailand) in 1811, were exhibited worldwide by circus ringmaster P.T. Barnum in the mid-1800s, married two sisters at age 31, fathered 21 children, and died at age 63.[16] The Bunkers' birthplace, Barnum's showmanship, and top circus billing gave the world the lay term "Siamese" twins, still commonly used today to describe conjoined twins.

The birth of conjoined twins remains an extremely rare event today that continues to fascinate physicians and the lay public alike. During the 1960s and early 1970s, recommendations for perioperative management of conjoined twin separation included preoperative planning sessions, dress rehearsals, and invasive intraoperative monitoring for blood and fluid losses. Although these earlier recommendations remain valid today, recent advances in diagnosis and management of conjoined twins were introduced in the 1980s. Improvements in obstetric ultrasound, fetal echocardiography, contrast tomography, magnetic resonance imaging, nuclear volume and flow studies, pulse oximetry, capnography, and extracorporeal membrane oxygenation now permit precise neonatal diagnosis, better evaluation of joining, and more extensive separation operations.

Conjoined twins may now be diagnosed prenatally, have their degree of joining delineated, and have a safe, elective delivery, usually by cesarean section. Planning for eventual surgical separation may also begin before delivery of the twins.

EPIDEMIOLOGY

Clear relationships among maternal factors, environmental exposures, and conjoined twinning are lacking.[17–19] However, there appears to be an increased incidence of stillbirths in mothers of conjoined twins.[9]

Chronic malnutrition and intrauterine hypoxia have been suggested as possible etiologic factors in conjoined twinning, which could explain higher incidences of conjoined twinning in underdeveloped countries.[19] Family history, paternal age, maternal age, and multiparity do not appear to influence the occurrence of conjoined twins.[7]

The exact incidence of conjoined twins is unknown. Estimated incidences in the United States range from 1 in 50,000 births to 1 in 200,000 births.[7, 13] An increased incidence of conjoined twins ranging from 1 in 14,000 to 1 in 25,000 births has been observed in Southeast Asia, especially India, Pakistan, and Thailand, and in Africa, especially East Africa, Nigeria, and South Africa.[7, 8] In the United States, 40% to 68% of conjoined twins are stillborn, and of the live births, 35% do not survive the first 24 hours of life.[19] As in separate twins, this high perinatal mortality may be partially attributed to prematurity and low birth weight.[20] Shared organs are often anomalous in conjoined twins and also contribute to high perinatal mortality.[19] Nearly 70% of conjoined twins are female.[21]

PRENATAL EVALUATION

Prior to the development of radiography, the prenatal diagnosis of conjoined twins was impossible.[21] Maternal polyhydramnios, twin gestation, unusual presentation, and labor dystocia with an adequate maternal pelvis suggested conjoined twins.[21, 22] Xiphopagus, omphalopagus, pygopagus, and craniopagus twins could often be delivered vaginally because of the pliability of the connecting bridges.[21, 22] Thoracopagus and ischiopagus twins had bony unions that caused severe dystocia and necessitated either abdominal delivery by cesarean section or fetal dismemberment with vaginal extraction.[21, 22]

With the introduction of pelvic radiography in obstetrics, the prenatal suspicion of conjoined twins could often be confirmed, especially in thoracopagus, ischiopagus, and craniopagus twins with bony unions.[22, 23] The limited degree of sternal fusion, incomplete ossification, and the extent of rotation permitted by flexible connecting bridges prevented the prenatal radiographic diagnosis of xiphopagus and omphalopagus twins in most cases.[22–24] Prenatal diagnosis was accomplished only twice (6%) in 36 sets of xiphopagus twins reported by Harper and others in 1980.[22]

In 1950, Gray and others[23] established the first set of radiographic criteria for antepartum diagnosis of conjoined twins. In the 1960s, radiographic contrast studies and amniocentesis were introduced to corroborate pelvic roentgenography in the antepartum diagnosis of potential conjoined twins.[24] Indigo carmine or methylene blue dyes were injected into the amniotic sac at one site and amniocentesis was performed at another site to confirm monoamniotic twins, either identical or conjoined.[24] By the 1970s, the risks of repeated fetomaternal irradiation and amniocentesis were fully recognized, and noninvasive ultrasonographic evaluation replaced radiographic evaluation in the prenatal assessment of conjoined twins.[25] In 1985, Sanders and others[26] correctly determined the extent of cardiac sharing in four sets of thoraco-abdominally conjoined twins studied prenatally by echocardiography. Postmortem findings in this study confirmed the usefulness of fetal echocardiography in the prenatal evaluation of thoracopagus twins with shared hearts and identified only two cardiac abnormalities commonly missed at echocardiography, anomalous pulmonary venous drainage and shared coronary circulation.[26] The authors suggested that conjoined twins could be more easily evaluated by echocardiography before birth than after birth since more three-dimensional views could be obtained in utero with less hindrance by commonly associated omphaloceles.[26]

Clearly, early prenatal diagnosis of many types of conjoined twins is now possible by obstetric ultrasound examinations. Later in gestation, echocardiography will accurately predict the extent of cardiac sharing in most thoraco-abdominally conjoined twins.[25, 26] Early plans may now be made for first- or early second-trimester termination of conjoined twin pregnancy in cases with extensive cardiac sharing and poor prognosis.[25, 26] Alternatively, early plans may also be made for surgical separation after cesarean delivery of conjoined twins with little or no cardiac sharing at fetal echocardiography.[25, 26]

At delivery, we and others recommend that space and personnel be available to provide immediate neonatal resuscitation, especially if separation of thoracopagus twins with a shared heart is being considered.[21, 22] With a limited number of trained personnel to attend each twin simultaneously, the less vigorous twin must be resuscitated first.[21, 22] Urgent operations shortly after birth may be indicated in conjoined twins with ruptured omphaloceles, damage to the connecting bridge, perforated viscus, or intestinal obstruction (see Fig. 13–1).[7]

PREOPERATIVE EVALUATION

The preoperative management of conjoined twins should be unhurried to permit infant growth, thorough diagnostic evaluation of visceral sharing, and creation of a multidisciplinary separation team from groups undertaking such operations for the first time. Depending on the type of conjoined twins being separated, a variety of diagnostic studies may be necessary to define organ sharing and demonstrate coexisting congenital anomalies (Table 13–2).

The training of a multidisciplinary separation team should include classroom discussion to delineate duplicate duties, define the degree of

Table 13–2. *Recommended Diagnostic Studies During Preoperative Evaluation of Conjoined Twins*

	Diagnostic Studies										
Type of Twin	CXR	ECG	ECHO	CARDIAC CATH	UGI	BE	LFT/ SCAN	IVP	ANGIO	CT	MRI
Thoracopagus	+	+	+	+	+	+	+	+	–	+	+
Xiphopagus	+	+	+	+	+	+	+	+	–	–	+
Omphalopagus	+	–	–	–	+	+	+	+	–	–	+
Ischiopagus	–	–	–	–	+	+	+	+	+	–	–
Pygopagus	–	–	–	–	–	+	–	+	–	–	–
Craniopagus	–	–	–	–	–	–	–	–	+	+	+

+ = highly recommended; – = optional; CXR = chest x-ray film; ECG = electrocardiogram; ECHO = echocardiogram; CARDIAC CATH = cardiac catheterization; UGI = upper gastrointestinal series; BE = barium enema; LFT/SCAN = liver function tests/liver–spleen scan; IVP = intravenous pyelogram; ANGIO = angiogram; CT = computed tomogram; MRI = magnetic resonance imaging.

Adapted with permission from Diaz JR, Furman EB: Perioperative management of conjoined twins. Anesthesiology 66:1039–1042, 1987.

circulatory admixture, diagram the extent of organ sharing, calculate blood and fluid requirements, and determine allowable blood losses.[15, 20, 27] In addition to anesthesiologists, the team should include circulating and operating room nurses, neonatal or pediatric intensive care nurses, respiratory therapists, pediatricians, and surgeons. Laboratory and blood-banking personnel should be notified of the separation and informed that numerous laboratory tests and large volumes of blood and its components may be necessary.

Simple but accurate diagrams of organ sharing and circulatory admixture based on radiographic and radioisotopic evaluation can be found in recent case reports on separations of thoracopagus[14, 15, 28] and craniopagus[10] twins. To estimate circulatory time and degree of admixture in conjoined twins, radioactive albumin, methylene blue, or indigo carmine dyes can be injected intravenously into one twin, and the first appearance of dye can be monitored in the other twin's blood and urine.[7] The rate of blood exchange can then be calculated.[29] Radioisotopic studies of blood volume are also very helpful in evaluating circulatory volumes and calculating allowable fluid and blood losses at separation.[29] Circulatory admixture is greatest in thoracopagus twins with a shared heart who may demonstrate complete blood exchange every minute.[7, 29]

During preoperative discussions, equipment operators should be designated and placement of personnel and machinery precisely determined to avoid crowding in the operating room. Necessary medical equipment will include operating tables, warming devices, infusion pumps, anesthesia machines, ventilators, a variety of electronic monitors, and possibly heart–lung machines. Some authors have suggested scheduling separation procedures on Sunday to minimize operating room traffic and congestion.[15] Besides operating room crowding, other major intraoperative problems to be discussed include choice of anesthetics, fluid management, cardiovascular monitoring, temperature preservation, and surgical techniques, especially skin closure.

Rehearsal of the separation procedure in the operating room can be very helpful in teaching personnel how to arrange needed equipment and coordinate their activities.[14, 15, 20] Rehearsal is especially necessary for a team performing its first separation of conjoined twins. A brief rehearsal is also recommended for experienced teams. We have also recommended that all personnel, equipment, monitoring leads, vascular lines, and records be color coded to identify at a glance with which twin they are associated (see Figs. 13–1 and 13–2).[27] Vascular lines, breathing circuits, and thermistor probes can be wrapped together with team-colored masking tape to form a single tangle-free "umbilical cord" for each infant (see Fig. 13–2).[20] The best dress rehearsal for proposed separation of conjoined twins is a palliative or diagnostic procedure that requires a general anesthetic, such as exploratory laparotomies or diverting colostomies (see Fig. 13–1).[10]

Due to circulatory admixture, drugs administered to one infant may have unpredictable effects on the other; therefore, light premedication, if any, is recommended for conjoined twins.[15, 20, 27, 29] Intravenous drug administration is preferred over intramuscular administration because of unpredictable drug absorption.[15, 20, 27, 29] The usual recommended intravenous dosages of premedicants, anesthetics, and adjuvants may be reduced by one-half and divided once again into equal doses for each twin. Using reduced incremental doses minimizes the dangers of compounding drug effects in one twin. The less vigorous twin should be premedicated first and incremental doses should be titrated to effect.[6, 15, 21] Steroid premedication has also been recommended before separation of conjoined twins as prophylaxis against adrenal insufficiency with hypotension in one or both twins.[30] Computed tomograms have detected the absence of adrenal tissue in xiphopagus, omphalopagus, and ischiopagus twins (see Table 13–2).[20] Magnetic resonance imaging may prove even more helpful than computed tomography in detecting the presence or absence of adrenals in conjoined twins (see Table 13–2). Intravenous hydrocortisone (1.5 mg/kg) may be administered to each twin at induction of anesthesia and again at separation, then tapered postoperatively. Thoracopagus, craniopagus, and pygopagus twins have all been separated successfully without steroid prophylaxis and without evidence of adrenal insufficiency or hypotension unrelated to blood loss.[20] Administration of prophylactic steroids to conjoined twins before separation remains controversial except in twins with demonstrated absence of adrenal tissue.[20, 30]

Some authors recommend establishment of airway and vascular access before the twins are transported to the operating room.[28] Others believe that dislodgement of tubes and lines is more likely during transport and

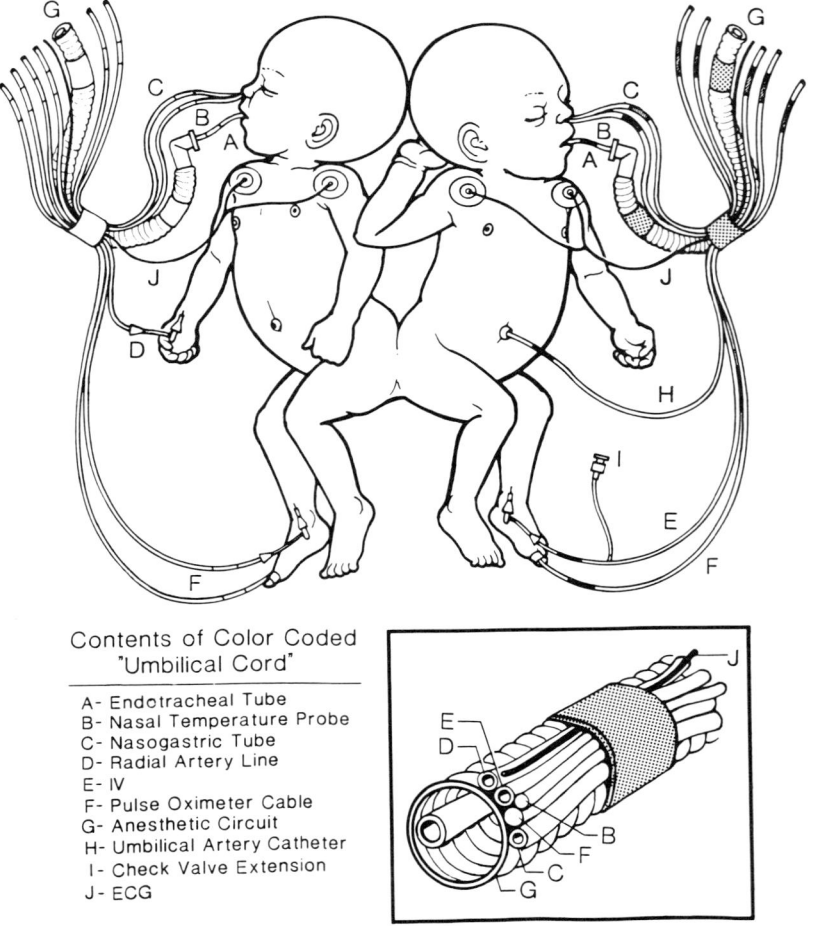

Contents of Color Coded
"Umbilical Cord"

A- Endotracheal Tube
B- Nasal Temperature Probe
C- Nasogastric Tube
D- Radial Artery Line
E- IV
F- Pulse Oximeter Cable
G- Anesthetic Circuit
H- Umbilical Artery Catheter
I- Check Valve Extension
J- ECG

FIGURE 13–2. Color coding of the breathing circuits, vascular lines, and monitoring leads in these pygopagus twins helped identify to which twin the lines belonged when the twins were draped for separation.[28] Personnel, equipment, and even anesthetic records should also be color coded to designate twin assignment at a glance.[28] Vascular lines, breathing circuits, and thermistor probes can be wrapped up together with team-colored masking tape to form a single tangle-free "umbilical cord" for each infant.[21]

prefer to wait until the twins are in the operating room to place monitors, intravenous lines, and endotracheal tubes.[20] We recommend that minimal transport monitors include electrocardiographs, skin or rectal thermistors, and pulse oximetry probes.

Normothermia can be maintained by transporting the twins in heated incubators or, preferably, in radiant warmers, which will permit better access and even surgery. We recommend transporting the twins to surgery (through cleared corridors) in the same radiant warmer in which surgery is to be performed to reduce risks of hypothermia and line dislodgement. As an option, two radiant warmers can be placed side-to-side or end-to-end (Fig. 13–3, *A*) in the operating room to permit the dual surgical teams to separate easily with their patients once the twins are disconnected (Fig. 13–3, *B*). The twins may be positioned parallel or at right angles to the long axes of the radiant warmers to provide for greatest surgical access (see Fig. 13–3, *A*). The problems of heat loss and surgical access must be individualized to the infants and to the separation operations, and they may be managed successfully with a variety of warming devices and operating tables.

The use of the same airway, breathing, and monitoring devices for transport and surgery can simplify transport duties and reduce confusion. To permit a continuum of care, certain anesthesia team members should also be designated as a transport team responsible for the twins' well-being, airways, vascular accesses, and monitors during transport as well as during surgery.

INTRAOPERATIVE MANAGEMENT

Conjoined twins may require general anesthesia for diagnostic and emergency procedures not involving separation as well as for urgent or elective separation and reconstruction of tissue defects (see Fig. 13–1). Many anesthetic management problems are similar regardless of operative procedures, including difficult airway establishment and maintenance, unpredictable drug responses from cross-circulation, thermal instability, and risks of extraordinary intravascular volume shifts or losses. Diagnostic procedures for conjoined twins may include endoscopy, invasive radiographic studies, or exploratory laparotomies.[7] Palliative procedures may include amputations, diverting colostomies, or ileal conduits.[7] As noted, urgent separations are recommended only for surgical catastrophes, damage to the connective bridge, or rapid deterioration of one or both twins.[7] Most separations can be carefully planned, organized, and executed by highly trained teams experienced in complex infant surgery. The intraoperative anesthetic management of conjoined twins requires a dual team of one or two anesthesiologists for each twin, with an additional anesthesiologist acting as anesthesia team coordinator.

Anesthetic Management

Analgesia and amnesia can be provided with inhalation and intravenous anesthetics. Muscle relaxants may be required to avoid cardiovascular depression from high inspired doses of inhaled anesthetics. We recommend percutaneous insertion of a 22- to 24-gauge intravenous catheter into each awake twin; larger vascular access lines can be established

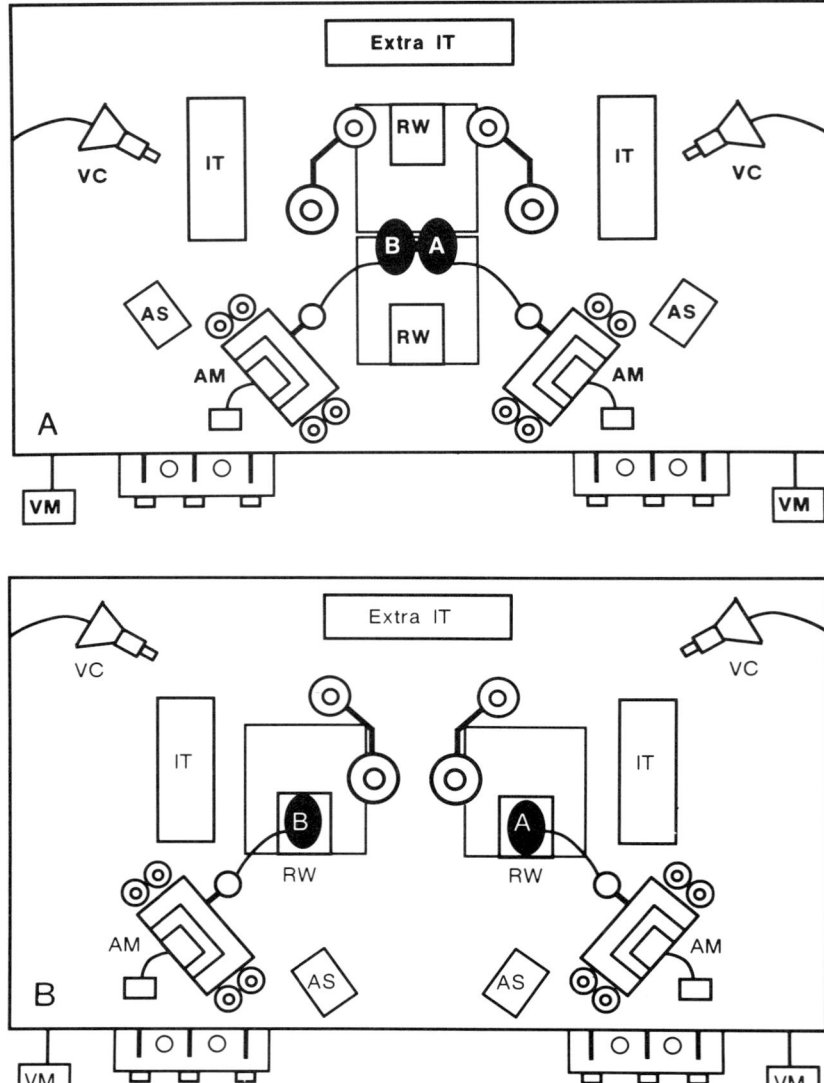

FIGURE 13–3. Two radiant warmers can be placed in the operating room either side-to-side or end-to-end (A), parallel to or at right angles to (A) the long axes of the radiant warmers to provide for greatest surgical access during separation. Adjoining radiant warmers (A) will permit the dual surgical teams to separate easily with their twins once the twins are disconnected (B). AM = anesthesia machine; AS = anesthesia supply cart; IT = instrument table; VC = video camera; VM = video monitor; RW = radiant warmer.

after induction of anesthesia. Frequent adjustments in levels of anesthesia and muscle relaxation may be necessary in each twin because of cross-circulation, cardiovascular depression, and unpredictable drug absorption and response.[27, 29, 30]

Monitoring

The intra-anesthetic monitoring of conjoined twins must be at least as extensive as that employed during routine infant anesthesia and perhaps more extensive, depending on the nature of the surgical procedure. Twins being separated require additional invasive monitoring, such as direct blood pressure monitoring by radial artery cannulas, umbilical artery catheters, or combinations (see Fig. 13–1). Right atrial catheters are indicated in separation surgery to provide reliable cardiac filling pressures and central circulatory access for vasopressors and volume restoration.[14, 15, 20] A pulse oximeter attached to a limb of each twin for continuous monitoring of peripheral perfusion and oxygenation will often sound the first warning if either twin is in jeopardy. We and others also recommend that urine volume be monitored for separation procedures and other major procedures lasting longer than 1 to 2 hours.[15, 20] Brown and others[15] have used low-dose continuous dopamine infusion (3.0 μg/kg/min) to augment renal perfusion and maintain a urine output of at least 0.5 ml/kg/hour during separation surgery. Blood loss is measured by suction traps calibrated to 200 ml and by weighing of sponges. Serial determinations of arterial blood gases, glucose, electrolytes, ionized calcium, hemoglobin, platelets, prothrombin time, partial thromboplastin time, and fibrinogen should be measured frequently during separations and other procedures involving major blood loss.

Airway Management

Endotracheal intubation is recommended for intraoperative airway management of conjoined twins and insufflation of O_2 and anesthetic gases during separation or nonseparation operations. In neonatal twins, awake tracheal intubation is recommended to prevent pulmonary aspiration and airway obstruction, which could complicate intravenous or mask inductions. Endotracheal intubation may be difficult in thoraco-abdominally conjoined twins of any age who are connected ventrally and facing each other. Spontaneous ventilation with 100% oxygen followed by awake tracheal intubation is also recommended in such cases. Nasotracheal tubes may offer more stability than orotracheal tubes in infants who require prolonged postoperative ventilation and may be substituted postoperatively for initially inserted orotracheal tubes. Insufflation induction of anesthesia and muscle relaxation, if indicated, can follow the awake establishment of a secure upper airway and auscultation of bilaterally equal breath sounds in each infant.

Ventilatory Management

As in all neonates, spontaneous ventilation is not recommended during anesthesia in conjoined twins because of anesthetic-induced depression of alveolar ventilation and widening of the alveolar to arterial O_2 gradient $(A-aDo_2)$.[31] Apparatus for administering gas anesthesia and ventilating conjoined twins during surgery should have minimal dead space and little resistance to breathing, should eliminate CO_2 adequately, and should provide for assisted or controlled ventilation. We also recommend that anesthesia breathing circuits allow for heated humidification of inspired gases and be compact and lightweight because of frequent positional changes during skin preparation, separation, and wound closures. To meet these needs, various nonrebreathing modifications of Ayre's T-piece system that require a fresh gas flow of at least twice minute ventilation to prevent rebreathing are recommended.[32-35] We prefer hand ventilation to mechanical ventilation during delicate stages of separation because hand ventilation affords better appreciation of subtle changes in lung compliance and lower airway resistance. Hand ventilation may also be timed with surgical techniques during delicate cardiothoracic dissections. The use of mechanical ventilation with these non-rebreathing circuits or with an infant circle system and CO_2 absorption is advocated for longer procedures and during tedious plastic reconstructions of tissue defects. Inspiratory and expiratory pressures must be carefully monitored and arterial blood gases measured at frequent (30-minute) intervals during intraoperative mechanical ventilation.

The adequacy of oxygenation and ventilation may be assessed by evaluation of color, breath sounds, chest excursions, transcutaneous O_2 saturation, and arterial blood gases. Cutaneous pulse oximetry provides more reliable noninvasive monitoring of oxygenation than transcutaneous O_2 tension because of frequent anesthetic-induced alterations in skin perfusion and fluctuating skin temperature.[36] Unlike transcutaneous O_2 tension, however, recent investigations have shown that transcutaneous CO_2 tension is a more reliable indicator of adequate ventilation than either intermittent arterial CO_2 sampling or end-tidal CO_2 monitoring by infrared or spectrometric analysis.[37] The small tidal volumes and rapid respiratory rates common among infants are now known to interfere with end-tidal capnograms and spectrometric analysis of both inhaled and exhaled gases.[37]

Fluid Therapy

Surgical fluid replacement will depend on the age of the twins at separation. Intravenous fluid maintenance with both dextrose-containing and isotonic solutions may be required throughout any surgical procedure. Acute care fluid requirements are 4 ml/kg/hour for twins 10 days old or older and 2 ml/kg/hour for the first 10 days.[38] Infants on appropriate preoperative intravenous therapy have no fluid deficits. Older infants and children accumulate deficits from the last oral intake. By assigning one-half the combined body weight to each child, the blood volume, fluid requirement, deficit replacement, and blood replacement can be determined.[27] We and others recommend that deficits be replaced 50% in the first hour of surgery and 25% in each subsequent hour until complete.[27, 38] Exposure of bowel to high-intensity lights causes fluid evaporation that can be replaced at a rate of 2 ml/kg/hour, and exposure of lung requires 4 ml/kg/hour of extra intravenous fluids.[38] Abdominoperineal separation often requires an extra 6 ml/kg/hour above the 4 ml/kg/hour basic replacement.[38] All fluid replacements may be made using balanced electrolyte solutions without dextrose, e.g., plain Ringer's lactate.[34] Infants needing glucose to maintain blood levels may be maintained on a separate infusion containing the appropriate dextrose concentration.[27, 38]

Blood loss and the need for replacement are assessed by obtaining serial hematocrits every 30 minutes throughout the procedure.[27] A predetermined low hematocrit level at which point red blood cells will be replaced should be chosen during the preoperative conference. Up to that point, we recommend that losses be replaced milliliter for milliliter with clear fluids.[27] It is critical to maintain circulating volume and avoid shock. In premature and newborn infants up to 10 days of age, a hematocrit of 40% is advisable.[38] In older infants, a hematocrit of 30% is acceptable.[38] In infants older than 6 months, hematocrits as low as 25% may also be acceptable.[38]

Packed red blood cells are used for replacement of lost blood when appropriate.[27] Exact quantities required to maintain a given hematocrit are injected via a syringe and stopcock using blood warmed to body temperature (see Fig. 11–3).[27, 38] If massive blood loss occurs at separation, the anesthesia team coordinator must determine which twin is losing the volume and direct replacement accordingly.[27] The initial need is to replace volume, using balanced electrolytes.[27] The hematocrit is then adjusted, using red blood cells.

Adequate fluid therapy produces urine at least 0.5 ml/kg/hour of specific gravity 1.012 to 1.018.[15, 27] Occasionally, when large quantities of clear fluid have been used, albumin may be required to restore the serum albumin level to 5 g/dl or greater.[27, 38] This is achieved by infusing

5.0-ml aliquots of "salt-poor" 25% albumin in divided doses.[27] When large volumes of replacement fluids have been infused, examinations of platelet counts and coagulation activity may be repeated. It is advisable to use blood from the blood bank that is as fresh as possible for all transfusions.[27] Cumulative graphic summaries of fluid and blood product administration directed by fluctuating hemodynamic and clotting status can be found in many twin separation reports.[20, 27, 28]

Anesthetic Pharmacology

Increased anesthetic requirements and greater sensitivity to the cardiodepressant properties of both inhaled and intravenous anesthetics apply to conjoined twins as well as to normal infants.[39, 40] In addition, limited energy reserves and reduced physiologic capabilities in shared systems help to account for the unpredictable responses to anesthetics in conjoined twins compared with normal infants.[20, 27, 29]

Inhalation Anesthetics. Combinations of N_2O, volatile anesthetic agents, muscle relaxants, barbiturates, and narcotics have now become the most widely employed anesthetic agents in infants.[31] During N_2O-relaxant anesthesia, additional analgesia with narcotics will be needed.[31] Narcotics or barbiturates added to N_2O may promote more cardiovascular instability and, if used, should be carefully titrated as to intraoperative effects (hypotension, hypoventilation) and postoperative effects (delayed emergence, respiratory depression).[31] As with resuscitation and premedication, the less vigorous twin should be anesthetized first.[6, 15, 21]

N_2O dilutes inspired O_2 concentrations, becomes a potent cardiovascular depressant when combined with narcotics, and rapidly expands air-containing cavities that are not being adequately decompressed, such as pneumothorax, congenital lung cysts, lobar and interstitial emphysema, or obstructed stomach or bowel.[41] Such obstructed air-containing cavities often complicate preoperative evaluation and surgical management of conjoined twins with duplicated respiratory and alimentary tracts.[7] Compressed air or helium may also serve as O_2-diluting carrier gases in neonatal conjoined twins at risk of retinopathy of prematurity or in whom N_2O is contraindicated.

Muscle Relaxants. Neuromuscular blocking drugs occupy a prominent place in infant anesthetic management for two main reasons.[31] First, muscle relaxants can provide optimal operating conditions and permit reduced doses of inhaled anesthetics with less cardiovascular depression.[31] Second, assisted or controlled ventilation of paralyzed, anesthetized infants provides better alveolar ventilation than spontaneous ventilation, with less mismatching of ventilation and lung perfusion.[31] Whether depolarizing or nondepolarizing, surgical muscle relaxants have distinct dosage requirements, cardiovascular effects, and elimination half-lives in normal infants that do not apply exactly to conjoined twins. As with all medications, dosage requirements, effects, and elimination are unpredictable and usually differ with each twin.[27] Variable responses to paralyzing doses of relaxants and resistance to antagonism of paralysis will be common in conjoined twins and may indicate the need for postoperative mechanical ventilation.[20, 27, 28] Hypothermia, hypocalcemia, and concomitant aminoglycoside antibiotic therapy will potentiate non-depolarizing neuromuscular relaxants and interfere with adequate reversal in conjoined twins as well as in other infants.

Intravenous Agents. Brown and coworkers[15] recently chose a single high-dose injection of fentanyl, 100 μg/kg, to anesthetize thoracopagus twins for separation. Such single-injection techniques may reduce pharmacologic manipulation; allow the anesthesia team more time to concentrate on thermoregulation, fluid management, and blood administration; and provide better cardiovascular support during separation.[15] In experimental animals, high-dose fentanyl anesthesia combined with atropine has been found to provide more hemodynamic stability than either fentanyl alone or inhalation anesthetics.[42]

Ketamine has proved most useful as an intravenous anesthetic in the sickest infants with cyanotic congenital heart disease who will require prolonged postoperative ventilation.[43] Intravenous ketamine titrated to effect could provide for safer induction of anesthesia in conjoined twins needing urgent separation or surgery for abdominal emergencies.

In summary, all intravenous anesthetics can produce unpredictable effects in conjoined twins and should be carefully titrated as reduced dosages at induction to avoid profound cardiovascular depression.[27] The reversible agents, like narcotics and muscle relaxants, may offer more versatility and less risk of postoperative apnea than the longer-acting irreversible agents like barbiturates, tranquilizers, and ketamine.

Termination of Anesthesia

At completion of surgery, several decisions must be made, including whether to reverse neuromuscular blockade, when to extubate the trachea, and what the course of postoperative pulmonary management is to be. Continued blood loss, systemic hypotension, hypothermia, and hypocalcemia are common after separation of conjoined twins and contraindicate reversal of nondepolarizing muscle relaxants.[15, 20, 27] Endotracheal tubes that are to remain in place postoperatively must be re-evaluated as to proper placement and patency and may need changing at the completion of surgery. Only when the infants are conscious and vigorous may endotracheal tubes be removed, usually several days postoperatively.[15, 20] Critically ill infants recently separated will certainly need controlled ventilation followed by a trial of spontaneous breathing with a T-piece and continuous positive airway pressure (CPAP) before tracheal extubation.[15, 20, 27] Reassessment of the adequacy of oxygenation and ventilation will determine the proper timing for tracheal extubation. Tight skin closures can restrict spontaneous ventilation and prolong the need for postoperative controlled ventilation.[44] Therapeutic pneumoperitoneum prior to planned separation or staged abdominal wall closures may reduce restrictive deficits following skin closure and permit earlier tracheal extubation postoperatively.[44]

POSTOPERATIVE MANAGEMENT

Postoperatively, separated twins should be transported to intensive care areas in warmed isolettes or radiant warmers and monitored for hemorrhage, hypotension, hypothermia, hypocalcemia, hypokalemia, hypoxia, hypercarbia, and acidosis.[7, 15, 20] Invasive cardiovascular monitoring of systemic blood pressure and central venous pressure should also continue, because unrecognized volume losses and cardiogenic instability occur commonly in separated twins.[7] Cardiovascular and respiratory failure remain the most frequent causes of death in the immediate postseparation period.[7] Prolonged inotropic support and continued mechanical ventilation of each twin are often required.[7, 15] Adrenocortical steroid therapy should be continued in infants without adrenal glands.[30] Further operations for wound dehiscences, secondary wound closures, and skin grafting of relaxing incisions are often necessary in the first few weeks postoperatively. Prolonged hospitalization and multiple operations will quickly consume peripheral intravenous access sites. Central venous lines will allow for prolonged intravenous fluid and nutritional support and permit frequent intravenous anesthetic inductions. Wound infections, pneumonia, and catheter sepsis from long-term vascular or urinary catheters may also complicate postoperative recovery of recently separated conjoined twins.[7]

CONCLUSIONS

Successful intraoperative management of conjoined twins undergoing surgical exploration or separation requires timing, teamwork, an appreciation of the risks involved, and a firm understanding of conjoined pathophysiology. Prenatal diagnosis of conjoined twins is now possible in a way that permits careful planning for delivery, for preoperative work-up if separation is possible, and for early mobilization of a multidisciplinary separation team. Delayed separation for weeks or months will allow the needed time for growth of the twins, thorough preoperative evaluation of the extent of joining, procedural planning sessions, and separation rehearsals. Urgent operations or separations may be necessary in conjoined twins (see Fig. 13–1). In these situations, rapid preoperative evaluation and management can be provided by precise noninvasive studies and cardiopulmonary stabilization before transport to the operating room.

References

1. Golladay ES, Williams GD, Seibert JJ, et al.: Dicephalus dipus conjoined twins: A surgical separation and review of previously reported cases. J Pediatr Surg 17:259–264, 1982
2. Diaz JH, Furman EB: History of conjoined twins. (Letter, in reply). Anesthesiology 68:824, 1988
3. Rockoff MA: History of conjoined twins. (Letter). Anesthesiology 68:823–824, 1988
4. Pentagalos GE, Las Caratos JG: A surgical operation in Siamese twins during the tenth century in Byzantium. Bull Hist Med 58:99–102, 1984
5. Baudouin M: Les monstres doubles autositaires operes et operables. Rev Chir 25:546, 1902
6. Towey RM, Kisia AKL, Jacobacci S, et al.: Anaesthesia for the separation of conjoined twins. Anaesthesia 34:184–192, 1979
7. Filler RM, Crocker D: Conjoined twins. In: Ravitch MM, Benson CD, Aberdeen E, et al. (eds): Pediatric Surgery, 3rd ed, vol 2. Chicago: Year Book Medical Publishers, 1979, pp 809–814
8. Bender C: Studies on symmetrical conjoined twins. J Pediatr 70:1010–1011, 1967
9. Milham S: Symmetrical conjoined twins: an analysis of the birth records of twenty-two sets. J Pediatr 69:643–647, 1966
10. Wong KC, Ohmura A, Roberts TH, et al.: Anesthetic management for separation of craniopagus twins. Anesth Analg 59:883–886, 1980
11. Grossman HG, Sugar O, Greeley PW, et al.: Surgical separation in craniopagus. JAMA 153:201–207, 1953
12. Wilson H, Storer EH: Surgery in Siamese twins: A report of three sets of conjoined twins treated surgically. Ann Surg 145:718–725, 1957
13. Eades JW, Thomas CC: Successful separation of ischiopagus tetrapus conjoined twins. Ann Surg 164:1059–1072, 1966
14. Synhorst D, Matlak M, Road Y, et al.: Separation of conjoined thoracopagus twins joined at the right atria. Am J Cardiol 43:662–665, 1979
15. Brown DL, Holubec DM, Towle DJ, et al.: Anesthetic management of thoracopagus twins undergoing cardiopagus separation. Anesthesiology 62:679–682, 1985
16. Luckhardt AB: Report of the autopsy of the Siamese twins with other interesting information covering their life: A sketch of the life of Chang and Eng. Surg Gynecol Obstet 72:116–125, 1941
17. Cox ML: Incidence and aetiology of multiple births in Nigeria. J Obstet Gynecol Br Commonwealth 70:878–884, 1963
18. Bankole MA, Oduntan SA, Oluwasanmi JA, et al.: The conjoined twins of Warri, Nigeria. Arch Surg 104:294–301, 1972
19. Edmonds LD, Layde PM: Conjoined twins in the United States: 1970–1977. Teratology 25:301–303, 1982
20. James PD, Lerman J, McLeod ME, et al.: Anaesthetic considerations for separation of omphalo-ischiopagus tripus twins. Can Anaesth Soc J 32:402–411, 1985
21. Rudolph AJ, Michaels JP, Nichold BL: Obstetric management of conjoined twins. Birth Defects 3:28–37, 1967
22. Harper RG, Kenigsberg K, Sia CG, et al.: Xiphopagus conjoined twins: A 300-year review of the obstetric, morphopathologic, neonatal, and surgical parameters. Am J Obstet Gynecol 137:617–629, 1980
23. Gray CM, Nix GH, Wallace AJ: Thoracopagus twins: Prenatal diagnosis. Radiology 54:398–400, 1950
24. Apuzzio JJ, Ganesh V, Landau I, et al.: Prenatal diagnosis of conjoined twins. Am J Obstet Gynecol 148:343–344, 1984
25. Koontz WL, Herbert WNP, Seeds JW, et al.: Ultrasonography in the antepartum diagnosis of conjoined twins: A report of two cases. J Reprod Med 28:627–630, 1983
26. Sanders SP, Chin AJ, Parness IA, et al.: Prenatal diagnosis of congenital heart defects in thoracoabdominally conjoined twins. N Engl J Med 313:370–374, 1985

27. Furman EB, Roman DG, Hairabet J, et al.: Management of anesthesia for surgical separation of newborn conjoined twins. Anesthesiology 34:95–101, 1971
28. Bloch EC, Karis JH: Cardiopagus in neonatal thoracopagus twins: Anesthetic management. Anesth Analg 59:304–307, 1980
29. Spencer RP, Rockhoff ML, Nichols BL, et al.: Radioisotopic flow studies in conjoined twins. Birth Defects 3:120–122, 1967
30. Aird I: Conjoined twins. Br Med J 1:1313–1315, 1959
31. Vivori E: Induction and maintenance of anaesthesia. In: Rees GJ, Gray TC (eds): Paediatric Anaesthesia: Trends in Current Practice. London: Butterworths, 1981, pp 101–114
32. Ayre P: Anaesthesia for intracranial operation. Lancet 1:561–563, 1937
33. Jackson-Rees G: Anaesthesia in the newborn. Br Med J 2:1419–1422, 1950
34. Mapleson WN: The elimination of rebreathing in various semi-closed anaesthetic systems. Br J Anaesth 26:323–332, 1954
35. Bain JA, Spoerel WE: Flow requirements for a modified Mapleson D system during controlled ventilation. Can Anaesth Soc J 20:629–636, 1973
36. Swedlow DB, Stern S: Continuous noninvasive oxygen saturation monitoring in children with a new pulse-oximeter (abstract). Crit Care Med 11:228, 1983
37. Severinghaus JW: Transcutaneous monitoring of arterial PCO_2. In: Spence AA (ed): Respiratory Monitoring in Intensive Care. New York: Churchill-Livingstone, 1982, pp 85–91
38. Furman EB: Blood and fluid replacement for paediatric patients. In: Steward DJ (ed): Some Aspects of Paediatric Anaesthesia. Amsterdam: Excerpta Medica, 1982, pp 79–100
39. Gregory GA, Eger EI, Munson ES: The relationship between age and halothane requirement in man. Anesthesiology 30:488–491, 1969
40. Cameron CB, Robinson S, Gregory GA: The minimum anesthetic concentration of isoflurane in children. Anesth Analg 63:418–420, 1984
41. Eger EI, Saidman LJ: Hazards of nitrous oxide anesthesia in bowel obstruction and pneumothorax. Anesthesiology 26:61–66, 1965
42. Shieber RA, Stiller RL, Cook DR: Cardiovascular and pharmacodynamic effects of high-dose fentanyl in newborn piglets. Anesthesiology 63:166–171, 1985
43. White PF, Way WL, Trevor AJ: Ketamine—its pharmacology and therapeutic uses. Anesthesiology 56:119–136, 1982
44. Chao CC, Susetio L, Luu KW, et al.: Anaesthetic management for successful separation of tripus ischiopagal conjoined male twins. Can Anaesth Soc J 27:565–571, 1980

14. Postoperative Critical Care Management of Neonates

Robert M. Arensman, M.D.
James H. Diaz, M.D.

INTRODUCTION

PARENTERAL HYPERALIMENTATION FOR NUTRITIONAL SUPPORT

EXTRACORPOREAL MEMBRANE OXYGENATION FOR NEONATAL RESPIRATORY FAILURE

CONCLUSIONS

INTRODUCTION

In the past quarter century, three major advances have helped to ensure good outcomes for high-risk neonates still struggling to complete their difficult transition from intrauterine to extrauterine life. These advances include (1) antibiotic therapy; (2) fluid, electrolyte, and nutritional replacement and supportive therapy; and (3) extracorporeal respiratory support by extracorporeal membrane oxygenation (ECMO). The preoperative management and basic techniques for operative correction of a number of congenital malformations are presented in Chapter 12. Neonatal fluid and electrolyte replacement and maintenance therapy are addressed in Chapters 10, 11, and 13. Postoperative neonatal nutritional support and respiratory support by ECMO are addressed.

PARENTERAL HYPERALIMENTATION FOR NUTRITIONAL SUPPORT

Postoperative nutritional support continues to have its widest application in neonates recovering from emergency surgery to close the common anterior abdominal wall defects, omphalocele, and gastroschisis. Such defects are generally large and difficult to close primarily and without intra-abdominal tension, a force that can restrict both alveolar ventilation and cardiac output (see Chapter 13).

Before the availability of synthetic silos, many large omphaloceles could be reduced but not closed primarily without cardiorespiratory compromise. Such defects were then allowed to slowly granulate over and to finally epithelialize. With the gastrointestinal tract intact, unobstructed, covered by a protective surface, and capable of normal absorptive functions, neonates with large omphaloceles were fed quickly and did reasonably well postoperatively if they had no associated anomalies. Mortality was related to associated anomalies and not to malnutrition.

In contrast to omphalocele, gastroschisis is usually a small anterior abdominal wall defect that can often be reduced and closed primarily. Even with primary closure, however, enteral alimentation is limited by a severe serositis that envelopes the involved bowel and limits peristalsis and nutrient absorption. In addition, many neonates with gastroschisis have foreshortened intestines with less surface area available for nutrient absorption, a condition now known as the short gut syndrome. Until recently, such infants often underwent successful primary reduction and closure of gastroschisis on the day of birth but became malnourished postoperatively despite oral feedings and were predisposed to frequent wound dehiscences. With the development of parenteral hyperalimentation, these infants now receive enough intravenous nutritional support postoperatively for normal growth and development, healing of surgical wounds, and adequate nourishment until normal feedings and bowel absorptive functions resume. Recent technological advances that now permit total intravenous alimentation or hyperalimentation include synthetic nutritional solutions, free-standing or implantable intravenous infusion pumps for their delivery, and long-term, indwelling intravascular catheters for chronic intravenous access and infusion.

Early investigations of total parenteral nutrition began nearly half a century ago with the intravenous infusion of hypertonic mixtures of glucose, amino acid, and oil. These early nutrient solutions were abandoned because of technical problems with emulsification and clinical problems with hypertonicity. Recently, renewed interest has led to the successful development and production of parenteral solutions that provide a balanced amount of the three nutrient substrates, amino acids, carbohydrates, and fats.

Amino acid solutions are now commercially available from most major suppliers of intravenous fluids as 8.5% solutions with about 1 g of protein per 12 ml and as 10% solutions with about 1 g of protein per 10 ml. Although these protein preparations differ slightly, each contains essential and nonessential amino acids, sodium and chloride as electrolytes, and phosphate and acetate as buffers. The pH of these solutions ranges from 5.0 to 7.0, and the osmolarity ranges from 750 to 1000 mOsm/L.

Large birth weight neonates and older neonates may receive the 8.5% and 10% solutions without difficulty because such mixtures adequately cover their dietary needs and provide excellent nutritional support without circulatory volume overloading. Recently released dilute solutions, such as Tropamine 6%, are indicated in very low birth weight and preterm infants whose renal excretory systems are too immature to handle concentrated intravenous protein solutions. The 6% protein solutions are designed to produce a plasma amino acid concentration consistent with that of a breast-fed preterm infant. In addition, these dilute solutions also contain cysteine.

Glucose-containing solutions for carbohydrate needs have been easy to prepare but difficult to administer through peripheral veins because 10% to 13% dextrose infusions will cause severe chemical phlebitis within 24 to 72 hours. Recent changes in hyperalimentation catheters and selection of central rather than peripheral venous routes now permit admininstration of up to 25% glucose solutions without local or systemic sequelae, provided a stepwise increase in glucose concentrations is employed. Higher glucose concentrations are rarely indicated unless fluid restriction dictates very slow rates of infusion of concentrated solutions or renal failure dictates the use of specially prepared hyperalimentation formulas. Even with moderate fluid restriction, central venous solutions of 20% to 25% glucose and 6% to 8.5% amino acids will meet the caloric and protein needs of most stressed, non-eating neonates. For peripheral intravenous hyperalimentation of neonates on restricted diets, less concentrated, 10% to 13% glucose solutions will meet only half of the neonate's caloric needs. The addition of concentrated fat substitutes will, however, permit peripheral intravenous hyperalimentation solutions to more fully cover caloric needs.

Concentrated fat substitutes, prepared from emulsions of soybean (Intralipid) or safflower oil (Liposyn) suspended in egg yolk phospholipids, will meet all neonatal dietary requirements for the major component fatty acids (linoleic, oleic, palmitic, linolenic, and stearic acids). These fat emulsions have tonicities between 250 and 275 mOsm/L, are buffered to a pH near 8.0, and contain chylomicron-like fat particles with diameters near 0.4 μ. Both Intralipid and Liposyn are available as 10% and 20% solutions providing 1.1 cal/ml and 2.0 cal/ml, respectively. As noted, these fat emulsions now permit high-caloric peripheral or central venous nutrition with minimal fluid administration and have been used extensively for total parenteral hyperalimentation in neonates with cardiac or renal dysfunction.

In addition to the three main nutrient groups, vitamins and trace elements are now available for intravenous alimentation. The most popular intravenous multiple vitamin preparation for neonates is multi-vitamin infusion (MVI), a lyophilized sterile powder reconstituted when added to the main nutrient infusion. MVI contains the water-soluble vitamins ascorbic acid (vitamin C), thiamine (vitamin B_1), riboflavin (vitamin B_2), pyridoxine (vitamin B_6), niacinamide, pantothenate, biotin, folic acid, and cyanocobalamin (vitamin B_{12}). MVI also contains the fat-soluble vitamins retinol (vitamin A), ergocalciferol (vitamin D), and alpha-tocopherol (vitamin E). The lipid-soluble vitamins are made water soluble for intravenous infusion by combination with polysorbate 80. Unlike adult MVI, pediatric MVI also contains phytonadione (vitamin K_1). MVI is hyperosmotic and should be reconstituted in no less than 100 ml of intravenous hyperalimentation formula. Multivitamin therapy is based on weight; a typical dosage schedule is shown in Table 14–1.

Besides vitamins, common trace elements are now available for addition to hyperalimentation solutions. These trace elements include zinc, copper, magnesium, manganese, and chromium in ready-to-mix preparations with dosages based on weight. Trace elements can be added to either central or peripheral nutrient infusions and can be supplemented with less common, individual trace elements such as selenium, as indicated.

Parallel with the development of intravenous nutrients was the design and development of intravenous catheters for nutrient infusions. Most intravenous hyperalimentation catheters are of the Broviac or Hickman variety. These catheters may have single or multiple lumens and are inserted percutaneously into the central venous system with their proximal ends connected to the infusion line. Such catheters can be used for continuous or intermittent infusion. With proper wound care and local line anticoagulation, hyperalimentation catheters can be left in place for long periods. These catheters are often inserted percutaneously into subclavian or internal jugular veins with local or general anesthesia.

The latest hyperalimentation catheters, such as the Medport, Lifeport, and Port-A-Cath, are totally implantable and may be accessed by

Table 14–1. Dosage of Pediatric Multivitamins

Infant Weight	Daily Dose
<1 kg	30% of full dose of 5 ml (1.5 ml)
1–3 kg	65% of full dose of 5 ml (3.25 ml)
>3 kg	A full dose of 5 ml

subcutaneous reservoir puncture. Multilumen catheters may have multiple reservoirs. Implantable hyperalimentation catheter insertions are now among the most common operative procedures in neonates and are usually performed under general anesthesia. Initial vein entry is by percutaneous venipuncture or venous cutdown. A venous guidewire is then inserted for catheter placement by the Seldinger technique; the guidewire is removed and the catheter tip is positioned within the central venous circulation with radiographic guidance. The distal end of the catheter is tunneled beneath the skin and connected to the reservoir, which is also buried in a subcutaneous pocket under the skin. The subcutaneous reservoir is accessible only by needle puncture.

The main disadvantage of implantable central venous catheters is the need for another minor surgical procedure to remove the reservoir and its connected catheter. This procedure is also performed under sterile conditions in the operating room during general anesthesia. Compared to externally exiting hyperalimentation catheters, implantable access systems have a lower incidence of infection and require less frequent catheter anticoagulation to maintain patency and central venous access.

When there is no need to restrict intravenous fluids, many neonates may receive total parenteral nutrition through peripheral rather than central veins. Peripheral hyperalimentation with combinations of 10% to 13% glucose solutions and 20% lipid solutions will require volumes of 150 to 175 ml/kg/day to provide adequate nutrition with 110 to 115 cal/kg/day. Peripheral hyperalimentation eliminates risks of catheter sepsis, venous air embolism, and central venous thrombosis with superior vena caval syndrome and can be administered for as long as 4 to 6 weeks by rotating the peripheral venous access sites.

For preterm neonates who require either fluid restriction or more than 4 to 6 weeks of parenteral nutrition, central venous hyperalimentation with a Broviac catheter or a small Hickman catheter is preferable to peripheral venous hyperalimention. When severe fluid restriction is indicated in such patients, glucose and lipid solutions may be concentrated and mixed to permit small volumes of hypertonic nutritional formulas to meet all caloric needs with little risk of circulatory volume overload. Such formulas, however, particularly low-volume solutions containing multivitamins, may present a hypertonic challenge to a contracted circulatory volume, raising serum osmolarity and predisposing preterm neonates to intracranial hemorrhage (see Chapters 8, 10, and 11).

For term neonates and larger infants requiring prolonged parenteral nutrition, small implantable venous catheters (Medport or Lifeport) with subcutaneous reservoirs may offer less risk of catheter sepsis and fungal contamination than exteriorized central venous catheters. Since many neonates will receive concomitant antibiotics during hyperalimentation, the risks of line sepsis with such opportunists as fungi and bacteria with multiple antibiotic resistances are magnified and demand central venous line placement under strictly sterile surgical conditions.

Soft Silastic hyperalimentation catheters are less likely to puncture thin-walled central veins or damage the tricuspid valve than stiffer polyvinyl chloride (PVC) catheters. In addition, Silastic catheters can be more easily telescoped over guidewires than stiffer PVC catheters. Once the central venous catheter is positioned, its location should be confirmed and pneumothorax from pleural puncture during catheter insertion should be ruled out by intraoperative x-ray study, preferably fluoroscopy. Catheter tips should be positioned in the middle of central thoracic veins (subclavian, internal jugular, innominate) and away from venous bifurcations, the right side of the atrial septum, the coronary sinus, and the tricuspid valve. Central venous and intracardiac perforations made by migrating or misplaced hyperalimentation catheter tips, if unrecognized, may result in hemothorax, intrapleural formula effusion, pericardial formula effusion, traumatic atrial septal defect, tricuspid valve damage, cardiac tamponade, and death. Thus, periodic catheter tip location by chest x-ray film is recommended for neonates receiving central venous hyperalimentation. In addition, catheter tips in the arms (axillary vein) or at the base of the skull (jugular venous bulb) may permit infusion of hypertonic solutions into the upper extremities or brain, increasing risks of phlebothrombosis, thrombophlebitis, venous thromboembolism, and cerebral venous air embolism. Misplaced hyperalimentation catheters should be repositioned with radiographic guidance in central thoracic veins before total parenteral nutrition commences.

In conclusion, recent advances in nutrient formulas and intravascular catheters permit prolonged total parenteral nutrition in neonates, thus eliminating the risks of malnutrition, starvation ketoacidosis, muscular wasting, and wound dehiscences. Many neonates undergoing emergency surgery will be candidates for total parenteral nutrition because of prolonged ileus, short gut malabsorption, or large surgical wounds (as in separated conjoined twins) that demand more nutrients for healing than enteral nutrition can provide (see Chapter 13).

EXTRACORPOREAL MEMBRANE OXYGENATION FOR NEONATAL RESPIRATORY FAILURE

Neonatal respiratory failure occurs commonly because of prematurity; congenital malformations of the heart, lungs, or diaphragm; pneumonia; congestive heart failure; or sepsis. Endotracheal intubation and mechanical ventilatory support were major early advances in the treatment of neonatal respiratory failure. In conjunction with surgical correction or palliation of cardiothoracic malformations and inotropic support of circulatory function, such advances have permitted life-saving surgery and prolonged postoperative mechanical ventilation. Prolonged mechanical ventilation, however, has its risks, including endotracheal tube accidents such as esophageal and endobronchial intubations, pulmonary barotrauma, and pulmonary oxygen toxicity. If unrecognized, any of these complications of mechanical ventilation could cause serious injury and death.

Over the past decade, heart-lung machines providing extracorporeal circulation during open heart surgery have been miniaturized to provide for pulmonary bypass and artificial oxygenation during respiratory failure.[1, 2] Extracorporeal circulation for total cardiopulmonary bypass can only be provided for minutes to hours, whereas ECMO for partial pulmonary bypass during heart-directed circulation can often be provided for days to weeks to support infants with respiratory failure.[3] Although originally developed for adults, ECMO has been most successful when applied to neonates and infants who cannot be effectively ventilated mechanically because of pulmonary barotrauma, congenital malformations, or pneumonia.

During ECMO, venous blood is drained from the body, oxygenated extracorporeally, and returned to the patient. Like the heart-lung machine, the ECMO machine includes a membrane oxygenator, a circulatory pump, and the necessary tubing and connections to permit its circuit to receive blood from and return it to the patient. Like cardiopulmonary bypass, lung bypass with ECMO will usually require both venous access for receipt of unoxygenated blood and vascular access for return of machine-oxygenated blood. Such veno-arterial ECMO, used most commonly, returns blood to the arterial circulation for distribution throughout the body. However, double-catheter and single-catheter venovenous ECMO circuits are becoming more common and, if they are employed before the onset of cardiac failure, may be quite successful in providing artificial oxygenation without the risks of arteriotomy (air embolism, stroke, or coronary or cerebral embolization).[4]

Venoarterial access for ECMO is usually obtained by separate cannulation of the internal jugular vein and the common carotid artery on the right side of the neck.[1-3] The venous drainage cannula is positioned in the right heart, and the arterial return catheter is placed in the aortic arch.[2] With dual venovenous access for ECMO, the internal jugular vein is cannulated for venous drainage and the femoral vein is cannulated for oxygenated blood return.[4] The latest double-lumen and single-catheter ECMO circuits require only a single and often percutaneous cannulation of a large central vein, preferably the internal jugular or subclavian vein.[4]

A venoarterial ECMO system is depicted in Figure 14–1.[3] In addition

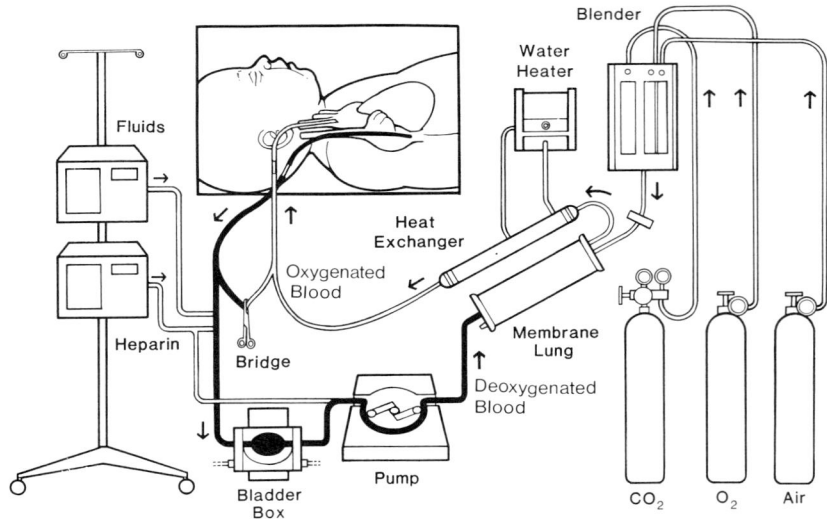

FIGURE 14–1. ECMO circuit.

to the cannulas previously noted, the ECMO system requires either a standard 5-inch roller pump, as depicted, or a newer centrifugal vortex pump, and an artificial lung or oxygenator/exchanger. The SciMed silicone membrane oxygenator is the most common membrane oxygenator in current use.[2, 3, 5] The membrane oxygenator receives an oxygen (O_2) source and often a carbon dioxide (CO_2) source since countercurrent flow through membrane oxygenators with large surface areas permits superefficient CO_2 removal. Without the addition of CO_2, the neonate on ECMO may become severely alkalotic and develop hypokalemia with cardiac irritability and/or cerebral vasospasm with brain ischemia or hemorrhage.[5] Since a major portion of the infant's circulatory volume is in the ECMO circuit at any given time, oxygenated blood is rewarmed by a heat exchanger on its return to the infant in order to maintain the most efficient thermoregulation during ECMO.

ECMO tubing surfaces are bioactive and will activate the coagulation cascade, quickly clotting the membrane oxygenator. Systemic anticoagulation with heparin is required for clot-free ECMO just as it is for cardiopulmonary bypass. However, overzealous anticoagulation with an activated coagulation time (ACT) several times normal often results in spontaneous bleeding, the major complication of ECMO. Bleeding may occur at incisional and puncture sites, in the gut, in the retroperitoneum, or intracranially. To avoid spontaneous and often uncontrollable bleeding during ECMO, the ACT is maintained at clotting times long enough to prevent intravascular coagulation and short enough to prevent extravascular hemorrhage, usually 180 to 220 seconds. In addition, frequent platelet transfusions are administered to maintain circulating platelet counts of 75,000 to 125,000 and to provide for effective platelet aggregation and hemostatic plugging. New heparin-bonded ECMO circuits may someday eliminate the need for systemic anticoagulation during prolonged ECMO and reduce the incidence of spontaneous bleeding, particularly intracranial hemorrhage, to which preterm neonates on ECMO are particularly predisposed (see Chapters 10 and 11).

The current major surgical indication for ECMO in neonates is congenital diaphragmatic hernia (CDH), an anatomic defect that is simple to correct surgically (see Chapter 12). Unfortunately, CDH repair does not correct coexisting pulmonary hypoplasia and postoperative respiratory failure. Despite concerted efforts to make an early diagnosis of CDH in utero and to perform rapid surgical correction at birth, the mortality from CDH did not improve substantially until the introduction of ECMO for postoperative respiratory failure. Future combinations of early CDH detection and surgical palliation by anterior abdominal decompression may offer even more hope of survival of neonates with CDH (see Chapter 5). At present, however, even when immediate death from bilateral pulmonary hypoplasia or associated congenital malformations is excluded, nearly one-half of neonates born with CDH die before reaching a pediatric surgical facility.[6–9]

With advanced life support, including tracheal intubation, mechanical ventilation, and inotropic therapy, neonates with CDH often arrive at tertiary treatment centers ready to undergo immediate subcostal laparotomy, reduction of the intrathoracic hernia, and repair of the affected hemidiaphragm by primary or prosthetic patch closure. Following surgical repair of CDH, one-half of neonates may be expected to survive the immediate postoperative period. However, in at least one-half of these short-term survivors, pulmonary hypoplasia and persistent pulmonary hypertension will result in progressive respiratory failure and death.[3] It is this group of neonates who should be considered for prolonged ECMO begun either before or after surgical CDH repair.[10]

When an infant with CDH is resuscitated and ultimately reaches a pediatric surgical facility, immediate surgical repair is performed in the hope that anatomic correction will permit the lungs to expand and grow during mechanical ventilation. Some patients may experience a transient period of respiratory improvement immediately following surgery, often referred to as the "honeymoon" period.[3] This period often leads to a phase of progressive respiratory failure and death. Now, as in the past, mechanical hyperventilation, often supplemented with pulmonary vasodilators,[11] is employed to prolong the honeymoon period or to treat bouts of respiratory failure and pulmonary hypertension. About 50% of the time, the hypoplastic lung on the side of the CDH begins to expand

and grow, pulmonary vascular resistance is lowered; and normal pulmonary gas exchange becomes possible.[11] Should standard management begin to fail, ECMO is indicated to prolong the honeymoon period and to buy time for growth and development of the hypoplastic lung(s) and the advent of pulmonary gas exchange without the barotrauma or hemodynamic compromise of prolonged positive-pressure mechanical ventilation. Often ECMO restores oxygenation, normocarbia, and neutral pH and lowers pulmonary vascular resistance. Whether lung growth or simply lung expansion occurs during the 1 to 4 weeks of ECMO is unclear at present; perhaps a combination of both growth and expansion occurs. In any event, the goal of ECMO is to establish a period of stability during which pulmonary growth/expansion can occur.

A major clinical problem at present is predicting who does and who does not need ECMO in order to survive CDH either before or after surgical repair of the defect.[12-16] Generally, if a neonate is markedly unstable with hypoxemia, acidosis, and hypercapnia, preoperative ECMO before surgical repair of CDH should be considered. Such a treatment sequence may allow for stabilization of the patient and, as indicated by our early report,[10] some reduction of herniated bowel from the hemithorax back into the abdomen. Preoperative ECMO may even improve pulmonary hypertension and allow weaning from ECMO prior to CDH repair. In addition, there is now enough experience to indicate that children can safely undergo CDH repair while they are anticoagulated and on an ECMO circuit.[9, 10] Such surgery involves careful attention to surgical hemostasis in order to avoid major bleeding problems. However, almost two dozen cases have been anecdotally reported in which repair of CDH was undertaken while the child was on the ECMO circuit, with surprisingly good results and survival well above previous national norms.[9, 10]

Bohn and associates[17] have described a relationship between $PaCO_2$ and ventilation parameters in predicting survival of neonates with CDH (Fig. 14–2). In their prospective study,[17] 58 infants with CDH within the first 6 hours of life who underwent surgical repair were analyzed in order to develop a reproducible index of severity of disease that would reliably predict eventual outcome. All infants in the study group were treated with muscular paralysis, mechanical hyperventilation, and intravenous isoproterenol for the first 48 postoperative hours. There were 30 survivors and 28 deaths for a 48% mortality. Using $PaCO_2$ values and correlating these values with an index of mechanical ventilation (mean airway pressure × respiratory rate), the authors clearly identified two groups of neonates with CDH based on their responses to mechanical hyperventilation (see Fig. 14–2). The first group, identified by triangles in Figure 14–2, developed CO_2 retention and stiff lungs and were unresponsive to mechanical hyperventilation, and most infants in this

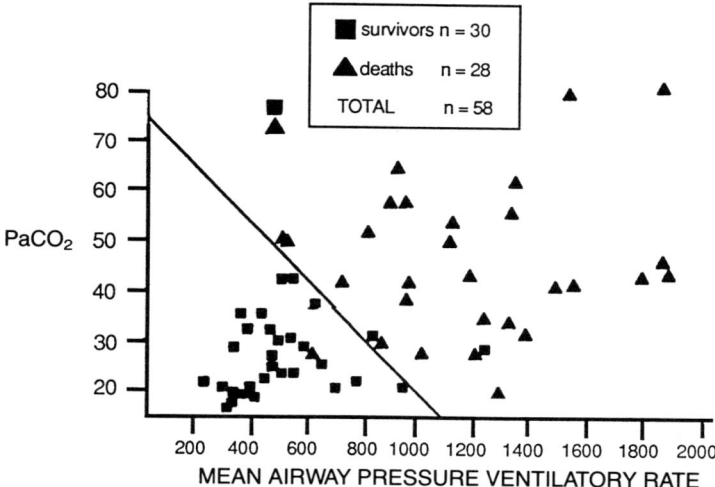

FIGURE 14–2. $Paco_2$ values (mmHg) plotted against mean airway pressure × ventilatory rate measured within 2 hours of surgical repair in 58 newborn infants with CDH. The diagonal line clearly separates the survivors (Group 2) (■) from nonsurvivors (Group 1) (▲). (Adapted with permission from Bohn DJ, James I, Filler RM, et al.: The relationship between $Paco_2$ and ventilation parameters in predicting survival in congenital diaphragmatic hernia. J Pediatr Surg 19:666–671, 1984.)

group died (90% mortality). The second group, identified by squares in Figure 14–2, responded well to mechanical hyperventilation, did not retain CO_2 or develop stiff lungs, and usually survived (survival 97%). Thus, for neonates with CDH satisfying the criteria for Bohn Group 1, ECMO may offer a better alternative for survival than mechanical hyperventilation with its 90% mortality (see Fig. 14–2).

At the Ochsner Foundation Hospital, ECMO has been available since Fall, 1983. Seventy-two children with CDH have been treated at this institution, either primarily for surgery and ECMO or secondarily after surgery for postoperative ECMO.[9, 10, 15] These infants were classified according to Bohn's criteria by $Paco_2$ and respiratory index and placed into the appropriate group (see Fig. 14–2). Survival increased among all ECMO-treated neonates with CDH by 15% over historic non-ECMO controls. For Group 1 patients at highest risk, survival with ECMO is now 50%.[9, 10, 15] For all groups, survival with ECMO is now 70%; mortality without ECMO is 50% to 100%, as in Bohn's original series.[17] Our overall results, depicted in Table 14–2, compare survival in neonates with CDH before (1978 to 1983) and after (1983 to 1989) the introduction of ECMO for all neonates with CDH.[9, 10, 15]

Gratifying results like these have been obtained by other institutions employing ECMO in CDH survivors. Even better outcomes have been

Table 14–2. *Survival of Neonates with Congenital Diaphragmatic Hernia (CDH) at Ochsner Foundation Hospital Before (1978–1983) and After (1983–1989) Introduction of ECMO for All Neonates*

1978–1983	1983–1989
CDH, n = 35	CDH, n = 37
Alive, n = 23 (survival = 66%)	Alive, n = 30 (survival = 81%)

achieved using ECMO in neonates with other less lethal conditions, such as meconium aspiration syndrome, beta-streptococcal sepsis, and persistent fetal circulation. Survival rates for neonates with these three conditions are now between 80% and 90% versus historic mortality rates before ECMO of 70% to 90%.[14–16] ECMO is now available to infants beyond the neonatal period and, although experience with infant ECMO is limited and survival rates are obscure, any infant with acute respiratory failure of any etiology or cardiac failure following complex open heart surgery should be seriously considered for temporary ECMO support of ventilation and oxygenation.

In conclusion, most neonates and infants with fulminant respiratory failure not associated with CDH may be successfully managed with tracheal intubation and mechanical ventilation. However, when such standard treatment modalities fail to achieve sufficient oxygenation and ventilation, ECMO may offer a temporary and often successful therapeutic alternative to otherwise lethal clinical conditions. Mounting clinical evidence continues to document that ECMO is an innovative and often highly successful temporary technology providing artificial oxygenation and ventilation that buy enough time for neonates and even older infants to recover from self-limited congenital (CDH) or acquired (meconium aspiration syndrome, near drowning) cardiopulmonary insults.

CONCLUSIONS

Parenteral hyperalimentation to restore metabolic balance and hasten wound healing and ECMO to restore respiratory gas exchange without barotrauma are now available to neonates recovering from complex operative procedures. Hyperalimentation has prevented starvation when enteral alimentation fails or is impossible, improving survival of neonates with extensive surgical wounds and inadequate nutrient absorption through the gut. ECMO now offers a better chance for survival to neonates with CDH and severely hypoplastic lungs.

References

1. Bartlett RH, Gazzaniga AB, Huxtable RF, et al.: Extracorporeal circulation (ECMO) in neonatal respiratory failure. J Thorac Cardiovasc Surg 74:826, 1977.

2. Bartlett RH, Andrews AF, Toomasian JM, et al.: Extracorporeal membrane oxygenation for newborn respiratory failure: Forty-five cases. Surgery 92:425, 1982.
3. Heaton JFG, Redmond CR, Graves ED, et al.: Congenital diaphragmatic hernia: Improving survival and extracorporeal membrane oxygenation. Pediatr Surg Int 3:6, 1988.
4. Andrews AF, Klein MD, Toomasian JM, et al.: Venovenous extracorporeal membrane oxygenation in neonates with respiratory failure. J Pediatr Surg 18:339, 1983.
5. Bartlett RH: Extracorporeal oxygenation in neonates. Hosp Pract 19:139, 1984.
6. Nguyen L, Guttman FM, de Chadarevian JP, et al.: The mortality of congenital diaphragmatic hernia: Is total pulmonary mass inadequate, no matter what? Ann Surg 198:766, 1983.
7. Holder TM, Ashcraft KW: Congenital diaphragmatic hernia. In: Ravitch M, Welch KJ, Benson CD, et al. (eds): Pediatric Surgery, 3rd ed, Vol 1. Chicago: Year Book Medical Publishers, 1979, pp 432–445.
8. O'Callaghan JD, Saunders NR, Chatrath RR, et al.: The management of neonatal posterolateral diaphragmatic hernia. Ann Thorac Surg 33:174, 1982.
9. Sawyer SF, Falterman KW, Goldsmith JP, et al.: Improving survival in the treatment of congenital diaphragmatic hernia. Ann Thorac Surg 41:75, 1986.
10. Redmond C, Heaton J, Calix J, et al.: A correlation of pulmonary hypoplasia, mean airway pressure, and survival in congenital diaphragmatic hernia treated with extracorporeal membrane oxygenation. J Pediatr Surg 22:1143, 1987.
11. Ormazabal M, Kirkpatrick B, Mueller D: Alteration of alveolar-arterial O_2 gradient (A-a) DO_2 in response to tolazoline (T) as a predictor of outcome in neonates with persistent pulmonary hypertension (PPH) (abstract). Pediatr Res 14:607, 1980.
12. Bartlett RH, Roloff DW, Cornell RG, et al.: Extracorporeal circulation in neonatal respiratory failure: A prospective randomized study. Pediatrics 76:479, 1985.
13. Krummel TM, Greenfield LJ, Kirkpatrick BV, et al.: Alveolar-arterial oxygenation gradients versus the neonatal pulmonary insufficiency index for prediction of mortality in ECMO candidates. J Pediatr Surg 19:380, 1984.
14. Beck R, Anderson KD, Pearson GD, et al.: Criteria for extracorporeal membrane oxygenation in a population of infants with persistent pulmonary hypertension of the newborn. J Pediatr Surg 21:297, 1986.
15. Graves ED III, Loe WA, Redmond CR, et al.: Extracorporeal membrane oxygenation as treatment of severe meconium aspiration syndrome. South Med J 82:696, 1989.
16. O'Rourke PP, Crone RK, Vacanti JP, et al.: Extracorporeal membrane oxygenation and conventional medical therapy in neonates with persistent pulmonary hypertension of the newborn: A prospective randomized study. Pediatrics 84:957, 1989.
17. Bohn DJ, James I, Filler RM, et al.: The relationship between $PaCO_2$ and ventilation parameters in predicting survival in congenital diaphragmatic hernia. J Pediatr Surg 19:666, 1984.

Index

Note: Page numbers in *italics* refer to illustrations; page numbers followed by t refer to tables.